# MANAGED CARE
## Strategies, Networks, and Management

Edited by

**Montague Brown, MBA, DrPH, JD**
Editor, *Health Care Management Review*
and
Chairman
Strategic Management Services, Inc.
Washington, D.C.

## HEALTH CARE MANAGEMENT REVIEW

AN ASPEN PUBLICATION®
Aspen Publisher's, Inc.
Gaithersburg, Maryland
1994

Library of Congress Cataloging-in-Publication Data

Managed care: strategies, networks, and management/edited by Montague Brown.
p. cm.

Articles previously published in Health care management review.
Includes bibliographical references and index.
ISBN 0-8342-0504-1

1. Managed care plans (Medical care)—United States. I. Brown, Montague. II. Health care management review.
[DNLM: 1. Managed Care Programs—organization & administration—United States—Collected works. 2. Health
Facilities—organization & administration—United States—collected works. 3. Health Facility Administrators—
collected works. W 275 M332 1993]
RA413.5.U5M363 1993
362. 1'0425—dc20
DNLM/DLC
for Library of Congress
93-20709
CIP

Editorial Resources: Ruth Bloom

Library of Congress Catalog Card Number: 93-20709
ISBN: 0-8342-0504-1
Series: 0-8342-0337-5

Printed in the United States of America

1 2 3 4 5

# Contents

## I  Managed Competition: The Future?

Managed care has clearly pointed the way to bringing health care costs under control. But the providers themselves, right now, must either take on the responsibility of more directly managing care, bringing utilization down, and sharing in the rewards, or they could find themselves asked to sacrifice while intermediaries prosper.

While Hillary Rodham Clinton and 500 experts toil over how to insert managed care disciplines into health care, people like Thompson have been working on the Nth generation of managed care products and services. Managed care in America has made great strides in payments, billing infrastructure, and contracting but the collection of good data and using it to make sound management decisions is lagging along with the sound use of data for clinical problem solving and treatment planning.

## II  Strategy, Structure, and Managed Care

A vertically integrated health care system is an arrangement whereby a health care organization offers, either directly or through others, a broad range of patient care and support services. This article discusses the market forces and strategic considerations driving the recent trend toward vertical linkages in health care markets and examines some of the managerial implications and issues associated with this vertical restructuring trend.

The history of vertical integration spans the Lord Dawson Report in England in 1920, the Committee on the Cost of Medical Care in the United States in 1932, the Regional Medical Program in 1966 to its more modern successor reports and developments. Who is moving in this direction, what forces drive integration, and a host of related questions, issues, and prognostications are discussed.

**55   The Economic Transformation of American Health Insurance: Implications for the Hospital Industry**

C. WAYNE HIGGINS AND EUGENE D. MEYERS

The economics of cost containment, growing competition, and the introduction of new technology are forcing major changes on the health insurance industry. This transformation will impact the hospital industry in significant ways, hastening its evolution from a cottage industry to a modern corporate structure.

**63   Health Maintenance Organizations: Improvements in the Regulatory Environment**

H. GLENN BOGGS

Health maintenance organizations (HMOs) can help slow rising health care costs. State regulatory statutes are needed that will protect critical interests of HMO members while freeing HMOs from needless statutory requirements. A model HMO regulatory law is designed to strike a balance between protection of members and freedom for HMOs to deliver programs that can reduce health care costs.

**79   Hospital-Health Care Plan Affiliations: Considerations for Strategy Design**

RICHARD A. REID, JULIE H. FULCHER, AND HOWARD L. SMITH

Hospital-health care plan affiliations are designed to use idle hospital service capacity while minimizing the resulting financial risks.

**III   Contractual Networks: Hospitals and Managed Care**

**91   Strategies Employed by HMOs To Achieve Hospital Discounts: A Case Study of Seven HMOs**

JOHN E. KRALEWSKI, ROGER FELDMAN, BRYAN DOWD, AND JANET SHAPIRO

This article is a summary of seven health maintenance organization (HMO) case studies focusing on strategies used to obtain favorable prices for inpatient hospital services. All of the HMOs stressed that the effort should be based on the local environment and should accommodate the special circumstances of organization of physicians' practices and hospitals, as well as the structure of the HMO and its strategic plan for growth.

**99   The Growth and Effects of Hospital Selective Contracting**

GLENN A. MELNICK, JACK ZWANZIGER, AND ALICIA VERITY-GUERRA

Since the passage of California's ground-breaking PPO legislation in 1982, enrollment in managed-care systems has risen dramatically in California and throughout the United States. This article charts the growth of selective contracting and presents data on the effects of these programs on hospital costs.

**185   The Secret of Medical Management**

JAMES E. ROHRER

A review of the research on group practices punctures the myth of physician autonomy in hospitals and opens the way for administrators to join in controlling the patient care process.

**193   Impact of IPAs on Fee-for-Service Medical Groups**

JOHN J. ALUISE, THOMAS R. KONRAD, AND BATES BUCKNER

Individual practice association (IPA) is the newest and most rapidly growing HMO model. Despite potential benefits, IPAs have experienced a variety of difficulties. A case study analysis of community practices in North Carolina revealed satisfactory results as well as concerns.

## V   Organization and Management Issues in Managed Care

**205   Determinants of HMO Success: The Case of Complete Health**

LINDA S. WIDRA AND MYRON D. FOTTLER

The health maintenance organization (HMO) industry has experienced a variety of difficulties and criticisms in recent years. Various hybrid models have been proposed to alleviate these problems. This article presents an in-depth case study of factors associated with the success of one such hybrid: an individual practice association (IPA)-model HMO affiliated with an academic health center. The major success factors identified include the plan design/structure, the strategic orientation/ practices, and the stakeholder management orientation practices.

**217   An Assessment of Employers' Experiences with HMOs: Factors That Make a Difference**

ARTHUR L. DOLINSKY AND RICHARD K. CAPUTO

This study investigated those factors that influenced employers' experiences with health maintenance organizations (HMOs). It examined a national cross-sectional sample of chief executive officers (CEOs) and benefits managers. Findings revealed that different administrative issues such as the volume of paperwork, confusion about benefits, and educating employees about HMO benefits were of primary importance in affecting management's experiences with HMOs. Differences were found between CEOs' and benefits managers' responses.

**225   Management Information Systems: Their Role in the Marketing Activities of HMOs**

DAVID B. ARONOW

HMOs are particularly dependent on their information resources in providing cost-effective, high quality, accessible care. Understanding the role of MIS in HMO marketing activities may guide administrators in evaluating information systems applications within their organizations.

# Preface

Health Care Management Review (HCMR) seeks articles that offer management insights for executives who set policy, design organizations, and operate the various enterprises making up the health care industry. Over the years, most articles dealt with generic management subjects applied to functional areas of management such as finance, human resources, and corporate strategy. At the same time, being a journal devoted to the health care industry, the organizational loci of the particular problems have been those populated by health administrators, and, for the most part, those formally trained in health administration and/or business. Many of those with such training and interest are employed in acute care hospitals and related organizations. Thus HCMR probably focused more of its attention on hospitals than most other areas of health care.

During the past 10 years, HCMR has seen a steadily growing stream of papers dealing in one way or another with managed care, vertical integration, and other issues that go to the core of health insurance and managed care. Some of these papers have dealt with the overarching issues of how best to tie the tools, methods, and goals of managed care into some kind of integrated organization whose main focus is on enhancing the health of a defined population. Of course, much of the actual development of managed care has more modest goals of meeting the short-term needs of market segment and doing this profitably.

This volume contains articles dealing with the very short-range issues of making existing product lines efficient while others deal with the policy logic of comprehensive, integrated systems. Opportunities remain for many more contributions to this growth of managed care techniques, organizations, linkages, and alliances.

From the HCMR perspective, managed care is a generic term that cuts across a wide spectrum of activities and organizations which currently offer services under one or more of the business concepts within that field. The term also means something much more fundamental in the way of applying management technologies to the entire range of issues between the perception of need, through financial strategies for meeting the need, and the care continuum involved when someone actually utilizes care. The need for concentrated focus on these functions has created a virtual industry.

Had HCMR set out to build a management handbook on managed care in the broadset sense, many other kinds of articles would be included here. Much more is needed by HCMR readers. Many opportunities exist for prospective writers to consider authoring interesting papers for future issues of *Health Care Management Review.*

We need more papers dealing with the management of risk that can be easily understood by general managers. Authors from the consulting actuarial field who work primarily for insurers need to rethink their contributions and make them available to general and specialized managers engaged in the overall process of managing care. Hospital administrators, marketing people, clinicians, and others would benefit from articles dealing with how actuarial estimates and techniques used to build insurance programs could be used to design and build care systems. Surely a powerful case can be made to apply risk concepts to help hospitals and other providers move more into the field of direct contracting with buyers. If risk is to be used as incentives for providers to shift practice patterns to lower resource modes, understanding risk and ways to hedge it without eliminating the acceptance of risk within ranges are essential.

The role and function of preferred provider organizations and third party administrators need greater scrutiny to show how information systems, control systems, and quality process management techniques can be used throughout the multiple and complex transactions network that makes up the totality of health care. There are schools that produce actuaries and insurance executives whose faculty and students will delve into these areas to see how the work of such groups can be made more effective in improving health care, its processes, and outcomes.

The international business and public administration literature speaks directly to the far reaching ways in which national and international businesses utilize strategic alliances. The long running examination of multihospital systems, shared services, and national alliances needs to be extended further into the nature and need for similar alliances between insurer and providers in health care. The history of health care and insurance is probably one of shifting alliances, the rise and fall of technologies, and varying patterns of ownership and control. More on those paradigms and how they work with new linkages between the world of insurance and the world of medical care delivery is needed in *HCMR.*

Much of the Hillary Rodham Clinton round of debates about changing the system deals with issues of taxation and its impact on consumer behavior. Some of the proposals for change include major alterations in the taxation of benefits. Some say it cannot impact cost in the

long run while others think that anything that ultimately raises or vastly alters the price of alternatives will in fact cause changes in behavior. Perhaps this belongs in economic and mathematical journals. Perhaps, but managers anxious to participate in the policy debate in an informed manner need to know what will happen as a result of some of these shifts. It is time to have more in journals such as *HCMR* and not just have various interest groups polled about their concerns.

Many health professionals work in managed care. We hear a great deal about the concerns of nurses and others in the clinical setting but less about those working out in the more administrative world. What happens to the professionals whose training and socialization took place in a care setting but is now utilized to control such settings from the outside? How do they network with and through their profession? How do the interactions occur between, say, physicians and nurses in the approval process for procedures compared with interactions within a clinical setting like a nursing unit? There must be some rich comparison studies waiting for the enterprising researcher.

Providers have developed health maintenance organizations that failed. Some of these undoubtedly came too early in their markets. Some sold out while still others are going into the business today. What is the history of such organizations and how can the many different strategic directions be reconciled?

Every article in this book raises questions that provide grist for the writer's quill. Perhaps some of you reading this volume will turn on your word processor to begin outlining your own paper on one or more of these subjects.

## MANAGED COMPETITION: THE FUTURE FOR MANAGED CARE?

As this is being written, Hillary Rodham Clinton has a cast of over 400 consultants and others working on a national health system transformation effort. At this stage, outsiders hear definitively that we will get managed competition, command and control price and resource regulation, a combination of the two and a buzz of other configurations. Whatever we ultimately get, this promises to be the year of attempts at major transformation. This effort is called reform although no one expects us to go back to anything resembling the past.

The current popular acronym for the likely package is *managed competition.* In this model, the state or federal authorities establish Health Care Purchasing Coalitions or Cooperatives. These entities contract with Accountable Health Plans that further provide or contract for the provision of services. The HCPC then signs up customers individually, small groups, governmental and other types of employees who chose to use the AHPs offered through the HCPC.

By whatever name and configuration, the future seems likely to be more heavily populated with concentrated buying groups, more tightly integrated managed care entities, and much more intense pressure on cost, access, and quality. It is this attempt to manage the variables of corporate, individual demand, and provider methods and processes that we think of as "managed care."

All of those things that currently come under the name of managed care seem to have a chance of growing rapidly during the next few years.

The articles in this section hit at many different facets of the overall problem set. Wolford et al. focus on a wide range of issues that need to be faced if we are ever to thoroughly transform the industry into a consumer friendly, cost-effective service. Most of the reforms recommended in that article for consideration will be difficult but all point in the direction of fundamental change. Part of that change will be the reduction of the administrative hierarchy between primary buyer and ultimate supplier of services. There is simply too much cost going to redundancy, transactional cost between entities, and protectionist cost associated with multiple cost and profit centers in and among managed care firms and providers.

The Thompson and Brown dialogue goes into a number of underlying fundamentals on just how does one get to the point when all of the players are seeking urgently to manage the purchase and delivery of care. Even the most sophisticated managed care firms, almost all of the third party administrators and other market intermediaries operate on global data without any highly developed budgeting and control systems. Thompson, a seasoned HMO operator, builds his data services around data useful to customers for actually asking and answering real management questions that can lead to meaningful change, a fact his numbers strongly support. Whoever ultimately gets the roles of managing care, information focused on decision parameters that can be used to truly improve the processes of the industry will be at a premium.

Still it seems that the industry is at the early phase of a buildup toward meaningful data. As the debate proceeds this year, the newspapers carry stories of how different managed care companies offer cost and quality indicators to their customers. Even the best admit to being at the front end of the movement.

Tom Weil in his piece on use rates adds a number of sobering factors to the transformation equation. A large number of people outside the system now have substantial problems. And those problems relatively unattended represent a backlog of work to be performed once they get coverage.

The next couple of years will offer many opportunities to critique what promises to be the major health care debate of the decade. Hill-Burton, Medicare, and Medicaid were high points with little else to compete with the intensity of the debate raging now.

Today we have at best a blue print for change. Some might even call it merely an artist sketch. It requires purchasing cooperatives not now in existence. It requires taxing benefits, something which hits hard at middle class workers along with many others. It requires or forces choices toward the most tightly run, closed panel types of plans (assuming that they continue to have the lowest cost). In short the utopia of regulated, managed "competition," puts many new and untried elements into a highly decentralized system. Aggregate or fail seems to be the message. Integrate to survive.

With a high probability that the current round of reform discussion will open up a deep and widespread debate to fully educate all sectors on the changes proposed, *HCMR* expects articles on this subject to increasingly dominate the space allocated to strategic concerns for health care management.

## STRATEGY, STRUCTURE, AND MANAGED CARE

The managed care process takes the relations between insurer, buyer, provider, and patient and begins to link them together in a manner to more rationally impact processes and outcomes, especially from the perspective of those at risk for paying the bill. Some of the pioneers in this movement sought an economical method of providing access through the use of prepayment and group practices. Most of the efforts in the 1980s sought profits from control of price increases and utilization. Providers sought customers through discounts. Ideally the earlier interest will emerge again to push for an overall transformation of the system to a more economical array of available quality health services promoting improvements in health status. This section deals with some of those ideals.

The last decade's growth of managed care activities is new in practice. It is not new in terms of scholarly attention. Paul Ellwood, MD, captured the spirit of prepaid group practice when he coined the term, *health maintenance organization*. We are still short of health maintenance, but we have gone irreversibly in the direction of systems of control and information gathering and use which begins to make it possible to envision tying together larger, more integrated systems of care for defined populations.

Provider groups seek to build multiple, comprehensive, and vertically integrated care systems that serve defined populations. For those self insured populations, the system provides documented control efforts and outcome data. For those populations that chose insurance it will be prepaid and the system will utilize the same control mechanism to gain the kinds of efficiencies that can be gained from deliberate development of mechanism to provide the insertion of standards and feedback loops into the system of care.

The managed care movement has systematically brought the use of population data to bear on individual care decisions. The pressure for such massive use came from cost concerns. However, much of the development of data for use in comparisons came earlier from quality concerns. No doubt the avalanche of pressure for cost containment will push this movement further. However, the national movement to embrace process management and its passion for statistical approaches to every process niche within health care will balance the concerns for cost and quality. This should lead us more closely to best value types of criteria. The methods being developed can be used by providers, buyers, insurers, and public agencies seeking to control the industry.

## CONTRACTUAL NETWORKS: HOSPITALS AND MANAGED CARE

Hospitals and the behavior of their subsystems, personnel, and practices are the focus of many of the tools and techniques of managed care. This section illustrates the many issues and concerns of general management of acute care hospitals as they grapple with the emergence of managed care as a force in the industry.

Kralewski et al. examine the strategy employed by HMOs to get hospital discounts. Hospitals generally unaccustomed to contracting over details in health plans have been slow to pick up on the many techniques, demands, and ploys used to gain advantage in this relationship. That is changing but remains a difficult issue for many hospitals even in 1993.

Other articles in this section deal with selective contracting by managed care plans and governments. Another deals with hospitals moving aggressively into case management internally. Marketing experts lay out the relationships between product line management and various forms of managed care buyers.

Much more could be written about the interactions between the care processes and modern managed care programs. Much can be learned from experiments not yet reported on generally in the health care literature.

In looking at many of the contractual relations developing between managed care firms, hospitals, and other providers, it appears that few are aimed at long-term partnership types of operations. It seems that the industry is still at a point where buyers seek advantage from price concessions from a provider sector with excess capacity, making it possible to get deals due to that fact. At some point in the future, it would seem desirable to build more win collaborative ventures with all parties trying to help the other to make the overall system more effective. Today it seems adversarial relations rule the day.

At what point might we expect managed care, especially when vertically integrated with providers, to begin to place the hospital and other such services into a cost center type of role versus its current profit center role? When will hospital trustees move their hospitals into ownership positions within managed care? Or will hospitals and other providers find it better to hang out and bargain with all types of intermediator organizations?

## PHYSICIANS AND MANAGED CARE

Physicians are necessary at every major juncture of managed care. Physicians lead the research effort that guides protocol development. They manage the care process. They manage other care givers, especially other physicians.

The articles in this section delve into physician motivation, management, leadership, and incentives. Much is being learned, much more needs to be discovered. What kinds of physicians make better managers, institutional and team leaders? How should physicians be compensated?

Many of the subjects in these articles will be familiar to those who follow the general management literature except for the fact that such questions are directed here at a professional group that is finding itself increasingly both object of and a critical component in managed care.

Future issues of *HCMR* will have more on these subjects. Physicians, like engineers and other professionals before them, will be moving into management, getting management education, and taking over the systems that seek to control their original professional domains.

## ORGANIZATION AND MANAGEMENT ISSUES IN MANAGED CARE

In this section mainstream management disciplines explore the application of their approaches to managed care operations. Operations research, information systems, marketing, finance, organizational behavior and other disciplines look at issues critical to understanding the new managed care operations.

Some look at systems, some customers, while others consider approaches to prevention and market segmentation. While this interesting collection offers major insights, it also points to the potential for more research that utilizes approaches found in most management disciplines.

## SUMMARY

*HCMR* seeks insight into management issues that arise in the efforts of insurers, health providers, businesses, and others as they seek to improve upon those processes that aid people to improve their health status. What does management have to offer to advance the purpose of health care? Hopefully the articles in this volume help. But overall it would seem to this observer that the industry is in its infancy when it comes to applying the full power of management disciplines to actually "manage care."

*—Montague Brown*
*Editor*

# Acknowledgments

This volume is dedicated to the authors. Many others contribute to bringing their work to fruition on these and other pages but it is they who drive us to see the merit of their ideas. Our volunteer editorial board helps, Aspen editors keep a sharp eye out for correctness, but the author brings order from chaos. We salute those who seek insight and thank them for sharing their thoughts with the rest of us.

Authors challenge editors to see what they see. The successful author learns to take their own love for their subject and present it in a manner which attracts and enlightens others who are interested in what they write about. As a consultant who thrives on looking at our industry in as many ways as possible, the authors represented here have helped me immensely. Every article adds something to our collective stock of knowledge. And, every one in some way reminds us just how much more we need to know and could learn by applying more of our management technologies.

This book is also dedicated to those who shared their ideas and work with the authors. Among those who contributed heavily to my own opportunities to explore managed care, I would like to thank Dick Stull, Pat Thompson, Barbara McCool, Kirk Oglesby, Larry Dozier, Helene Pellet, Jon Jaeger, Rodney Wolford, Chuck Lindstrom, Joe Lammers, Mike Abell, Jim Boyle, Howard Veit, Frank Pinckney, Charlie Boone, Bill Yates, and many, many others in managed care, Blue Cross, and other such organizations whose work provides grist for the writers mill.

PART I

# MANAGED COMPETITION: THE FUTURE?

# Getting to go in managed care

G. Rodney Wolford,
Montague Brown,
and
Barbara P. McCool

*Managed care has clearly pointed the way to bringing health care costs under control. But the providers themselves, right now, must either take on the responsibility of more directly managing care, bringing utilization down, and sharing in the rewards, or they could find themselves asked to sacrifice while intermediaries prosper.*

The American health care system operates on a commodity and commerce basis in a marketplace that does not respond to classic market principles of supply, demand, price, or quality. The system is bloated with unaffordable insurance packages and services. It is also heavily burdened with good intentions, overindulgence, and self-interest, all serving to increase societal cost for care that is considered a right by many and directly paid for by few. While new technologies flood the market, less incremental improvements occur in our overall health status. The fix, because of lack of national direction, could be long and painful, but there will be a sigh of relief when it is over.

The panacea emerging as the most touted for our salvation is managed competition, which, in essence, is a comprehensive use of managed care organizations in the marketplace. Managed care in its existing and likely emulated formats means many things including the micromanaging of consumer choice, consumer selection of providers, providers' use of procedures, diagnosis, and treatment. Coupled with this new set of micromanagement tools are myriad financial incentives presumed to alter the behavior of physicians, hospitals, and other providers.

Will managed care in the form that has emerged be capable of delivering a more efficient, competitively managed health care system? Have we lost a sense of

*G. Rodney Wolford, C.P.A., M.B.A., is President/CEO of Alliant Health System in Louisville, Kentucky.*

*Montague Brown, M.B.A., Dr.P.H., J.D., consults on health care strategy and structure and is Editor of* Health Care Management Review.

*Barbara P. McCool, R.N., M.H.A., Ph.D., consults on health care strategy and structure and is Associated Editor of* Health Care Management Review.

This article was initially written for a speech made before the Health Systems Section of the American Hospital Association. Many of the thoughts expressed here were developed and tested during several years of work by the authors in attempting to put together more integrated systems of services that go beyond the traditional separation of managed care from provider networks. This work continues and has included attempts to merge and joint venture with insurers, development of networks of providers who own and operate full-fledged managed care operations, and other related strategies designed to reduce the layering between consumers and providers and to build organizations more attuned to long-term community interest.

In the process of development, this article has been reviewed and critiqued by dozens of reviewers. It is also the product of many years of building vertically integrated systems, both by the authors and their many colleagues too numerous to name, who refuse to accept the system as given and strive to wrest change from it.

Of course the faults remain with the authors. We readily admit to wanting far more from the field than we can expect any time soon. Still we remain optimistic and intend to work with any and all who aspire to do better for the community than we have accomplished so far.

community sharing in the risk of health care with the growth of our current system of managed care? Can insurers and providers come together to form organizations focused on community health? Are there structural barriers that virtually prohibit us from making those positive changes? This article explores these and other issues.

## HISTORICAL PERSPECTIVE

Our traditional financing methods gave us nearly unlimited license to overspend. Third party financing and marketing of health insurance and financing created third parties to collect and dispense monies to purchase health care as needed. For many years this worked well; growing risk pools making it possible to meet the big needs of the few from the small payments of the many. But contained within the payment system were the seeds of its destruction. Costs plus for hospitals, fee-for-service for physicians, and other incentives to use resources provided the impetus to spend, but not to be efficient. Neither providers nor insurers had strong incentives to meet health care needs within a budget.

Medicare adopted this spendthrift approach to financing against the advice of some, but with the approval of many who feared fixed budgets or prices. Faced with unlimited demand, the prospect of unlimited payment for the likely sickest of our population, the race was on. The commercialization of the field began in earnest.

Little time elapsed before growing health care cost burdens caused employers and governments to demand change. The first major round of attempts to control came shortly after Medicare and Medicaid passed. The nation turned to centralized planning to allocate capital resources. This strategy failed in the face of demand increases fueled by a flawed payment system that kept usual and customary treatment patterns that rewarded health professionals handsomely.

While the national health planning strategies were failing, the concept of managed care began to develop through the creation of health maintenance organizations (HMOs), preferred provider organizations (PPOs), and through health insurers who began to manage more closely their payments for health services. The early round of HMOs, financed largely with federal grants, were later converted to public market–financed commercial entities, pushing to expand and produce profits. In markets where indemnity payment had heavily bloated the system, these new managed care insurance entities could produce profits with even the most minor changes in benefit structures and with price discounts from pro-

viders who could easily pass on the cost of discounts to others less able to get discounts.

The emergence of HMOs came at a time when health insurance companies were moving away from community-rated insurance to corporate or group-rated insurance. The sense of community sharing of health care risk was being lost as corporations and other groups chose to reduce their health care cost by extracting themselves from the community pool. The focused marketing of HMOs toward young, healthy groups exacerbated the flight from the concept of community health. The results are massive cost shifting among buyers of health services and massive displacement of potential buyers of health insurance who are either deemed an unhealthy risk or insufficient in group size to be offered affordable health care rates. Selective underwriting has left millions of Americans uninsured.

Providers of care responded well to a growing but false sense of price competition. Huge discounts were offered to the HMOs, insurers, or employers who had large numbers of purchasers. As a result, the displacement of the uninsured or underinsured became even more severe. Providers had slipped unwittingly into the mode of discriminatory pricing. Those individuals who were good insurance risks or employed by the wealthiest corporations now paid less for the same health care service than those who were uninsured, underinsured, or employed by smaller, less wealthy corporations.

Without major structural changes, will this evolution of insurance markets, preferential risks, and discriminatory pricing continue? With these structural and behavioral flaws, will managed competition with more extensive use of managed care work, or are we just laying down another facade of bandages?

For those who count on making the market system work more effectively some cautions are in order. If we could go to a system where the user paid everything out of pocket, then providers could offer anything anyone wanted to buy. But when average major encounters with the medical care system can run around $20,000, who can pay?

If we use collective buying and government payments, can we leave the ultimate choices to patients?

---

*Reform proposals in the Clinton era will most likely call for national and state boards, managed care networks, more protocols, and greater discipline on the part of customers.*

---

When the payment comes from the collective pocket, the product must meet community or societal standards of efficient, good and needed value criterion. Unbridled use of health services paid for by collective means cannot stand.

Reform proposals likely to pass muster in the Clinton era will most likely call for national and state boards, managed care networks, more protocols, and greater discipline on the part of customers who must, early in seeking health care, make broad choices that link them into a more narrow range of choices, if and when they might actually need medical care.

Health care providers must be restructured and managed in a manner that recognizes provider accountability and reward efficiency, quality, and value. If this restructuring is to happen, the distance between buyers and providers must be shortened to make the providers more direct sellers with nothing between them and the buyer to alter incentives for efficiency or the certainty that success or failure is felt directly by providers. An extra layering of micromanagement of care systems adds cost and helps providers avoid the necessity for taking on the responsibility for their own management systems.

Current reform proposals fail to recognize this fundamental issue. If we go with the emerging managed care companies and place other layers of control systems on top, we can look forward to the world's most expensive and micromanaged health care system with an increasing share of cost going into the battles between the experts and accountants.

## PROVIDER ACCOUNTABILITY

It is time for real reform that puts resources and accountability directly with provider organizations. Make them responsible and accountable through their own management skills and recognition of value and quality. The worst possible approach to ultimately mastering cost-effective care would entail reliance on outside control, second guessing, micromanaging of essentially professional tasks and duties by outsiders.

On the other hand, none of us is naive enough to believe that providers would have realized the need for or been willing to make the necessary changes without outsider intervention. Purchasers and insurers have done us a favor, but now we need to move to ensure that the job is done properly. Having recognized the need, do we need to continue to support an army of micromanagers in order to get the job done?

Everyone must change. Our communities have suffered from this dysfunctional system and the powerful efforts put forth to ensure the survival of providers in their current organizational forms, along with their management and boards of directors. Today we need leadership for radical reform, but the radical reform we need originates at home, not in Washington, in big towns, small towns, medical practices, hospitals, and especially in regional systems of care.

In recent months, proposals have been stacking up in Congress to reform the health care system. With Clinton's election, interest groups are in high gear producing these proposals. Moreover, major newspapers are calling for quick action. There are so many patchwork proposals that government is paralyzed and likely little or nothing will be done except for minor adjustments to a flawed delivery model.

It will take more than "simple tweaks" to the system to modify the culture and the behaviors of the current players. To achieve the level of services and value our society needs and to remain competitive in a worldwide economy, more dramatic action is needed.

Signals from Clinton suggest new, more powerful, "managed competition" models that will take the best of competition and of regulation. These models, however, keep the separation between insurer and network micromanagement and provider systems of care. Maintaining this separation will further postpone necessary reform.

The challenge for physicians, hospitals, and insurers—the power brokers of the health care system—is to radically rethink our organizations and construct delivery models. Can there be any doubt that this is true?

Currently our health care system reels from chronic schizophrenia. When we ask, "Does everyone have the right to basic health care?" we respond by saying "Yes," but our system fails to deliver to millions of Americans who are simply priced out of the market. When asked if the health care dollar is a limited scarce resource, most in society say "Yes," but we practice "No" by making few "value judgments" as to the right level of health services.

Far too many businesses have opted out of the community solution to health care financing. Larger businesses, including most of America's hospitals, now self-insure and thus take themselves out of the community health risk pool, which only adds to the difficulty of smaller firms and individuals who need insurance and access to health care.

Competition is not working either. When we encourage a good dose of adversarial competition as a solution, we find that basic self-balancing economic fundamentals are not present, and the costs continue to spiral upward. Competition merely makes it easier for larger businesses and governments to shift further cost to the smaller businesses and individuals with no power to obtain discounts. Self-insurance and insurance company competition on rates to employers was first in line to destroy the community rating risk pool. Today, managed care, HMOs, PPOs, and other methods of getting price breaks for a select few further burdens the uninsured, the small businesses, and the individuals who must self-pay. And, in the process, a mountain of administrative cost overburdens the care that is given.

This flight from responsibility must stop. We would do well to heed Clinton's call for us to be Americans again, recognizing that we are all in this together and need to pull ourselves through it together. Health system leaders can do something to turn this shameful tide of irresponsibility. But we cannot get anyone, except perhaps ourselves, to rejoin the community unless we move aggressively on utilization and cost. We must master efficient care. We must organize to prevent unnecessary duplication. And, we must move to deal directly with our customers, at risk and with full responsibility and accountability for results.

Our goal should be to build health care financing and delivery models aimed at "community good" versus the good of individual providers, individual businesses, or individual insurance or managed care businesses. Some fear that no one will come back into the game on behalf of the greater community. We may well be pleasantly surprised when individual patients and their families understand that much of what can be done often does little good and may be counter to their supposed goals.

Do we need to just wait for the perfect model? No! The most challenging reform for each of us is to stop passing the buck for what happens. We must take a stand and lead our own organizations step by step to reform at the local level. If the ideal of community is ever to mean anything in this country, then community institutions need to stop whining and get on with leading the grass roots revolt for change.

One place to start this revolt is with managed care. The concept of managed care in the hands of fiscal intermediaries falls far short of the capabilities of the fully integrated organizations such as Kaiser, Group Health of Puget Sound, and others. Something can be learned from the vast differences between the success of one form, and the failure of the other. One uses an external agent or fiscal intermediary third party to micromanage; the other form accepts risk from the buyer. One works, the other does not. We must learn what is critical to this success and failure.

Why must we learn? Because most professional policymakers and certainly every "get on the wagon" policymaker are offering managed care as a solution without making the critical distinction made here. We are about to embrace the wrong kind of managed care.

For those who believe that only an integrated form of managed care will ever work well, the challenge is "getting to go" in managed care.

## MANAGED CARE: HAS IT WORKED?

In the early 1970s, the concept of managed care was introduced as the magic pill to cure the growing health care cost problem. While Kaiser and Group Health of Puget Sound provided an integrated type of managed care, the concept was not given much attention until Paul Ellwood with the Interstudy think tank group championed it as a solution for the future. Dubbed health maintenance organizations, few have become the solid foundation of economically based health care of the early models and have successfully adopted a solid approach to wellness and health maintenance.

*Health maintenance organizations and their modern day clones—managed care businesses—have rarely come close to the concept from which they sprang.*

Since the launching of HMOs in a blizzard of promotion, health maintenance organizations and their modern day clones—managed care businesses—have rarely come close to the totally dedicated, vertically integrated concept from which they sprang. Most of the managed care movement is in fact aimed at making sure that vertical integration and whole organizations at risk never happen.

The concept of organizing hospitals, physicians, and other services to provide health care for a given population for a fixed price seems simple, but it has not happened. Insurers going into the business act more as brokers, not integrated organizations. Providers shy away from what they view as strange territory of insuring and processing claims. Insurers are comfortable with contracts, pricing, and processing, but not with delivering care. Therefore they stay away from the responsibilities of giving care. As a result, professional autonomy, financial independence, and fee-for-service flourish under the guise of concepts of managed care.

Thus we have insurers attempting remote-controlled micromanagement of providers, risks underwriting, and a national call for "managed care" without an effective model to do the job. Providers must ultimately do the job, but are we prepared to move aggressively in that direction? Are we instead preparing for another round of policy being implemented with failures likely to cost more and destroy what is left of the strong organizations that might build vertically integrated systems of service?

Is there room for pessimism? If what is today called managed care has the flaws noted here, can we survive a decade of more of the same or a more modern version with the added regulatory features called for in "managed competition"? Managed competition proposals, fragmentary as they are and probably must be at this stage, call for roles for all the old players and the same distancing between controller managers and provider systems of the earlier varieties.

Have the existing managed care approaches solved our most pressing problems? Hardly. Managed care and indemnity underwriters have pursued aggressive underwriting techniques leading to groups and individuals at the highest risk of needing health services being left uncovered by insurance. Groups lose their insurance, people with chronic health problems cause their group to lose their insurance, or people are locked into their job because of insurance. In short, insurance for those in need only goes to those in very large organizations who can spread the risk internally within the group. Organizations with aging work forces who sought escape from community rating, now find their own groups caught in the squeeze. They want back in now that they too need subsidy and support from a still larger and younger group. In short, nearly everyone wants change. How does managed care differ from the more traditional insurance? It is sharper and more determined to profit from the many ways one can use to avoid people who may need large amounts of care and keep down the amount given to those who get into their plans. Is this an exaggeration? A bit perhaps, but who really doubts the larger truth of it? We do not get many chances for major reform. And, major attempts have been made to secure health care for all in America. If we are to do it with any hope of not bankrupting the country, we need to get it right on this go around.

Uwe Reinhart of Princeton University, an active policy critic and frequent "talking head," says managed care is simply a new snake oil that has come down the pike that has done nothing so far and has just a few local victories. Mainly it has shifted cost. If we expect managed care to be the savior of the health care delivery system, the start has not been good. If there are local victories, these organizations should show the way. Vertically integrated organizations delivering managed care do an outstanding job. Can we emulate the best and abandon the worst of managed care?

## MANAGED CARE EVOLUTION

What does our present system of managed care look like? How has it evolved from traditions of the past and, more specifically, where must it go in the future if we are to "get to go"? Figure 1 outlines the progression from the past through the future. The past and the present generally describe the system as it has progressed. Obviously exceptions can be made to any of these specifications. The future outlines the conceptual elements necessary to "get to go."

### Past (traditional)

In the traditional health care model, government provided capital and generous payments to allow ample profits to fuel access and provider growth. Purchasers hired insurers from a relatively homogeneous market to insure, process, and pay their bills. Physicians and hospitals provided services and collected a charge. The employer gave little, if any, choice of insurer, and the patient had little knowledge of health care treatment options and regarded his or her hospital and physicians with great sanctity. Traditional patterns of care prevailed. These times were great. Everyone seemed to be happy, but the components of the system were increasing their capability to consume more dollars. A form of fiscal hypertension was developing.

### Present (traditional and managed care)

Elements of the past still exist, but many varieties of managed care have taken root in the market. Government no longer provides capital and certainly does not provide profits through Medicare and Medicaid rates. The purchaser (employer and government) function with a great deal of self-interest, wishing to pay only cost (less if possible), for only the people for which they are directly responsible. Pure self-interest by the powerful has placed greater financial burden on the private pay, uninsured, and underinsured. Many small employers are out of the insurance market; one big claim ends their prospects for insurance.

Insurers have moved from merely processing and paying bills to seeking ways of using market power and

# FIGURE 1

## MANAGED CARE EVOLUTION

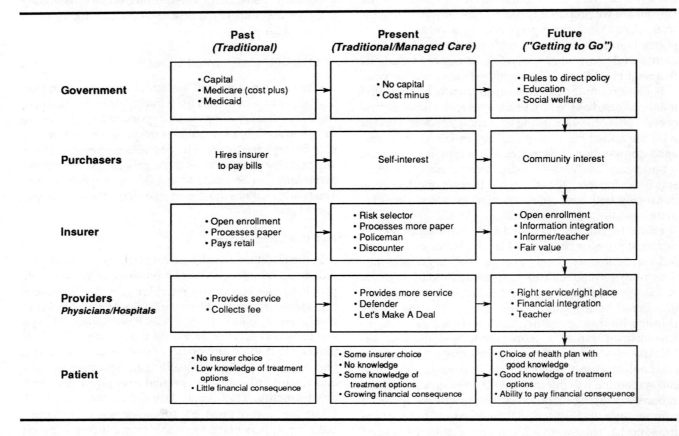

| | Past (Traditional) | Present (Traditional/Managed Care) | Future ("Getting to Go") |
|---|---|---|---|
| **Government** | • Capital<br>• Medicare (cost plus)<br>• Medicaid | • No capital<br>• Cost minus | • Rules to direct policy<br>• Education<br>• Social welfare |
| **Purchasers** | Hires insurer to pay bills | Self-interest | Community interest |
| **Insurer** | • Open enrollment<br>• Processes paper<br>• Pays retail | • Risk selector<br>• Processes more paper<br>• Policeman<br>• Discounter | • Open enrollment<br>• Information integration<br>• Informer/teacher<br>• Fair value |
| **Providers** *Physicians/Hospitals* | • Provides service<br>• Collects fee | • Provides more service<br>• Defender<br>• Let's Make A Deal | • Right service/right place<br>• Financial integration<br>• Teacher |
| **Patient** | • No insurer choice<br>• Low knowledge of treatment options<br>• Little financial consequence | • Some insurer choice<br>• No knowledge<br>• Some knowledge of treatment options<br>• Growing financial consequence | • Choice of health plan with good knowledge<br>• Good knowledge of treatment options<br>• Ability to pay financial consequence |

provider competitive fear in order to become a super discount payor of services. The cost shift problem has been exacerbated.

Providers have accepted this change by assuming this is real and productive competition and pursue a "Let's make a deal" mentality. The high level of payor inspection of ordered services has caused providers to spend enormous resources defending their actions. The past had no controls to moderate increases in cost. The present has seen insurers with managed care leading the way to cultivate onerous inspection controls that have not proven to be effective in moderating cost, while causing administrative cost to explode in growth. Estimates for administrative costs built into our health care system now range up to 25 percent and is climbing. And no doubt this cost represent thousands of jobs, a powerful lever when it comes to political maneuvering to give everyone a role in the changed system. Whatever savings might have come from managed care have easily been

consumed by the heavy administrative load of managed care businesses and related expenses by providers.

The endpoint consumer (predominantly employees) is now given some choice of insurers, but with relatively no knowledge as to the quality of the options. Frankly, most people do not have the energy to consider complex networks, much less the qualifications of the hundreds of physicians and hospitals on such a list. Given the variety of possible medical needs, it is totally unrealistic for anyone to expect that individual consumers can make such decisions rationally, especially when the many needs that might have to be faced in a lifetime do in fact only occur once or twice in a lifetime. Choose a network to meet such possible needs whose probabilities would require cosmic numbers to express? Just who is kidding whom about making real choices of networks? Through enhanced media attention, and growing individual awareness of health needs, consumers seem to be gaining knowledge of treatment options, but most are certainly not informed enough or sufficiently sensitized economically to make rational cost and quality decisions of selected insurers or providers.

### Future ("getting to go")

Neither the past traditional health system nor the present attempts at managed care appear to be viable. Let us assume, however, that some form of managed care is a solution that should be pursued. In fact, some fully integrated models do work. If we are to direct our attention toward this goal, then we must begin to create a vision of a managed care delivery system that can work.

First, the ideal managed care delivery system will be an organized body of health services and financial mechanisms. It will operate in an integrated and systematic fashion to manage and provide the right wellness, medical, and related services at the right place and time. The system's organizational goal will be to improve the long-term health status of the community.

Moreover, the ideal organization will be designed to function as a seamless system of services. Information will flow freely between the organized parts to provide a basis for customer convenience, provider and consumer learning, continuous improvement in delivery processes, avoidance of medical duplication, and containment of costs. Incentives will exist to focus the organized parts on the long-term improvement of community health status. The organized parts will be related through ownership and collaborative incentives to optimize the system versus optimizing the individual parts. Furthermore, mechanisms will be in place to assure community accountability and responsibility.

Step back and compare this vision with the present health care system, and you will find that most of the key elements do not exist. There are pieces that may be found randomly in various geographic areas, but no system embodies all of the elements.

The goal of long-term improvement in community health status is the most noble element. One might even argue that it is elusive, even unattainable. While most health professionals hold this goal as an ideal, there is growing concern that the present system is incapable of being modified to accomplish this goal. Such a goal is almost totally absent in our independent organizational and individual goals. We lack systems. We lack a wellness focus. We lack incentives for resource conservation or prudence in resource use. We profit most from waste. Our paradigms, regulations, incentives, and adversarial competition combine to form high-growth, self-optimizing units of health delivery and financing. Reverse synergism occurs resulting in costs that are out

of control. How many organizations, managed care companies, insurers, providers, or others in the overall business have an ongoing, long-term interest in just one major community?

The key question becomes, Can we create an organized system that has the goal of improving the health status of the community and encouraging prudence in resource use? Given our inherent lack of trust for government, the more important question is, Can we accomplish this in the private sector? The authors believe we can if government pursues it as a policy, and providers constructively embrace the goal.

---

*The key question becomes, Can we create an organized system that has the goal of improving the health status of the community and encouraging prudence in resource use?*

---

The American Hospital Association (AHA), in its most recent reform scenarios, proposes the formation of community networks that integrate health care services with accountability and responsibility to the community. The community network proposal is just beginning to evolve in its conceptual state at the AHA. While the many conflicting interests in the association will batter and mold the concept, what is most important is that it represents the potential for a radical departure from the past and a brave proposal for the future.

By comparison, the managed competition approach apparently assumes at least two systems per community. Many communities simply are too small to afford more than one full-fledged system of services. This issue of size is especially a factor if one assumes that tertiary and referral services are to be contained within the overall system.

If the AHA community networks and managed competition models are to have some hope of working out, then one may well need to carve out some level of referral services and have those designated nationally or at the state level and not allow them to be duplicated. In this fashion, community care networks and managed competition will be left to provide more primary, preventive, and long-term services. Any attempt to have truly comprehensive networks and competition will create tremendous pressures to differentiate networks by more and more esoteric service offerings. This differentiation means costly duplication.

Underlying our ability to achieve this future is the notion that our behaviors, rules, and incentives as purchasers and consumers must change if we are to develop the ideal health care system. Without being encumbered by these learned or regulated behaviors, the future portrayed in Figure 1 outlines the attributes of our system described in the vision that could "get us to go."

The delivery model that would "get us to go" will have citizens, including professionals, ready to demand that government tackle existing laws, regulations, and policies to pave the way for productive change. Provisions such as malpractice, antitrust laws, and guild restrictions are all well entrenched, leaving the health system with great inflexibility for change. A government wishing to promote positive change must modify or remove existing regulations and establish new rules to achieve the desired policy. Furthermore, the government must play a very significant role in changing attitudes and promoting actions necessary for health prevention using educational devices and incentives. Finally, the government must provide for the social welfare of the overall population through appropriate financing for that part of the population that is unable to obtain health care services through their own financial means.

Health insurance purchasers must change their purchasing philosophy. Through an intensely individualistic and competitive system, we have conditioned ourselves and corporate America to put self-interest first. Health insurance purchasers of the future must place the needs of the community first. Only then can they ensure their own long-term survival.

To insure against routine and catastrophic health care costs, we must all recognize that we live in the same life boat. However, the costs that go into this pool must be truly affordable and insurable. Optional, opulent, discretionary, and wasteful practices and procedures cannot be allowed in the pool. To work, careful attention to ethics and need must be incorporated into designing the basic coverage plan.

The insurer must become a part of the system, but as a function, and not as a totally discrete entity. Joint ventures might work, but over the long term the separate goals of brokers and suppliers must mesh.

The insurer function must experience a transformation from a paper-bound, health policeman seeking to pay discount fees for selected risks to a more community-oriented organization known as a "health plan." The health plan must make open enrollment available to all businesses and individuals at community rates. The only allowed price adjustment would be to adjust for company or employee actions to learn and practice healthy life styles. Use of data systems must eliminate most paper

transfer, while assembling an electronic medical record that will follow the patient throughout the system.

The information collected on treatment and outcome must be assembled to inform and teach the public of the most efficient and appropriate use of resources. It must also provide data tools for the providers to foster continuous improvement in quality and value, with little or no inspection required by the health plan. Finally, the health plan must seek to optimize the system of quality providers through integration of finances and incentives, where possible, and by establishing fair values for the services provided by those not consolidated into the system.

Ultimately the insurer role must merge with the provider role. Where Blue Cross and Blue Shield plans still have a strong community service ethic, mergers or amalgamations of these units with providers may well occur. In states with multiple regions, farsighted plans may well find ways to merge by region, perhaps keeping some of the technical support services needed by the regions in cooperatives as service bureaus. We need innovation in this arena. As long as Blue Cross and Blue Shield plans adhere to their policeman role and do not see themselves as part and parcel of the delivery system such change will not occur. Over the short term, providers must integrate further. Some may well build their own managed care machinery in order to go direct to customers and bypass the third parties.

The providers—physicians, hospitals, and others—must collaborate and integrate to develop a system that delivers the right service at the right place for the right value. Guild restrictions must be modified to allow manpower capabilities to be fully utilized. Multidisciplinary group practices integrated with a health plan must be the dominant form of physician organization. Financial integration must provide incentives for each provider to be sensitized to overpriced, inappropriate, or poor quality care. Finally, the provider must be armed with information and have the incentive to teach the patient of appropriate treatments and preventive care.

The patient must be a knowledgeable consumer, possessing information gained through lifelong learning. Adequate information must be available to the consumer enabling quality and value judgments regarding the selection of health plan (insurer) and providers. Choice of health plans must be limited to two or three in major metropolitan areas. In rural and smaller communities, it may only be a single choice. Furthermore, the knowledge consumers gain must give them the ability to make choices relative to needed treatment, taking into account both cost and quality-of-life considerations. Finally, the consumer must have financial obligations for the health services received, based on the individual's ability to pay. Discretionary use, overuse, and misuse must have individual financial consequences. The common pool cannot be wasted and still retain the confidence of the broader community.

The vision therefore comprises a system of parts working together, each having an interest in the success and outcome of the other's action. The provider and insurer component under ideal circumstances would be a single integrated unit that is directed at creating a healthier community instead of a fragmented, suboptimized system of multiple providers and insurers that strive for their own individual success.

## CHANGES REQUIRED

"Getting to go" will require significant changes in the financing and organization of health services. This level of change can only be achieved through leadership that is willing and able to do what is necessary to achieve the vision. Figure 2 outlines the transition in leadership, financing, and organization required to "get to go." A snapshot of our present behaviors and structures would place us between the "old way" and "getting there." Thus, many leadership challenges remain ahead.

## Leadership

The speed of change and the ultimate ability to achieve our vision are in the hands of leadership. Years and years of the American management paradigm has left us with learned and comfortable habits to lead with command-and-control techniques with a self-interest focus for the short-term financial success of the organization and the leadership itself. A management leadership revolution is beginning to occur in America's battered, intensely competitive industries that compete in world markets. There are lessons to be learned from their experiences.

Deming and Juran, who brought great change to postwar Japan, are being heard by American industry. Their philosophies of organizational design to optimize the system and managed and collaborative competition have great applicability to the American health system. Many health care organizations have adopted quality initiatives that are leading to organizational redesign, increased value, and a recognition that cooperative collaboration is required if the community (system) is to be well served.

---

## FIGURE 2

CHANGES REQUIRED TO "GET TO GO"

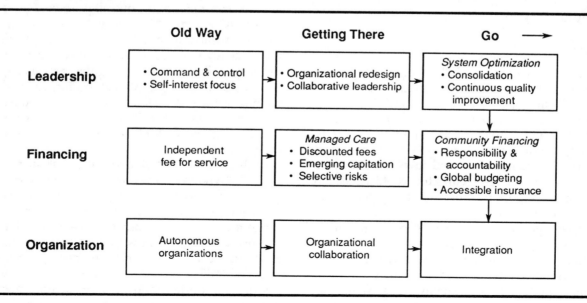

*Refocusing from institutional loyalty to community loyalty is a lofty demand of the vision, but essential and certainly not impossible.*

Management, however, is not the only component of leadership that must play a part in this chain. Boards of directors, volunteers, staffs, and concerned members in the communities are the best links with the needs of the community. They must be informed and lead in their own external circles. More important, they must ultimately inform management and other professionals of what the consumer, the patient, and the community want from health care leaders.

External leaders have not been given an appropriate role in helping us change the system. We must be accountable to our community links. While we must provide them with professional advice, education, and guidance, these external leaders must ultimately be the masters of a change paradigm requiring vast changes in organizational and political circles far beyond our own narrow professional domains.

Leadership, both internal and external, will arrive at "getting to go" when we all speak passionately for achieving maximum value for the community, not for the individual organizations. Most professionals demand institutional loyalty from trustees, not community loyalty. To progress, we must refocus this loyalty. Refocusing is a lofty demand of the vision, but essential and certainly not impossible.

## Financing

The adage that where the dollars go, so goes the mind applies to health care. Consequently the financing system must change if we are to "get to go." The struggle between independent fee-for-service payments and discounted fees and capitation used in managed care has been long and miserable. Adversarial relationships and loss of trust between provider and payor have prospered and the likelihood of correcting this conflict seems remote. Again, suboptimization of the system occurs through self-interest incentives provided to each of the parts. "Getting to go" will ultimately require merging of the finance and delivery mechanisms.

"Getting to go" will require a broader community perspective with both provider and financing systems having some community responsibility and accountability. Global budgeting for defined populations has been sug-

gested as a means to assure that health expenditures stay within some reasonable value limits for the community. A major departure from our present system, global budgeting conjures up images of onerous government control. Examples of successful structures such as state or community utility commissions may provide some direction or examples of the solutions, but we must recognize that they are diametrically opposed to the prevailing paradigm.

Furthermore, some portion of the health care dollar must begin to be invested for future improvements. Wellness prevention, community education, research on best demonstrated clinical processes and outcomes must receive an appropriate and ongoing investment. In a system with heavy constraints on costs, it would be easy to avoid investing in the future. We must not repeat the mistake of only investing in technology.

## Organization

Finally, the organization of the health care system must change to "get to go." Our health care system at a community level predominantly consists of autonomous organizations conditioned to compete for resources, survival, and growth. Some examples of provider collaboration have emerged but only after purchasers have proposed a system and community philosophy and exerted the necessary economic pressure to force collaboration.

Financial integration is integral to functioning as a system. Financial integration requires all of the provider and insurer parts to focus on delivering services within the financial constraint of the overall price paid by the purchasers in the form of insurance. Fee-for-service (piecework payment) is the antithesis of this concept. The natural tendency embedded in any piecework payment system is to revert to optimizing the parts, as measured by individual or organizational income, as opposed to optimizing the system. Kaiser and other well-developed, closed panel, staff model HMOs serve as examples of the "systemness" created when piecework payment is removed.

With calls for consolidation, the first question that arises is "Who owns the system?" In the existing "system," many owners exist. Few, however, have the range of resources needed to take on the comprehensive job suggested by the vision proposed here. Only the major metropolitan areas possess a population base sufficient to have more than two or three competing systems.

In a pluralistic economy, there will not be one right answer. Not-for-profit and for-profit, investor-owned organizations may emerge. As our analysis here indicates,

America pays a high price for its pluralistic amalgam of providers, insurers, and consumer methods. Perhaps we must think more boldly and take none of the current modes of insuring and caring as the starting point for reform. Whatever form of ownership and control that is chosen, it must be yoked to strong incentives that give the entity a long-term incentive to pay attention to wellness and community health status.

If a sense of community is to be achieved, the concept of consumer cooperatives should be considered as a method of bringing the community into the role of defining, using, and building the policies and programs that will help them to help themselves. Managed competition calls for consumer cooperatives, but it makes them mere intermediaries between consumers and the more traditional insurers and providers. In our version of the cooperative, it might be desirable to convert existing Blue Cross plans, voluntary hospitals, and other community health resources into property of the consumer cooperative. Put people back in the loop through ownership via the consumer cooperative! The separation of people from the institutions is undoubtedly one of the core problems. It might be reversed, in part, through consumer cooperatives.

## STRUCTURAL IMPEDIMENTS

Even with national policy consensus it will be difficult to "get to go" swiftly or efficiently. Our health care system is constructed around structures created or protected by incentives, laws, and behaviors learned and established over many years. These structures and incentives will act as impediments to a positive evolutionary change unless they are identified and changed or removed. The following sections discuss some significant impediments that should be evaluated.

### Consumer information

The best way to create positive change in the health system is to develop knowledgeable consumers. The more consumers know about price, quality, and medical alternatives, the more effective the private competitive market will be in delivering a continuously improving, high-value product. Consumers are generally confused and unknowledgeable relative to health care prices and quality. Providers have resisted dispensing information based on claims of professionalism, patient confidentiality, or a variety of other excuses. Consumer information and action are keys to positive change.

*Solution:* Information should be collected and disseminated by the government if not voluntarily and system-atically done by providers and insurers. User groups, self-help groups, and other modes of consumer involvement should be fully exploited in this process.

### Community philosophy

The current health system is not geared toward health care as a social responsibility of the community. Insurers have turned to aggressive selection of the best risks in the market, and business purchasers of health insurance want no part of community responsibility. The result has been low rates for some and unaffordable rates or unavailability for others. A return to the traditional community rating with open enrollment would be far superior to the current practice.

*Solution:* License only those insurers who agree to provide open enrollment with community rating to businesses and individuals in specified geographical regions. No licensed insurer may turn away any person or group for a pre-existing condition or risk factor. Insurers, however, can obtain reinsurance for extraordinarily high individual health care costs through a state or national pool funded by a revenue tax on all health insurers.

Second, providers have created an insidious form of discrimination through pricing systems. Discounts given to insurers who market to large business and good risks are balanced by charging extraordinarily high retail prices to those who cannot obtain insurance through mainstream insurers or who cannot afford insurance. This "reverse Robin Hood" principle is working to exacerbate the growing problem of access to health care.

*Solution:* Prohibit excessive or discriminatory price discounting.

### Guild laws

Over the years, the health professions have crafted laws with the purported purpose of protecting consumers seeking their services. A second, and many times more powerful motivation, is the protection of the professional status, supply of manpower, and income of the profession. Many states protect the independence of the physician through corporate practice of medicine laws. These laws, plus inappropriate Medicare fraud and abuse regulations, limit the ways physicians, hospitals, and other providers can band together as a group or system. If we are to achieve systemness, such artificial constraints must be removed.

Also, physicians and other health professionals have created restrictions as to who may provide certain services. These restrictions sometimes serve as barriers to more efficient, alternative practices. Removing these re-

> *Much of the micromanagement and utilization review that exist today are an outgrowth of the piecework payment inherent in fee-for-service structures.*

strictions would allow quality alternatives to be explored thereby increasing value and accessibility.

*Solution I:* Repeal laws that inappropriately protect physicians or other health care providers.

*Solution II:* Repeal laws or regulations that deter financial relationships between physicians and other providers.

*Solution III:* Repeal or amend professional work protections not necessary to protect the consumer.

*Solution IV:* Establish a national program of research, experimentation, and demonstration to work toward more efficient ways to use medical manpower to deliver health care. Provide federal exemptions for such projects. When amply demonstrated, disallow federal funds to any state that bars the use of the procedures demonstrated to be more efficacious.

### Fee-for-service

Piecework payment is an insidious deterrent to achieving an optimized system. It represents an incentive to provide (consume) more. Much of the micromanagement and utilization review that exist today are an outgrowth of piecework payment.

*Solution:* Systematically move away from fee-for-service payment structures. A powerful first step toward this objective would be modifying Medicare and Medicaid payment policies to adopt capitated or global payments.

### Ownership

For years the voluntary not-for-profit hospital has been the backbone of hospital services. The remaining providers in the system have been proprietary tax-paying organizations and individuals. The sanctity of the tax-exempt community ownership acts as a barrier to uniting tax-exempt and for-profit, proprietary interest— an essential element of creating systems. Furthermore, tax exemption has many times shielded economic decisions that would have been made differently if proprietary ownership interests were involved. Tax exemption has served a very valuable part in building our system, but it should not be allowed to serve as a deterrent for change in the system.

*Solution:* Careful and rational examination of not-for-profit laws and modifying them to achieve desired public policy purpose.

There may be many possible ownership combinations for promoting community interest in a health care system. Neither not-for-profits nor for-profits should be excluded from the opportunity. In some areas of the country public hospital systems have worked exceptionally well. Many of the public authorities in California, the Broward Hospital District in Ft. Lauderdale, the Greenville Hospital System in South Carolina, and others are outstanding systems. Public ownership may be distasteful to many due to the widely held belief that the government should only do what the private sector cannot do for itself. Many models work well making one model for all an unlikely option for provider systems. Therefore, new models must be developed to bridge the concerns.

The creation of community health cooperatives could bring a broad section of the community into play with providers, workers, and industry participating in a community-type ownership. Existing not-for-profit and public models along with Blue Cross plans could be integrated under a cooperative model. And, for community responsiveness, an ownership model that vested control in the people of the community could be a powerful incentive to put prevention first, a goal worth trying.

*Solution:* Examine and change regulations to ease the formation of community health cooperatives and encourage and allow not-for-profit providers and mutual insurers to contribute their assets to these cooperatives.

### Antitrust laws

The antitrust laws, now used so much in health care, were written in a different time for a different purpose. The desires of the communities and policymakers seem to differ from the application of these laws. The laws perpetuate a fractionated system that avoids integrating, while fearing expensive scrutiny or prosecution from a schizophrenic government policy.

A counter to this argument is that until the health care industry finds methods of truly putting the community and consumers into effective power positions so that accountability is restored, it will remain difficult to abolish or significantly change antitrust laws that are designed to punish anticonsumer behavior. To the extent that we keep professional control of health care, we are more likely to have antitrust laws to regulate our behavior. If we want change in antitrust laws, we must accept much more public accountability as the price for that change.

*Solution:* Revise antitrust laws and their application to health care but provide specific exemptions for monopoly-like consolidations when public accountability is assured by its structure and appropriate governmental oversight.

## Opportunities

Whether the solution is public or private, massive consolidation needs to take place in the health system to create integrated health systems combining provider services and financing mechanisms.

If one concurs with the vision, and the structural impediments begin to fall, what are some of the practical opportunities available?

*Opportunity 1: Voluntary consolidation.* With some change in the antitrust laws and a newfound community purpose of health provider leadership (managers and board), renewed efforts could be made to create managed care corporations that overarch the various provider and insurance parts. Authorization to create such entities would only be granted after assurances of public accountability have been made through a formal contract with the community.

*Opportunity 2: Consumer cooperatives.* New organizations such as the consumer cooperative, Puget Sound, could be promoted and formed. Proper clearances and existing laws would be required to allow not-for-profit assets to be contributed to these consumer cooperatives and to Blue Cross mutual insurance organizations that may be converted to consumer cooperatives.

*Opportunity 3: Utility commissions.* Communities could take charge of health care financing and operate in a utility commission fashion, establishing rates and demanding service integration. Demands made by the utility commission would encourage a natural consolidation among providers to protect their solvency and ownership interests. As in existing utilities, these organizations could be investor owned or not-for-profit (community owned).

*Opportunity 4: Give your assets to those most likely to use them to promote the goals enunciated here.* Not-for-profits who simply do not want to struggle with changes coming about in health care could give their assets to another not-for-profit organization on the condition that these assets be used to build a new vision of managed care in a community health system.

*Opportunity 5: Declare defeat and nationalize the system.* The system could be financed on a budgetary basis, forcing everyone into some national bargaining over roles, allocations, and the like. Having no enthusiasm for this opportunity, we offer no further details.

•   •   •

The challenge for leadership and the required changes are great. Our personal limitations include a limited view of the world and the threat of an overwhelming risk if one gets too far out on the limb. "Getting to go" will open up new and strange territories that will provide opportunity and failure for leaders. Capable leaders will pursue the opportunity. Threatened leaders will resist the change.

For those leaders who feel that the managed care existing today provides the most cost-effective, quality outcome for the individual, his or her sponsor in the community, they will go no further. Unfortunately for many of us, managed care means a third party trying to micromanage patients (deductions, authorizations, and so on), employers (claims, incentives, and so forth), and providers (approvals, forums, payment, tricks, and the like). Providers need to go ahead and master efficient care. We owe that to the community and the third party nightmare of administrative overkill must be laid to rest.

For those healthcare leaders who believe that managed care as a system focused on improving the health status of our communities is superior to our existing system, their individual goals and leadership focus must be changed accordingly. We cannot sit by idly and wait for the system to change us. Instead our obligation is to lead our organizations toward a new era in health care.

# HCMR dialogue: Managed care

Patrick A. Thompson
and
Montague Brown

*While Hillary Rodham Clinton and 500 experts toil over how to insert managed care disciplines into health care, people like Thompson have been working on the Nth generation of managed care products and services. Managed care in America has made great strides in payments, billing infrastructure, and contracting but the collection of good data and using it to make sound management decisions is lagging along with the sound use of data for clinical problem solving and treatment planning.*

*Health Care Manage Rev*, 1993, 18(2), 87–93
© 1993 Aspen Publishers, Inc.

**MB: *Pat, I'd like to have a conversation with you today about managed care and managed competition as they relate to health care reform. We've got a new administration in Washington with Mr. and Mrs. Clinton developing health care policy. They are pushing for health care legislative proposals within the first 100 days. Clinton recently renewed his pledge for a bill before the Congress in the first 100 days. There is a lot of action on this issue. But before we get into the details of that story I'd like to ask you to tell us a little bit about your background and where you're coming from in the health care field so the readers will have a sense of Pat Thompson.***

PAT: My professional background is primarily in managed care. I have been involved in the managed care industry in many different roles over the last 15 years. I have danced across the spectrum of managed care health care financing, built and managed health maintenance organizations [HMOs], preferred provider organizations [PPOs], third-party administrators [TPAs] and utilization review companies, and combined those into multi-option companies. The focus has always been managed care, however. Because of this diversity in my career, I'm probably not easily niched: Can't say I'm an HMO guy, can't say I'm a PPO guy. The current business that I'm in is described or defined as health plan risk management, but it has evolved over 15 years of my career and specifically the last 8 years with Cost Management Technologies (CMT). I founded CMT, Inc., in 1985 because I could see that the so-called managed care market was about to become more diversified. In the mid 1980s, CMT was focused on building and managing multi-option companies. In the late 1980s, as a result of what we had learned in the multi-option business, we decided to refocus on transporting managed care technologies to self-funded employees.

This interview was conducted by Montague Brown, Editor.

MB: Well let's take it from the top. What do you think are the main problems that need to be addressed in the health care field? What are the issues that must be addressed?

PAT: Cost and access are the two issues that are clearly on the front burner. And I think that these two issues reflect, at least from my perspective, what is the fundamental issue that's creating this breakdown in the health care system. And that issue is market failure. Market failure in the sense that both the buyers, those who purchase health care services, and the sellers, health care providers, transact in ways that violate classic market theory. Over a period of time we just simply managed to construct a health care system (including delivery and financing of subsystems) that makes it very very difficult for the health care market to develop in a rational way. And I believe that the issues of cost and access both flow from that fundamental failure.

MB: That fundamental failure is pretty complicated. It is easier to say cost and access than it is to say exactly what fundamental failure is.

PAT: Oh it is. That's why we all say cost and access.

MB: It seems to me that on the insurance side, insurance is dead. I don't know anybody who can buy insurance anymore. I don't know anybody who sells it anymore. If they do sell it and they have to pay out or suffer a loss, they want their money back the next year. So the premium is raised or changed in a way that insurance does not transfer risk. It seems to me that we've lost any semblance of insurance in the marketplace.

PAT: Yes. Insurance in the sense of . . . .

MB: Spreading risks.

PAT: Yes. Spreading risks without management systems, good or bad.

MB: Yes. We started out without any management systems.

PAT: That's right.

MB: Health insurance really started out as a not-for-profit venture. It didn't start out in the profit sector, and community ratings were used so that everybody could get into one big pool. Those who needed insurance got it, and everybody paid roughly the same amount.

PAT: That's right. It is called Blue Cross.

MB: Broad risk sharing is gone. How about the provider's side? I can tell you for a fact that on the provider side the incentives force providers to try to provide as many services as they possibly can because they get no revenue from most patients unless they do something for the patient. So doing things for patients is what they try to maximize. And that practice drives costs up.

PAT: Yes, I would agree.

MB : Providers may try to minimize the cost of doing something. But many payors also try to make their payments related to costs. So they have had incentives to raise the costs and raise gross revenue, which is a disastrous combination. Now what can managed care do about that? Can it change that fact? Is managed competition managed care going to change that situation?

PAT: Managed competition will only change those patterns if buyers and sellers—whose money is at stake on both sides of the transaction—are truly tied in fundamentally different ways. There are failures both on the side of the buyer and the seller. Managed care will not be able to make a substantial contribution to the resolution of cost and access issues unless the buyer's side of the market actually begins to behave rationally, and the key to rational behavior or decision making is better decision-making information. In other words what we've got is an irrational system. Webster defines irrational as not endowed with reason or understanding. And that's what we have. Now to some people it may look crazy but health care now represents 14 percent of the gross domestic product. On both the buyer's side and the seller's side we are not going to address the market failure issues that have contributed to the cost and access issues until we create a rational market.

MB: Well, one step toward a rational market would have to be a change in people's awareness of costs. If you ask them whether or not they are aware of the costs involved when they are selecting a hospital for a heart operation they are not going to look at costs very closely. At that point they are asking "My God, get me to a hospital that does good work." At the point of delivery cost cannot be the major issue. Most people make their buying decisions when they make their insurance decisions. And, at this point, employers play the largest role in such decisions. In effect, with health insurance we have a company store mentality. Except for health care, company stores have disappeared. Today many seem to want to put the responsibility on the really big company store, namely, Washington.

PAT: No you can put the big dollar decisions at the patient level.

MB: Well, patients don't buy. They're not real customers. They're not making dollar decisions at that point. They don't think the way they probably should. They really make their decisions back there at the insurance level. Most of the dollar decisions are made by employers, the company store.

PAT: That's right, the employee benefits package . . . the health benefits program.

MB: During World War II, companies didn't report benefits as compensation and the Internal Revenue Service [IRS] found out and ruled that insurance was compensation. Where there's money, there's value coming to the government and it is going to be taxed. Employees got upset. Congress said well let's not tax health benefits, let's drop it. It did and forever after we've masked the costs to the employee. Do we have to change that tax? That is a big issue in Washington.

PAT: That's right. Yes, we do need to consider it. Current tax policy is an extension of the irrationality of the market such as it is. Those incentives have financial consequences that I believe are basically societal reflections of the absence of a healthy market dynamic in the health care industry. Those tax policies only serve to give incentive to further irrationality.

*MB: So it really is a systemic problem.*

PAT: That's right.

*MB: So anybody who tries to tinker with it probably isn't going to change very much are they?*

PAT: No. Tinkering around the edges won't get it done.

*MB: Let's go in a slightly different direction. There are many pieces of the puzzle, and we're not going to cover them all in one conversation. But one of the trial balloons coming out of the Clinton administration is the prospect of cutting Social Security benefits. He would use retiree benefits to shore up the deficit problem. It's a way of getting some of the money that goes to retirees under Social Security back into the federal treasury. A cost of living adjustment [COLA] freeze will cut down on the outlays in future years because every single COLA compounds over the years. So stopping the COLA for one year is a savings that accrues again and again. It is big money. That principle could be applied to Medicare as well. What do you think about that? Is that fair? Is there fairness or equity in doing something like that? People are retired; they have made their financial decisions years earlier. Is it the right thing to do? the wrong thing to do? Will it "incentivize" older people if their Social Security benefits are taxed a little bit? Will that make the market more rational?*

PAT: No. I don't think it would make the health care market more rational.

*MB: Such a tax would help pay for more access for more people. Is that correct?*

PAT: That's right. But in the presence of the fundamentally irrational market system, we would simply be pouring gasoline on the fire.

*MB: Okay, let me ask you another question. Should we tax benefits over some basic level?*

PAT: That would presumably cut down on consumption. It raises the price to the employer and in doing so encourages the employer to become a better buyer.

*MB: And it basically raises costs to the employee because it adds to labor costs that employers will either recoup through lower wages or higher prices to consumers.*

PAT: It would also serve to reverse the unhealthy market dynamic that began after World War II with health benefits not being taxed.

*MB: Yes, it would start to bring the consumer back into the loop.*

PAT: That's right. The individual patient and the employer are both brought into the loop. You need to have the individual patient and the group purchaser involved.

*MB: But the tax issue would occur at the group purchase level. It goes on the pay stub.*

PAT: Yes.

*MB: Taxes get paid or withheld or whatever.*

PAT: That's right.

*MB: And that could be applied both with the employer and the employee.*

PAT: That's right. In the absence of some kind of tax policy that supports rational market systems, we will still see an extension of the irrationality.

*MB: It seems to me that these payment mechanisms are not necessarily going to help this rationality issue. Taxing benefits would be a step in that direction. At least that's fairly straightforward but likely to be resisted. Everything is likely to be resisted.*

PAT: Right.

*MB: We've got 37 million people uninsured. And, it's hard to tell exactly what their needs are, what services they require, and what the costs would be to cover them. How do you think the administration could pay for that 37 million? Out of the savings to be achieved from better management? We're talking managed competition as the method that's supposed to generate savings that the government can then use to bring more people into the system. What do you think of that proposition?*

PAT: Well, I think it is unrealistic to expect savings in the first few years.

*MB: Clinton heard the same response from his professional advisors. It's unrealistic to expect savings to do this job without creating a bigger deficit. When Clinton heard that he pushed them aside and put his wife in charge. He didn't buy that argument. He wants to cut costs sufficiently to pay for greatly improved access.*

PAT: I don't think it is necessarily unrealistic over the long term. I think it is unrealistic over the short and intermediate term. In other words, Monty, what I'm saying is that undoing the irrationality in the market system is not going to happen overnight as a result of legislation or restructuring into a managed competition model. It is not going to happen overnight. If we move progressively toward a more rational market system, then it may be possible to absorb the 37 million uninsured on the differential cost savings. As a matter of fact, today other major industrial, competitive countries are at 7 percent instead of 14 percent of the gross domestic product.

*MB: So if we spend twice as much on health care, we should be able to find savings someplace if we want to be competitive.*

PAT: Yes, absolutely. The difference between or the multiple of the 14 percent over the 7 percent would tell you that somehow in a rational system that differential of 7 percent [14 percent minus 7 percent] ought to provide enough resources to take care of 37 million or roughly 15 percent of our population.

*MB: There are many professionals who argue that the resources that we have are quite adequate if used more rationally. It would, however, require that the savings achieved actually stay in the system to support access. Government wants all of the savings. Thus, private business and consumers would get lower cost care at the old, high price.*

PAT: Right. I believe that incentives alone won't carry the day. So we cannot turn this into some kind of tax policy chess game and stop there. I don't believe that will get the job done.

*MB: Correct.*

PAT: In addition to a tax policy (i.e., incentives), we need better management both on the seller side and on the buyer side. We have to introduce rational decision making by informed management.

*MB: Pat, you've spent the last 8 to 12 years working on these issues. Tell us what do we need to do? What can we do short of major reforms? Or even with major reforms, how do we get to the point where people are making rational decisions? Data drive decisions. So what do we need?*

PAT: About four years ago CMT decided to redefine what business we were in and then move in that direction. We basically moved out of the HMO segment into the large self-funded group segment.

*MB: Which is still the growing segment, right?*

PAT: That's right. The percentage of employees covered by self-insured employee health benefit plans increases each year. In the process of making some of our business decisions, a number of things occurred to us. First it occurred to us that the language of the health care, insurance, and managed care industries was sufficiently arcane to keep health care purchasers in the dark. I can remember one specific discussion we had while redefining where we wanted CMT to go as a company. In specific terms, we wanted to be a health care cost management company. We were talking then about health care cost management and all the language that we were hearing from ourselves, from the marketplace, and from our competitors was health care, not cost management. This problem was a fundamental one. How are we going to meet our primary objectives working with clients in such a way in the self funding market that we could help them become informed decision makers? How could we do that if we were using language that they couldn't understand? We said

let's do a search of the literature and let's look at our own internal experience in terms of managing the business of this corporation, especially the cost side. Let's look for language that is business expense management language rather than health care language. Along the way, Monty, a number of things became very clear to us. What occurred to us then was that using fundamental business expense management tools—tools used by businesses in every other expense category but health care—was the most effective way to go.

*MB: Give me some examples.*

PAT: Well, a primary example is the use of a budget. Virtually every corporation focused on managing its expenses in this competitive economy prepares a benchmark or a baseline against which it can measure its actual performance.

*MB: Well, the companies that have budgets know they have x number of people and they know the amount of their premiums, so they budget enough for the premiums. That's a budget, isn't it?*

PAT: That is too broad to manage. Break it down a little bit more. Indeed, employers don't know what their premium should be. Corporations that self-insure do not know in advance what their "premiums" will be. They will pay the bills as the health care expenses are incurred. What a corporation pays for employee health care services will be a function of the average unit cost per service and the volume of services the corporation buys. From an insurance perspective, the insurance company establishes a premium by reviewing what an employer has paid in the past. For its self-funded clients, CMT prepares an employee health plan budget based on what an employer should be paying for health care services, not how much it has paid in the past.

*MB: You came into the HMO business first, and you priced the market based on a fairly detailed, actuarially based net of possible cost. You were probably 10 times more sophisticated in building a budget in the HMOs. Therefore, is that what you are now building for the buyers?*

PAT: Yes, that is exactly what we are doing.

*MB: So that they can get deeply into expectations from a much more sophisticated database development.*

PAT: We sure do. We use an actuarial base, region by region, company by company, to provide a company-specific or a group-specific target.

As we prepare this basic management tool, this benchmark budget, for our large self-funded employer clients, the budget is based on the specifics of that client's health plan. In other words, we take into consideration not simply the number of employees and the number of dependents, but we look at their age-sex mix, the region they're in, and the industry our client is in.

*MB: So you're bringing actuarial tools to the table for the employer.*

PAT: For the manager, right.

*MB: For the manager, and coupling that with the kind of budgetary detail that you used in the HMO.*

PAT: That's correct.

*MB: And then you're tracking their experience and providing them with what?*

PAT: Providing them with the information that they need to know regarding what is going right and what is going wrong, and of those things that aren't going right, the reasons why they may be varying negatively.

*MB: You're using your insight in managing care the HMO way, knowing what things can go wrong and where they're most likely to go wrong.*

PAT: We combine that insight with the specific data, cost accounting data so to speak, that we generate from our claims payment system.

*MB: Don't all TPAs do that?*

PAT: No, all TPAs pay claims, but very few TPAs—in fact we don't know of another TPA in the country—actually take the raw data that come from each claims transaction and in effect convert that data into a highly organized cost accounting system that allows analysis of variance against the budget. We can identify patterns based simply on the cost accounting system that we are using. When we combine the results of the cost accounting system with the experience that the personnel in this company have built up over a number of years in managed care, we are then able to identify and make recommendations or provide employers with options on how they can deal with the identified variance.

*MB: Fascinating. Now, you're doing this for businesses. What do you do for health care organizations? Are they just on the other end of the stick? You show employers how to cut their costs and that means cutting the revenue going back to providers doesn't it?*

PAT: As a matter of fact, among our large clients are some major health care providers in the Kansas City area. Specifically, these clients are hospitals. In this situation, the client is both a buyer and a seller.

*MB: So they're learning a lot from you about how to manage their own health care benefits?*

PAT: Yes.

*MB: And at the same time they're learning exactly how a sophisticated managed care company would evaluate them as a provider, I presume.*

PAT: In other words, what we give them is a glimpse of what a rational market system would look like. When they're wearing their provider business hat, they can in effect bounce back to those buyer discussions we've had with them. Now some of these conversations about performance—financial performance of the hospital employee health plan—can become schizophrenic because these clients—hospitals—are both the buyer and the seller at the same time. But the client learns. This approach introduces the client to a view of how the market works in some situations or how it can be made to work.

*MB: I know one or two of your clients, and I have talked with them. It is my impression that their level of sophistication is growing as to what's going on and how care can be managed by buyers and for buyers; that is, how managed care can and should work. Their sophistication is growing by leaps and bounds. They should be much better prepared to sell to HMOs.*

PAT: Yes.

*MB: As a matter of fact, I can almost see them taking your product and having you monitor other HMOs with whom they're working. Couldn't they do that? Then they could provide you with the same form that goes to the HMO or the PPA and then have you monitor that. You could probably enable them to make reports to buyers faster than their own PPAs could.*

PAT: In many ways that is right.

*MB: That is possible. I don't know that you've made a business of it, right?*

PAT: As a matter of fact, we are having discussions with some hospital clients that would in effect have us transport our technologies again, this time from the buyer's side over to the seller's side.

*MB: You're really at your best, it seems to me, when you serve both sides and provide each with opportunities to gain insight into how they could better serve one another.*

PAT: Absolutely. We're committed to that, because part and parcel of the market failure issue that we highlighted earlier is that both the buyers and the sellers must behave rationally. Therefore, we must have a baseline of information on which to make decisions on both sides of the transactions.

*MB: Well it seems to me that anything that comes across as managed care has to be at least as sophisticated as the level you've achieved so far. I'm not saying that to denigrate your level of sophistication, but I know that you're at the front end of this effort and not at the back end. It's not as though you feel you've gone all the way or that you're ahead of everybody else, but that you probably still have a long way to go.*

PAT: Absolutely, and what we are learning on a daily basis, Monty, is that each new refinement that we add does not come from great conceptual quan-

tum leaps but from day-to-day transactional lessons that we learn. Indeed, we are at the very beginning, both on the seller side and on the buyer side. There's also a strong element of many of the same dynamics of total quality management or continuous improvement that we have built into our products and our company.

*MB: I know you have in fact used total quality techniques to help you in the past.*

PAT: That's right. One of the health care reform issues is better management, which, as we said earlier, is the supplemental piece of rational tax policy. We're moving our clients, the buyers, away from the notion that assessing financial performance of their health plan is a once a year event. It's a continuous process. Previous to doing business with us, our clients only knew how they had performed financially at the end of the year. Generally, they didn't know why they had done what they had done.

*MB: Let me ask you the bottom line question, Pat. You've been doing this for several years now. What's happening to the health care costs for your clients? What kind of experience are you having? Most people I talk with experience 15 to 20 percent cost increases per year, and I see brokers and health care plans talking about trying to limit or guarantee results. It may be somewhere in the 10 percent cost increase per year. What are you getting for your clients?*

PAT: Your numbers about the market are right-on, Monty. Currently, 18 percent increases are the accepted trend. We did a comparison of 1992 claims and administrative costs on a per employee per month basis for all of our clients. Each one saw an actual reduction, a net reduction of costs in an absolute manner of about 7.5 percent in 1992.

*MB: So if the average increase is running 15 percent and you're running a 7.5 percent decrease, you're talking about a 20 percent difference or gain.*

PAT: Right, a swing of 20 percent. That's the average for all of our groups over 1,000 employees.

MB: *Is that because you got the groups that were the easiest to handle and with the most to save, or are you getting more sophisticated ones? Are they really ready to manage?*

PAT: No, cour clients reflect a great deal of diversity, and, yes, they're ready to manage.

MB: *Using the data, they're actually taking the advice and making the changes.*

PAT: That's right. They love being empowered, and what CMT does is to empower health plan managers to manage. A key element of our relationship with our clients is that we serve them by making them better managers. Frankly, a lot of our competitors have positioned themselves with large employers, self-funded employers, in such a way that the employers feel that it's the responsibility of the TPA to manage. TPAs are the ones who have all the tools. We say, no, wait a minute, we should help the managers manage.

MB: *You use our tools to obtain the data you need to make the decisions.*

PAT: Yes, absolutely. CMT will give the health plan manager the information in a form that is understandable and actionable on a timely basis. We do a budgeted versus actual assessment, a written analysis, an on-site briefing every quarter with each client. It's continuous, Monty.

MB: *I don't think I've every gotten any report like that. Most people don't.*

PAT: It can't be done once a year, it has to be continuous. Our ability, given the budget models that we use to spot negative variances, is very, very strong. We budget unit cost and volume expectations. In other words, CMT defines what your unit cost and volume per type of service should be, and we budget and track approximately 50 categories of health services.

MB: *That's a lot of detail right there.*

PAT: An awful lot of detail, but it's that kind of detail that allows us to serve the client and identify the anomalies, the variances.

MB: *And you get their data, and you also have data from the actuarial firms that collect this data on an action basis?*

PAT: That's correct.

MB: *So you have norms, some kind of reason to know what's in range and what the normal versus abnormal variation is.*

PAT: That's right. We also can establish norms across our book of businesses by comparing the performance of a particular client to the performance of all of our clients. In addition to the unit cost budget we also build a volume of services or a frequency of services budget using the same 50 categories. In other words, what we say is this: At a fundamental level, health care costs really originate from only two factors. One, how much you are paying for a service. Two, how many services you are buying. So we budget 50 separate categories, and we trend each of those categories separately, because inpatient hospital costs are not rising at the same rate as outpatient diagnostic costs.

MB: *You must be giving people 20 times, 30 times more information than they've ever gotten before.*

PAT: Well, yes, but I'd like to qualify that, Monty. Each of our quarterly reports are restricted to a maximum of four pages in terms of the executive summary. We noticed as we moved into this particular field that our competitors—third party administrators and insurance companies who administered self-funded plans—pumped volumes and volumes of data in literally 10 inches of computer paper each month. We decided clients needed actionable information. That's right, understandable, actionable information. So those 50 line items are actually collapsed down into six major subcategories. Then we move through each quarter of the analysis of what the performance was against what we had budgeted for a particular item, identify the variances, and then we move into our cost accounting system and we "peel the onion."

Our ability to peel the onion through that cost accounting system is substan-

tial. Let me give you an example. We have a client that is a financial services company with about 1,600 employees spread throughout the entire continental United States. In the second quarter of doing analysis of actual versus budgeted for this firm, we identified that there was a substantial negative variance in the area of cardiac surgery. As we peeled the onion, we narrowed 80 percent of that variance down to one single medical group, a small group of cardiac surgeons in a Midwestern state. Boom! Problem identified. If you are unable to identify the problem, you have no chance to resolve it.

MB: *How extensive is this approach to managing these claims and data systems for employers? How extensive is it across the industry? How many people are doing it?*

PAT: We know of no other company in the country that is using this tool.

MB: *Sounds to me like you've got room for explosive expansion.*

PAT: We do.

MB: *Networking? Chain?*

PAT: Possibly. Not out of the question.

MB: *Let me switch gears just a little, get off the microlevel and go back a little to the macrolevel. You've been in government, you've been in the private sector. You've worked for not-for-profit and for-profit institutions. You've got a good sense of the industry. What changes do you think we'll be able to implement in health care reforms over the next two years? What's possible, what is the most likely scenario?*

PAT: I think the most likely scenario is that we will end up with the core elements of what is currently being described as the managed competition model, and the structure will resemble what has been put forward in that particular model. I think that model will be supplemented beyond the structure—it will be supplemented with some fundamental changes in tax policy. I think relative to the issue of the uninsured there will be a phasing in rather than a push to cover all 37 million up front. I believe any attempt to cover all 37 million would fail, because the structural capacity at the beginning would not produce the kinds of savings that would be needed to extend the coverage.

*MB: What about these buyer's co-ops? Do you expect that they will be one of the major elements? I'm part of a small business that buys its health insurance, which is basically an HMO plan, here in Washington, D.C. The plan is bought through a cooperative arrangement with an organization, located in Boston, that acts on behalf of smaller employers. After contacting some of the local plans I don't think the firm would ever have gotten in if it had had to fill out all the forms, give all the guarantees, get all the blood tests, and so on. By going through this quasi co-op and paying a very small fee, the firm got in for at least 40 percent less than what is being quoted to individuals. It was amazing.*

PAT: Yes. A good solid example of the value of the cooperative purchasing agent function. I also believe that we will see a substantial reduction, Monty, in the existing exclusions and restrictions with regard to coverage and eligibility.

*MB: As far as I can tell, the underwriters have mastered the art of the "nth degree" and destroyed health insurance. The good news is they can make a profit, no matter who sent them, because they'll figure out that charge. The bad news is there's no more risk sharing, and we've got to get back to some risk sharing.*

*Okay, we've got phase-in of the enrollments, we've got cooperatives, which are buying groups of some sort. Actually, co-ops could actually own the systems from as far as I can tell. The one in Puget Sound is a very fine consumer co-op. They would not be bad owners for providers as well, would they, although Clinton is not anticipating that role.*

PAT: No, he's anticipating that the competition will come from a diversity of AHPs, accountable health plans.

*MB: So you've got that competition. Let me throw out another factor. On the provider side, I was told the other day that Aetna is buying physician practices. Baxter buys physician practices as well as CIGNA and Kansas City Blue Cross. Are we seeing the beginning of a vertical integration on the part of insurers into practice via primary care?*

PAT: Yes.

*MB: How far will it go?*

PAT: I don't think it will go as far as some people might think. I do believe that a number of insurance companies will continue that trend. I feel that ultimately what will happen, however, will be that the dynamic of group practice will become a much more dominant dynamic than insurers owning physicians.

*MB: Well, there are companies out there that are buying group practices.*

PAT: Yes, that is right. What I'm saying is that, from a market perspective, it is the multispecialty group practice that will create change in behavior and change in movement—whether it's owned by an insurance company or not.

*MB: It doesn't really matter.*

PAT: Actually, from my perspective, the opportunity for some providers can be substantial in managed competition. There clearly are some potentially significant threats in the managed competition model and the focus that is now being put upon health care delivery. Nevertheless, I believe that certain providers—the early innovators—are going to lock in on the idea that improved quality actually produces decreased costs. It will be the providers who manage themselves within that context who wind up winning.

*MB: Providers need data, and they need people like you to provide the data to employers so employers know the difference. Right now no one knows the difference.*

*Let me switch gears again and ask you another more general question. If you were advising young people about health care and managed care and whether to get into this field today, what would you tell them?*

PAT: Interesting question.

*MB: Think of your daughters.*

PAT: Well, as a matter of fact, my older daughter, Beth, is in health care. She works for CMT as our Client Services Manager. So I've thought about those types of issues. I would say that there's some good news and some bad news in the future for young people coming into the industry. I think that the net result of so-called reform will be a tightening of the labor market, the exponential growth in jobs in the health care sector that we have seen over . . . .

*MB: Some say a million jobs will be lost.*

PAT: Remember, Clinton said at his economic summit that growth of the health care industry is "bad growth."

*MB: We shouldn't be growing jobs in a sector that's wasting money.*

PAT: That's what he's saying. So industrywide I believe that there will be a severe loss of jobs and that is a real downside for young people entering the industry. Yet I believe that young people coming into the industry will be able to select employers, either on the buyer or the seller side, who are geared to efficiency. Frankly, this era in health care could turn out to be the most exciting.

Part II

# STRATEGY, STRUCTURE, and MANAGED CARE

# Vertical integration in health services: Theory and managerial implications

Douglas A. Conrad
and
William L. Dowling

*A vertically integrated health care system is an arrangement whereby a health care organization offers, either directly or through others, a broad range of patient care and support services. This article discusses the market forces and strategic considerations driving the recent trend toward vertical linkages in health care markets and examines some of the managerial implications and issues associated with this vertical restructuring trend.*

*Health Care Manage Rev*, 1990, 15(4), 9–22

The health services market is undergoing radical transformation, a transformation that began with extensive horizontal integration and multisystem formulation in the 1970s and has been followed more recently by extensive vertical integration and diversification in the 1980s. We believe that these recent trends in vertical linkages in health care markets will continue throughout the foreseeable future. There are definite economic and clinical benefits associated with such vertical structuring. Our goal is to try and understand the market forces and strategic considerations that are driving the vertical reorganization of the health care system and to present some of the managerial implications and issues associated with this vertical restructuring.

The article proceeds in 4 parts:
1. definition of vertical integration,
2. presentation of a theoretical framework that sets out the underlying determinants of vertical integration and its associated benefits and costs,
3. examination of inter- and intraorganizational forms responding to those underlying determinants of vertical integration, and
4. managerial implications and issues associated with development of vertically integrated health care systems.

We draw on microeconomic theory, particularly the literature on transaction costs and competitive strategy that emerged in the late 1970s and early 1980s, as well as on empirical evidence and insights concerning practical managerial and organizational issues. Those managerial and organizational issues translate into agenda for future research and investigation by both the academic community and the fields of practice. This research needs to be informed by collaboration among management practitioners, clinicians, and academics working within the frameworks of their basic scientific disciplines.

## DEFINITIONS

A vertically integrated health care system is an arrangement whereby a health care organization (or

**Douglas A. Conrad,** *Ph.D., is a Professor in the Department of Health Services, University of Washington in Seattle. He also serves as Director of the University of Washington's Graduate Program in Health Services Administration in Seattle.*

**William L. Dowling,** *Ph.D., is Vice President for Planning and Policy Development at Sisters of Providence health system. He is also a Clinical Professor in the University of Washington's graduate program in Health Services Administration in Seattle.*

closely related group of organizations) offers, either directly or through others, a broad range of patient care and support services operated in a functionally unified manner. The range of services offered may include preacute, acute, and postacute care organized around an acute hospital. Alternatively, a delivery system might specialize in offering a range of services related solely to long-term care, mental health care, or some other specialized area.

Full functional integration requires both administrative and clinical integration. As a corollary, the management and operation of vertically integrated services will tend to be closely coordinated or centralized. The major purpose of such integration is to enhance the system's overall effectiveness or profitability, not necessarily the effectiveness or profitability of each individual service line.

Clinical integration of the health care services provided to individual patients implies geographic proximity, since both the delivery of patient care and, consequently, the geographic boundaries of a vertically integrated delivery system are generally local or regional. These boundaries conform to natural patient care service areas or markets.

The importance of particular health care services being coordinated within a local or somewhat larger regional market—as opposed to a national or large regional area—will depend on the geographic scope of the market for the relevant services. For example, an individual receiving specialized cancer care might well be served by a tertiary referral hospital far from his or her residence. The tertiary hospital care could be augmented by home health care and long-term care for the cancer patient in his or her local market. If the various elements of the individual's care were integrated within a single health care system, organizational and clinical integration could still exist even though the various levels of the patient's care were delivered in physically distinct settings. This highlights the need to define the geographic nature of the market for a given service before judging whether the patient care functions are integrated.

Put simply, vertical integration is the coordination or linkage of businesses (service lines) that are at different stages in the production process of health care. For example, an acute care hospital vertically integrates when it acquires or establishes different levels or types of care such as ambulatory care, long-term care, or home care. The principal aims of vertical integration are to enhance coordination among the elements or stages of the production process (Porter[1] has called this proc-

*The primary purposes of vertical integration in health care are to enhance the comprehensiveness and continuity of patient care and to control the sources of patients or other users of a delivery system's services.*

ess "the value chain") and to control the channels of demand for, or distribution of, a firm's core services. In the case of the hospital, the core service is acute inpatient care. Control and coordination of ambulatory care, long-term care, home care, medical products supply, and even wellness and health-promotion activities serve either to promote referrals to the hospital's core (inpatient) service line or to improve its distribution (as in the example of postdischarge care).

In short, the primary purposes of vertical integration in health care are to enhance the comprehensiveness and continuity of patient care and to control the sources of patients or other users of a delivery system's services. In the past, vertical integration in health care focused on closing gaps in the availability of services and improving the continuity of patient care. In today's competitive and reimbursement-constrained environment, controlling the flow of patients to an institution is often the key to maintaining market share. The emphasis on controlling demand and/or channels of distribution has increased as competition has intensified.

## DIMENSIONS OF VERTICAL CONTROL

In defining vertical integration in general, one can distinguish four dimensions of the vertical control continuum, which is a more general way of describing vertical integration.[2] These four dimensions are

1. the breadth of the integration; for example, the range of diagnosis related groups (DRGs) cared for by the vertically integrated system;
2. the degree of within-firm purchases and internal sales of vertically related services, as contrasted with the use of external sources ("outsourcing") for inputs and sales to other firms of one's service outputs;
3. the number of stages in the vertically related value chain integrated or explicitly coordinated by a single organization; for example, the health maintenance organization (HMO) that provides a wellness program, ambulatory care, acute inpa-

tient care, long-term care, and home health care, as well as the full continuum of primary and specialty care for given clinical conditions, would be integrated at many stages in the value chain; and

4. the form of integration, that is, the nature of the coordination or ownership arrangements that link related services.

The breadth of vertical integration is a strategic decision for the firm, one that balances the firm's efficiency and effectiveness in delivering services among different product (e.g., DRG) types. For example, the firm that chooses to offer a wide array of service types—for instance, from comprehensive mental health services all the way through specialized cancer care and sophisticated trauma services—has presumably made a conscious decision that it can function efficiently and effectively across that wide array of services. An organization can vertically integrate in one product stream (e.g., cancer care) without necessarily integrating vertically or even offering significant services in other areas.

The decisions about breadth depend on synergies across service types, just as decisions about "depth" turn on the efficiency and effectiveness of an organization across different levels of a vertical value chain. For instance, there are cross-benefits between offering general medical-surgical services and possessing a trauma care capacity. Similarly, the chemotherapy and radiological services required in a comprehensive oncology program also serve to support the delivery of general medical-surgical care.

The degree to which a single level of a vertically integrated firm purchases all of its inputs from internal sources and provides the outputs of its level exclusively to other divisions or levels within the firm also involves a strategic balance. The use of external sources in addition to internal sources for inputs stimulates competition within the firm as to the source of supply of drugs, laboratory tests, and other inputs to the delivery of services. Outsourcing also maintains strategic flexibility in the event that the firm's own capacity is compromised by external events, such as staffing shortages or declines in demand for the organization's primary output.

The business knowledge gained through provision of one level's service to another level within the same organization can be used to develop outside markets for the organization's services. For example, the in-house pharmacy or laboratory that supplies the needs of a hospital could also arrange the sale of those products to other organizations such as physician practices.

This strategy serves to enhance the prospects for internal vertical integration by raising the scale of output at any one stage (through enhanced numbers of markets for that stage of production), and thus may justify the integration by creating gains through economies of scale.

The number of stages in the value chain that a single firm decides to control—so as to better coordinate its contracts and other arrangements—will be driven by consideration of the cost savings from coordinating input and output flows as well as of gains in the continuity and quality of patient care derived from more closely controlling the different stages of service. For instance, the provision of health promotion and disease prevention services within a health services organization that also operates a hospital provides a base for the hospital's activities in acute patient care, either by generating referrals or by providing advance information regarding patient needs that aids in coordinating these patients' later care. A key to the decision to vertically integrate a series of related stages is an organization's conscious commitment to serve a population base. The depth of integration is thus driven both by the ability to share information, physical capital, and patient care human resources across different levels of health services activity and by the gains to continuity of care that result from doing so.

The organization can add or gain control of a product or service line through many different means:

- internal development of new services
- acquisition of another organization or service
- formal merger
- lease or sale/lease-back arrangement
- franchise
- joint venture
- contractual agreement
- loan guarantee
- informal agreement or affiliation

Each of these different forms of vertical control has different risks, costs, and benefits. An organization's decision to vertically integrate is not a simple zero-to-one choice, but rather, involves a continuous balancing act among these different forms of vertical control.[3]

In addition to the four generic dimensions of vertical control discussed above, a unique "fifth dimension" in health care exists—the potential integration of health insurance with health services delivery.

At one level of analysis, the linkage of the source of health care payment with the source of health care delivery simply seems to represent decisions along each of the four dimensions already discussed:

1. It represents the addition of a new stage in the production of process—backward integration into delivery from the viewpoint of the third party payer, or forward integration into payment for its own services by the health care delivery organization.
2. A third party payer who hired or purchased its own physician services network would be choosing the "common ownership" form of backward integration into delivery, whereas the payer who signed a long-term arrangement for physician services with a single multispecialty group practice would be integrating by contract.
3. Given the decision to integrate backward by contract, the third party payer increases its degree of vertical integration by forming exclusive contracts with physicians rather than preferred provider contracts.
4. Similarly, a local multihospital system with a broad service line (e.g., mental health, cancer care, cardiac specialty care) might sign an exclusive contract with a third party payer to deliver service to that payer's enrollees. If the payer previously offered only psychiatric coverage, such a move would increase the breadth of the insurer's integration with delivery.

Insurance/delivery system integration involves a fifth dimension in that the fundamental "ethos" of the business is changed. The insurer now manages the care process directly rather than just paying the bills. On the flip side, the delivery system changes its perspective from a "revenue center" for itself to that of a "cost center" to the integrated health delivery and financing system. The integrated delivery and financing system both manages the economic risk of health care and assumes that risk.

Accordingly, integration of financing and delivery calls for new management expertise. This movement into previously "foreign territory" by both payers and providers requires different competitive strategies than those of providers. The competition between integrated financing and delivery systems is over premium dollars, not prices; that is, the control of utilization, not the maximization of volume, becomes crucial to success. Prepaid health plans compete for persons, not procedures.

## THEORETICAL FRAMEWORK

The box entitled "Determinants of Vertical Integration" summarizes what we believe to be the fundamen-

### Determinants of Vertical Integration

Production cost savings
  Shared fixed inputs
  Synergies between vertical stages
Transaction cost savings and service coordination benefits
  Information economies
  Savings on costs of negotiating and administering contracts
  Coordination of services among related stages (continuity of care)
Overcoming market imperfections
  Regulatory constraints
  Monopoly power on buyer or seller side
Management and internal organization factors
  New organizational forms
  Organizational "culture"
Environmental conditions

tal determinants of, and benefits sought by, vertical integration. Since there exists little empirical research that assesses the costs, risks, and benefits of vertical integration under different conditions, these determinants are justified conceptually rather than empirically. The major drivers of vertical integration are

- production cost savings;
- transaction cost savings and improved coordination of services (i.e., continuity of care);
- overcoming market imperfections;
- responding to management and internal factors; and
- responding to environmental changes that alter market conditions, production technologies, and transactional relationships.

### Environmental forces

We begin with observations about some of the environmental conditions influencing vertical integration. In our judgment, the two critical environmental forces behind the rapid evolution of vertically linked systems are (1) new prospective payment arrangements that significantly alter the interdependencies between economic agents at different levels in health care delivery—hospitals and physicians, payers and providers (both institutional and individuals)—and between informational intermediaries and those parties responsible for paying for and providing health care services; and (2) dramatically increased cost and price sensitivity by purchasers of health care services, which has given rise to a demand for increased organizational efficiencies and price reductions.

The increased price sensitivity of purchasers has tightened the interdependencies among hospitals and their physicians, physicians and their support professionals, medical products and informational technology suppliers, service providers themselves, and among third party payers and individual and institutional providers. Backward integration by employer groups and insurance companies into the delivery of care is just one symptom and response to these increased interorganizational interdependencies.

Prospective payment is perhaps the single most important contemporary example of an environmental shift that alters the interdependencies among stages in the health services value chain. Movements to more closely integrate hospitals and their medical staffs through employment relationships, strict probationary periods prior to the granting of full admitting privi-

---

*Prospective payment is perhaps the single most important contemporary example of an environmental shift that alters the interdependencies among stages in the health services value chain.*

---

leges, and preferred provider contracting between insurers and providers and between institutional and individual providers, each respond to the increased interdependencies forced by prospective payment. Hospitals are also moving to coordinate their relationships with their physicians and to structure enhanced predischarge care and referral relationships, together with better postdischarge care, by employing or exclusively contracting with groups of physicians to provide the full range of inpatient and outpatient services. This form of vertical integration is increasingly being forced on the delivery system by the payer side.

Another factor fostering vertically integrated arrangements is the aging of the population. Heightened attention to the treatment of chronic diseases encourages organizations, particularly hospitals, to develop pre- and postacute care arrangements for facilitating the care of a given person over time. Chronic disease involves long-term care and long-term rehabilitation, which requires coordination of many different services. A key decision for many organizations will be how to structure enhanced continuity of care between different

levels in the process of caring for individual patients. The increased prevalence of chronic disease, brought about by the aging of the population, reinforces the need for an integrated delivery system.

At the same time, the aging of the population has increased the relative importance of the Medicare program to the overall delivery system. Both the nature of chronic disease and the growing significance of the Medicare population, already under a per case form of prospective inpatient payment, are pushing the system toward capitated payment structures. Within capitated structures, the providers quickly learn to reduce transaction costs among different parties in the system by entering into contractual arrangements or by devising closely coordinated networks. These moves bring about integration in one form or another at both the clinical and the administrative levels of the organization.

### Efficiency and effectiveness "drivers"

The key to production cost savings does not seem to be at the unit-cost level, but rather in relation to the utilization of inputs between different stages in health care delivery. If HMOs have shown us one thing, it is that the principal gain from vertically structured arrangements flows from substituting the use of less-expensive treatment modalities for acute inpatient care. Organizations increasingly will need to focus on finding synergies between different levels of the care process, and these will depend on using the talent in one part of the business, for example, ambulatory care or prevention/wellness, to economize on utilization at other stages in delivery (most typically, the hospital or nursing home levels).

Transaction cost savings center on economies in the transfer and use of information between different levels of care. For example, the nursing home that coordinates its admissions with an integrated hospital and physician clinic system can design supportive acute inpatient care arrangements for those episodes that require hospitalization within the context of a single linked system. A common organization may save on the cost of entering into and enforcing contracts between different care providers as it substitutes internal management and organizational culture for pricing incentives as mechanisms for organizing services at different levels in the care process.

Tighter linkages between different levels of care (e.g., through combining skilled nursing home care with hospital acute inpatient care in a common organization) not only save transaction costs, but also should yield improved coordination and continuity of care. Systematic preadmission and postdischarge planning save on the transaction costs of "errors" between steps in the value chain while also improving the quality of services delivered at each point in the process.

### Regulatory constraints and market imperfections

In addition, vertical integration can be a means to work around regulatory constraints or market power on the buyer or seller side. For example, a hospital might form its own HMO, along with a physician group, as one means to avoid hospital rate-setting restrictions in a particular state. By doing this, the hospital substitutes disclosure and regulation of its HMO premiums by the state insurance department for control over its rates as an acute hospital by a state rate-regulation agency. The regulatory control in this case is moved up from an intermediate stage (the hospital rates) to the final stage of production (total premiums to the buyer), thus potentially economizing on the costs of regulatory compliance. Vertically integrated systems are also one means of exerting countervailing power against groups (such as organized physicians in a local area) that charge above-cost prices to hospital producers. Similarly, the physician group that integrates forward into its own preferred provider organization (PPO) arrangement through coordination with other physician groups can overcome strong market power exerted on the buying side by a sole community hospital or other monopoly provider of hospital services. In both cases, whether the monopoly is on the buyer or seller side, the integration serves to eliminate the social inefficiencies that result when any one player in the marketplace can control the transaction prices for health services.

## INTEGRATIVE MECHANISMS

A key to the success of vertical integration rests with the nature of the coordinative mechanisms crafted to support that integration. These mechanisms merit emphasis in this article, and we now turn to a discussion of integrative instrumentalities, which fundamentally determine the success of vertically linked strategies.

### Administrative coordination mechanisms

The first step in developing a vertically integrated delivery system is the building of administrative mechanisms to coordinate and integrate services. We

focus first on administrative mechanisms at the interorganizational level. The box entitled "Administrative Coordination/Integration: Interorganization or System Level" illustrates the variety of these interorganizational mechanisms, which range from tapping the benefits of single ownership to utilizing the advantages of proximity among different organizational units.

Given the different mechanisms for achieving interorganizational coordination, an integrated delivery system does not have to own or even provide every service itself; it may enter into cooperative relationships with other entities to achieve the desired degree of coordination among services. An example of such a cooperative relationship would be the use of a transfer agreement between a hospital and a nursing home that specifies incentives for bringing nursing home patients back to the hospital for subacute care. Through the use of such innovative contracting arrangements, the organization can manage other elements of the delivery system without accepting the final business risk for its operation. An HMO or a PPO that contracts with providers of all the different levels and types of care illustrates an extreme example of this coordinative mechanism.

### Intraorganizational administrative coordination

Administrative mechanisms are also required within the organization (intraorganizational) to more closely link different stages in the production process of health services. The box entitled "Administrative Coordination/Integration: Intraorganization or Program Level"

---

**Administrative Coordination/Integration: Interorganization or System Level**

| | |
|---|---|
| Single ownership | Informal agreement |
| Internal development | Coordinating/steering |
| Acquisition/merger | committee |
| Lease | Planning |
| Franchise | Budget and operations |
| Shared ownership | Marketing |
| Joint venture | Shared coordinator/manager |
| Partnership | ager |
| Management contract | Governing board participation |
| Contractual agreement | pation |
| External party (e.g., HMO) | Management participation |
| Interorganizational | Proximity |
| Affiliation agreement | |

---

**Administrative Coordination/Integration:
Intraorganization or Program Level**

Program/product line form of organization
Matrix organization
Program coordinator/manager
    Extent of authority?
    Physician, nurse, manager head?
    Single individual, team?
Liaison roles to link departments
Program steering committee/team
    Authority?
    Membership?
Program planning committee/task force
Program budgeting
Program data
    Integration of financial and patient data around pro-
    grams
Administrative policies and procedures
"Culture"
    Encourage direct communication/problem solving
    across departments

---

displays a spectrum of these linking methodologies. We pinpoint a few examples here for further discussion. These internal administrative integrating processes may take the form of assigning the responsibility for coordinating different components to a program manager, using program planning task forces, and integrating clinical and financial information around specific clinical programs or services.

A study of Japanese management in the last several years (e.g., in the works of Ouchi[4])has revealed the importance of multidimensional and multidivisional organizations in responding to the changing health care market place. The matrix organization illustrates one such innovation, wherein a manager is alternately responsible to both a functional manager (e.g., marketing, finance) and a product-line manager (e.g., surgical services).

Some of the most important vertical linkages in health services will not involve the integration of the entire organization's complete product line or service mix, but rather the design and implementation of vertically integrated programs (e.g., a heart center organizing the comprehensive spectrum of primary, secondar, and tertiary cardiovascular services for a defined patient population). A new set of administrative coordination "technologies" may need to be established to make these programs work. The vertical integration of

programs raises questions not only concerning product management and matrix organization models, but also regarding
- the appropriate mix and locus of function and program authority and accountability;
- the nature and composition of steering committees and program planning task forces;
- the integration of clinical, financial, and sociodemographic information; and
- the crafting and nurturing of new organizational "cultures" and the administrative policies and procedures that support "vertically linked," direct communication and problem solving across interrelated subunits of the organization.

### Patient care coordination

Although such administrative mechanisms are necessary conditions for cost-effective vertical integration, they are hardly sufficient. For a system to be fully integrated, patient care itself must be coordinated and its continuity assured. Sample approaches to this critical step are outlined in the box entitled "Clinical Mechanisms for Patient Care Integration."

The common thread running through these different mechanisms for patient care coordination and integration is their emphasis on connecting patient services at different stages in the care process. The managed care plan does this by developing HMO and PPO products, using exclusive or preferred contracting with a defined set of providers as the means for linking different levels of patient care, as well as their financing. Case management—whether directed by a primary care physician, nurse specialist, or interdisciplinary team—integrates

---

**Clinical Mechanisms for Patient Care
Integration**

Managed care plan
Case management
Case manager (e.g., physician, nurse)
Interdisciplinary team
Primary care "gatekeeper"/case manager
Medical director
Clinical coordinator/clinical nurse specialist
Single medical record
Discharge planning
Program-oriented quality assurance activity
Continuing medical education and in-service training
Consumer information and referral program

*The managed care plan develops HMO and PPO products, using exclusive or preferred contracting with a defined set of providers as the means for linking different levels of patient care.*

by explicitly managing and assuming responsibility for the care of individual patients and by coordinating patient care with the various social and financial support resources needed over the course of an individual's illness. Case management models hold particular promise for integrating the care of chronically ill persons, for whom the case management team functions much like a "personalized HMO."

To elaborate on just one other example, the single (integrated) medical record that would follow the patient over time and across delivery settings offers an important opportunity for coordinating patient care. The integrated record would serve three critical functions; it would

1. link information on illness episodes over time;
2. capture diagnostic, treatment, and health status information sufficient to provide an intertemporal health assessment for the patient; and
3. record outcomes of the nursing and medical interventions applied to the patient.

These different coordinative mechanisms serve to reinforce a variety of intra- and interorganizational forms, each of which is adapted to fit a particular set of environmental, market, and organizational managerial circumstances. Our next task is to examine these organizational forms under the terms of our conceptual framework.

## A MATRIX OF ORGANIZATIONAL FORMS

Table 1 matches the determinants of vertical integration (as suggested by our conceptual framework) with different intra- and interorganizational forms of vertical integration observed in the marketplace. This is by no means an exhaustive list of integrated arrangements, nor does it represent an ordered (i.e., from more to less integrated) continuum of vertical structures. Instead, Table 1 gives a series of examples that are meant to provide a "reality test" of the relevance of our conceptual framework.

We discuss each of the examples in Table 1 briefly and only to emphasize key insights, since the detailed analysis is contained within the table itself. First, the development of the closed-staff-model HMO has been a response to the environmental pressures of cost sensitivity on the part of health care purchasers and to the supply and mix of physicians in local markets. The production and transaction cost benefits of the closed-staff-model HMO are driven by strong internal utilization management and organizational integration of hospitals, ambulatory care facilities, and physicians.

Individual practice associations (IPAs) and PPOs are somewhat newer organizational forms, created primarily to balance the tradeoffs between purchasers' access to a broad range of providers and the production cost and transaction cost efficiencies that result from tighter integration. These more "loosely coupled" arrangements are capturing increased market share relative to closed-staff HMOs (although both are gaining relative to "unmanaged" fee-for-service arrangements) because consumers are attracted by the large numbers of participating providers they offer.[5] It remains to be seen whether the utilization controls of IPAs and PPOs will be as effective as the more tightly structured closed-staff HMOs.[6]

The integrated hospital-multispecialty physician group practice model, which predates the HMO and PPO models, developed in a market context different from that of managed care plans. In Seattle, a multispecialty physician group practice is one of four core organizations making up the vertically linked Virginia Mason Medical Center: the physician group practice partnership, the hospital, the fund development foundation, and a research center.[7] The hospital–clinic integration was in place even before Medicare and Medicaid ushered in retrospective cost-based reimbursement in 1965. The primary "drivers" behind this organizational form appear to be the desire for closer coordination of referral and patient care relationships between specialty and primary care physicians and the benefits of convenience to physicians and continuity of care to patients from the integration of ambulatory and inpatient care. The internal management culture promotes this integration through several mechanisms, such as

- a single set of written objectives relating to patient care, education, and research for all the core organizations;

- maintenance of "medical center discipline" by top managers; and
- overlapping management responsibilities for organizational components (e.g., the executive administrator of the Mason Clinic is also vice president of the hospital).

The hospital-based, primary care group practice is described by Shortell and Zajac as a "hybrid" organizational form, one that combines features of a joint venture (i.e., a shared equity investment by initially autonomous physicians and a hospital) with those of an internal corporate venture (i.e., the closer linkage of a hospital with the primary care physicians who admit patients there).[8] In this case, the venture is knitted together by a joint equity investment of physicians and the hospital and by internal staffing of a semiautonomous unit (i.e., the group practice itself). Consistent with our conceptual framework, Shortell and Zajac posit that resource scarcity (prospective and restricted payment to doctors and hospitals) and competition (e.g., due to the increasing supply of physicians and to excess hospital bed capacity) are the primary environmental stimuli for these ventures. Their survival and success in the marketplace will be determined by their ability to craft performance-based incentives, overcome medical staff resistance to new referral and admitting practice patterns, and structure sufficient operating autonomy for the group practice, while at the same time maintaining both the strategic importance of the group practice and its integration with the hospital's and the physician members' core services.

The managed care product is an innovation of the 1980s that reflects the competing pressures for autonomy and control experienced by today's health care organizations.[5] The example, Pointer, Begun and Luke (referred to in Table 1) comprises four hypothetical organizations operating in the same local market. These organizations form a "strategic alliance" to offer a managed care insurance product that covers physician services, hospital care, and skilled nursing services.[9] Depending on the circumstances of a particular market environment, these organizations would use a combination of arms-length contracting and joint ownership to design, deliver, and market the managed care product. The members of the alliance come together for a specific strategic purpose, but remain parallel and, in some cases, competing organizations in other local markets and other service lines.

Finally, the McKesson Corporation, a large distributor of drugs, health care products, and other consumer goods illustrates the notion of a value-adding partnership (VAP).[10] All five determinants of vertical integration are germane to this example, as shown in Table 1. While the primary technologic innovation behind the VAP between McKesson and the independent drugstores it serves is a computer information system, the key to McKesson's success in prescription drug services is its management's commitment to monitoring and strengthening each link in the value chain from product supplier, to distributor (McKesson itself), to drug store, to final consumer. The history of this VAP illustrates that such partnerships develop first between adjacent stages in the value chain (e.g., distributor and independent drug store), but are then reinforced at stages close to the final consumer (e.g., in the form of computerized information on the effects of different drug combinations).

## MANAGEMENT ISSUES

We close with a series of questions for those who do, and those who would, manage vertically integrated health care systems. Although we do not know the answers to all of these questions, we believe that they must be addressed if vertical integration is to be pursued efficiently and effectively in specific situations. The issues raised by these questions fall into five categories:

1. The fit of the vertical integration strategy with the core mission of the organizations involved.
2. Capital requirements and capital financing approaches.
3. The design of organizational processes, incentives, and responsibility/accountability mechanisms in support of vertical integration.
4. The amounts, types, and sequencing of the expertise and resources required to effectively carry out vertical integration.
5. The need to broaden both clinical and managerial perspectives on case-mix management and quality assurance.

### Fit and mission

1. What can an organization do to ensure that diversification into areas other than traditional patient care services does not threaten its basic character, identity, and values?

This question emerges with particular force as the organization seeks to integrate different levels of patient care and "population-based services" (e.g., home

---

**TABLE 1**

---

## THE "INTEGRATIVE BALANCE": INTRA- AND INTERORGANIZATIONAL FORMS

| Form of vertical integration | Determinants Production cost savings | Transaction cost savings |
|---|---|---|
| 1. Closed-staff-model HMO (common ownership, fully integrated value chain) | Primarily through utilization management of inpatient care | Continuity of care through integration of facilities and medical staff |
| 2. IPA-model HMO (separate ownership; contracting between the "plan" and physicians, hospitals; contract-based integration of value chain) | Utilization management; less-rigorous utilization management incentives than in closed-staff HMO | Still essentially market in contracting between plan and physicians, hospitals |
| 3. Insurer-sponsored PPO (separate ownership; contracting on preferred vs. closed-panel or exclusive basis; contract-based integration) | Minimal; achieved primarily through unit cost reductions stimulated by price discounting | Replaces repeated contracting with one-time costs of establishing preferred provider network |
| 4. Integrated hospital-multispecialty physician group practice (shared governance of the hospital and clinic; partially integrated value chain) | Not a prominent factor | Continuity of care benefits; referral and practice network; increased congruence of hospital and physician goals |
| 5. Hospital-based ambulatory primary care group practice (shared-equity investment by hospital and physician group; internal staffing of semi-autonomous unit; partially integrated value chain) | Minimal factor | Some continuity of care gains due to tightened referral network between the hospital and primary care physicians (PCPs) |
| 6. Local-market-based managed care product (formation of "quasi-firm" by short-term general hospital, multispecialty physician group, skilled nursing facility, and insurance carrier; partially integrated value chain) | Primarily through overall "case management" of utilization | Managed care via case manager; partially supplants arms-length market contracting; enhanced pre- and postdischarge services (visit, planning for hospital, ambulatory care, and long-term care); link to insurer enhances continuity between delivery and financing of care |
| 7. McKesson's "value-adding partnership" (VAP) (with manufacturing, distribution, retailing, third party insurance, and consumers for prescription drugs) (separate ownership of value chain components, contract-based integration) | Dramatic reductions in cost of order processing; reduced costs of restocking orders through conscious redesign of shelves | Enhanced monitoring through computer database of clinical-biological effects of alternative drug combinations |

| Overcoming market imperfections | Management and internal factors | Environmental conditions |
| --- | --- | --- |
| Response to physician market power | Internal "culture" linking organizational and physician interests | Cost sensitivity of purchasers; necessary supply of physicians |
| Potential for more competitive physician pricing through contract and capitation incentives | Contracting largely supplants internal hierarchy | |
| Simulates competitive market's price network | Minimal | Similar to Form 4 |
| Minimal factor | Internal culture linking hospital and physician interests | Minimal factor |
| Minimal factor | Example: an internal corporate joint venture | Excess hospital bed capacity; increasing supply of PCPs |
| "Backward" integration by insured into delivery; exerts buyer bargaining power on providers to reduce costs of services | Can deliver the product through variety of tightly or loosely "coupled" market or ownership mechanisms | Cost sensitivity of purchasers; excess supply of physicians; limited reimbursement for long-term care; (health) insurance underwriting cycle |
| Minimal factor | Create management culture that monitors competitive dynamics throughout value chain and fixes weaknesses as they occur; use of computer systems and information technology for order entry, packing, shipping, shelf design (e.g., for quality assurance) (drug combination) | Increasing competition from large drug store chains; eroding market share of independent drug stores served by McKesson |

*What can the organization do to ensure that diversification does not threaten its basic character, identity, and values?*

health, long-term care, health promotion) with its core activity (e.g., acute inpatient care), rather than simply diversify into new product lines.

2. What explicit criteria should be employed in evaluating major potential diversification and vertical integration opportunities? Are different criteria pertinent to diversification, as contrasted with vertical integration?

For example, might diversification initiatives be expected to earn greater profits than services added to enhance vertical integration? Which criteria should be used to decide when to divest, as well as when to add services?

Criteria could be developed in such areas as

- compatibility with mission and image;
- fit with system priorities;
- availability of expertise, management time, and other crucial resources;
- reporting relationships;
- financial return;
- evidence of demand/need; and
- prospective specification of integrative mechanisms.

### Capital requirements and capital financing

The available literature tells us little about the following capital formation issues posed by vertical restructuring:

- The size, scope of services, or geographic distribution of facilities required for a delivery system to achieve an adequate degree of dominance or identity in its local or regional market (especially if it is located in a major metropolitan area) may necessitate a considerable amount of growth. Is the health services organization willing to make the major investments that may be required to build a dominant local and regional delivery system?
- Assuming that it would be desirable from the delivery system's perspective to add a particular business or service, where should the funds come from? Can mechanisms be developed to transform a portion of the economic benefits flowing to one component of the system to finance or subsidize another? In short, should

one look at interunit financial incentives? Alternatively, how will the capital markets respond to demands for equity and debt capital to support the development of such comprehensive systems?

- Will the creation of better control and coordination of referral flows and channels of distribution (e.g., postacute care in the case of the hospital) lower the total business risk of the vertically integrated system relative to that of single-product or single-level organizations (e.g., home health, long-term care, primary care physicians, multispecialty groups)? If total business risk in the system is lowered, to what extent will the consequent reduction in the cost of capital (required return on assets) be passed through in price benefits to payers rather than ploughed back into new investments in facilities and services?

### Organizational processes, incentives, and responsibility/accountability

To integrate previously separate stages in the health care value chain, the system must develop a supportive organizational "culture" reinforced by communication processes (e.g., between clinical service line and functional managers), incentives, and a framework for responsibility and accountability. The key aim of such a culture is to promote the effectiveness, efficiency, and long-run return on capital of the delivery system as a whole, rather than only individual units making up that system.

How should the system address conflicts between systemwide (global) optimization and suboptimization by the individual units? For example, the cost-efficient size, scope of services, or location for a nursing home may not be what would best meet the needs of the system. Another example is the hospital that, to minimize DRG losses, seeks to discharge patients needing more intensive care than the system's nursing home wants to provide, given the level of reimbursement available to the nursing home. An extreme example is managed care plans where the factors required for success go far beyond the interests of the individual hospitals that first sponsored the plans. In fact, the basic goals of managed care and hospitals may conflict in very fundamental ways. This difference reflects the need to clarify the locus of responsibility for delivery system as well as individual unit results. Another related issue is the visibility of the performance of individual units that are part of a larger delivery system (e.g., the skilled nursing facility unit of an acute hospital).

What should be the reporting relationship of the administrators of the different types of facilities and programs that make up a vertically integrated delivery system in a given region? Should they report to the administrator of the hospital that serves as the organizational hub of the regional delivery system? To a regional administrator? To program specialists in the corporate office? To the corporate executive vice president for operations? Should the integrated system consider some form of matrix organization structure?

How should the system and/or components of the system respond to the fact that full or optimal integration may call for fundamental changes in operating systems and organization structures at the corporate or institutional level, or at both levels, that are difficult to implement (e.g., program budgeting, program versus functional organization structures, integration of clinical and financial data systems, and greater participation of physicians and other clinical professionals in management decision making)?

When a vertically integrated health care system is formed that bridges several previously freestanding levels of care (e.g., primary and specialty physician care, home health care, long-term care, and acute hospital inpatient care), what sorts of internal transfer pricing mechanisms are most appropriate between those different levels of care: short-run marginal cost of production, long-run fully allocated (with overhead) average cost, cost plus, or market prices for comparable services? Nonprice transfer arrangements (e.g., guaranteed swing bed capacity in the hospital for long-term care patients requiring subacute care) must also be designed among organizational units in the integrated system.

How can the organization encourage physician acceptance and support of mechanisms that contribute to clinical coordination and functional integration of patient care programs and services? Physicians tend to resist, for example, the establishment of medical director or other clinical administrative positions that act to integrate and provide leadership for programs that cut across specialties. Physicians often see specialists in integrative fields like geriatrics and rehabilitation as a competitive threat. Physicians may also resist such concepts as case management and interdisciplinary patient assessment teams. Finally, because hospital medical staffs are organized along traditional medical specialty lines, they are not well structured to deal with many of the issues and needs of vertical integration (e.g., interdisciplinary program planning).

How can an adequate degree of administrative coordination and integration be achieved in a delivery system where some components are under neither common management nor common ownership? In effect, this question challenges the organization seeking to develop and maintain a vertically linked system to shape contracting and pricing incentives and "good will" relationships between separately owned entities that can substitute effectively for the authority and control structures embedded in a system whose components are all under common ownership.

### Sequencing of expertise and resources

Because many of the organizations considering vertical integration are acute hospital systems, expertise may be lacking at both the corporate and institutional levels with regard to nonacute care programs and services. Yet expertise—in evaluating and negotiating acquisitions, joint ventures, or other arrangements, and in managing new services—is often the single most important ingredient in success. The system must ask itself: do we need to make a special effort to develop or assure the availability of expertise in areas other than acute care? How, and in what areas? One needs to recognize the great amount of management time required to acquire or start up a new service, especially one outside the scope of management's normal responsibilities.

Can the organization define priority areas such as ambulatory care, long-term care, or managed care to be acquired or established first in building vertically integrated delivery systems?

There may be significant "free-rider" problems in initiating vertically integrated delivery systems. In the long run, and over a sufficiently large population base, there are likely to be patient care benefits and total cost savings from a better coordinated comprehensive delivery system. The cost savings may be realized not only in direct production costs, but also in transaction costs (e.g., administrative costs, travel time, waiting time, and other "side costs" of patient care). Unless the organization leading the drive to integrate delivery can capture direct market share and financial gains to justify

*Because hospital medical staffs are organized along traditional medical specialty lines, they are not well structured to deal with many of the issues and needs of vertical integration.*

the costs of devising coordinated health care arrangements, efforts to implement vertical integration may be impeded because of concentrated costs and diffuse benefits. This reasoning suggests two corollary questions:

1. In areas where the organization has neither a dominant hospital nor sufficient resources to develop a dominant vertically integrated system, and so must collaborate with other organizations to this end, what strategies for allocating costs and benefits among "strategic partners" might work best?
2. What bargains can be struck between the dominant institution and the nondominant institutions involved in a nascent, vertically integrated system for sharing risks, costs, gains, and fixed-capital investment outlays?

### Clinical and managerial perspectives on case mix measurement and quality assurance

The vertically integrated delivery system encourages a fundamental shift in clinical and managerial focus from (1) caring for and billing transactions for whichever patients present themselves to the organization's door at a given point in time, to (2) accepting broader responsibility for the continuity and coordination of patient care for a defined population. This population-based perspective applies to clinical and financial management, and raises the following questions:

- How does the organization measure and manage case mix and the quality of patient care processes and outcomes for persons over time, in contrast to the more familiar measures of case mix and quality, which are defined for discrete episodes of care?
- What is the relationship between the costs borne by the integrated system (which, in the case of an HMO, should be recouped in premiums charged) and the process and outcome quality of patient care?

### CONCLUSION: THE INTEGRATIVE BALANCE

We do not have the knowledge to answer these managerial questions definitively at this point, but we can articulate many of the crucial challenges for vertically integrated arrangements. The key to success is to strike the "integrative balance," that is, to adopt the intra- or interorganizational forms that optimize the mix of strategic flexibility with production and transaction cost-efficiency, given the market conditions facing the organizational decision makers.

Management analysts of vertical integration have been discussing the strategic flexibility/cost control tradeoff for years, so to state the need for integrative balance has not been the thrust of this article. Rather, we have presented a fresh synthesis of the theory and have articulated the managerial implications of developing and sustaining vertically integrated health care systems.

## REFERENCES

1. Porter, M.E. *Competitive Strategy.* New York, N.Y.: Free Press, 1980.
2. Harrigan, K.R. "Formulating Vertical Integration Strategies." *Academy of Management Review* 9 (1984): 638–52.
3. Mick, S.S., and Conrad, D.A. "The Decision to Integrate Vertically in Health Care Organizations." *Hospital and Health Services Administration* 33 (1988): 345–60.
4. Ouchi, W.G. "A Conceptual Framework for the Design of Organizational Control Mechanisms." *Management Science* 25 (1979): 833–48.
5. Pointer, D.D., Begun, J.W., and Luke, R.D. "Managing Inter-organizational Dependencies in the New Health Care Marketplace." *Hospital and Health Services Administration* 33 (1988): 167–77.
6. Conrad, D.A., et al. "Vertical Structures and Control in Health Care Markets: A Conceptual Framework and Empirical Review." *Medical Care Review* 45 (1988): 49–100.
7. Ross, A. "Organizational Challenges and Linkages Associated With Vertically Linked Health Organizations." In *Vertically Linked Health Organizations: The 1978 National Forum on Hospital and Health Affairs,* edited by B.J. Jaeger. Durham, N.C.: Department of Health Administration, Duke University, 1978.
8. Shortell, S.M., and Zajac, E.J. "Internal Corporate Joint Ventures: Development Process and Performance Outcomes." *Strategic Management Journal* 9 (1988): 527–42.
9. Hamel, G., Doz, Y.L., and Prahalad, C.K. "Collaborate With Your Competitors—and Win." *Harvard Business Review* 89 (1989): 133–39.
10. Johnston, R., and Lawrence, P.R. "Beyond Vertical Integration: The Rise of the Value-Adding Partnership." *Harvard Business Review* 88 (1988): 94–101.

# Vertical integration: exploration of a popular strategic concept

Montague Brown
and
Barbara P. McCool

News headlines continue to proclaim the virtues of vertical integration, networking, regionalization, cluster markets, and other methods of organizing health care.[1] With insurers entering major joint ventures with providers (Aetna with Voluntary Hospitals of America [VHA]; Provident and Transamerica Occidental with American Healthcare Systems [AHS]; Equitable with Hospital Corporation of America [HCA]), it would seem that something fundamental is occurring that might presage a more vertically integrated health care delivery system.

The idea of vertical integration in health care easily stirs the imagination and holds the attention of policy makers, health administrators, and, increasingly, entrepreneurs. Those seeking to regulate expenditures want vertical integration to avoid duplication of services. Those seeking to ensure quality and efficiency attempt to own or control whatever resources a patient might need within an episode of illness or even a lifetime. More pragmatic people seek to bring downstream services and upstream services under their wings for many reasons: to stabilize markets, to use excess capacity, to secure profits from related services, and, from time to time, to capitalize on the prestige one hopes will enhance an entire line of services.

The concept of regionalization of health care services for a particular population, territory, or trade area has a long history: the Lord Dawson Report in England in 1920[2]; the Committee on the Cost of Medical Care in the United States in 1932[3]; the Commission on Hospital Care in 1956[4]; the Regional Medical Program in 1966[5]; and AHA's Ameriplan proposal[6], which sought some form of integrated care for a geopolitical region.[7-10] Since these ideas seem to surface frequently, one can reasonably question whether the current enthusiasm will lead to major change or whether it merely represents another fad.

One should remember that earlier calls for regionalization and vertical integration came during times of physician and hospital shortage. Access and comprehensiveness were big issues. Today, there is a sur-

**Montague Brown,** *M.B.A., Dr.P.H., J.D., is Chairman and CEO of Strategic Management Services, Inc., in Washington, D.C., and Editor of* Health Care Management Review.

**Barbara P. McCool,** *R.N., M.H.A., Ph.D., is President of Strategic Management Services, Inc., in Washington, D.C., and Associate Editor of* Health Care Management Review.

*Health Care Manage Rev, 1986, 11(4), 7–19*

plus of hospitals, beds, and physicians, coupled with high cost and overuse. If these old ideas fit today, it will have to be for different reasons than those cited in earlier days.

The literature on the regionalization of health services discusses many, if not all, of the underlying reasons for vertical integration. However, the literature and rationale for regionalization go beyond the ideas of economy and medical efficiency to endorse political governance.

Many proponents of regionalization basically are seeking a way to govern. For those who prefer governance within the framework of the political system, regional health care systems can be directed by elected and appointed government officials and institutions. For others who prefer private, voluntary institutions, regional systems can work under a governmental charter or framework, but can be essentially self-directed by their own voluntary governing bodies. Those who sit at the supposed apex of a vertically integrated system seem to think it equally natural and desirable to have such a system governed and controlled by the medical elite at the academic health science center. In a pluralistic system such as the United States, regionalization represents a move toward greater vertical integration and centralization of control.

Whatever the motive, proponents of vertical integration generally share the arguments of economy, efficiency, quality, and access associated with the concept.

## WHAT IS VERTICAL INTEGRATION?

Vertical integration is a term used in marketing and economics to describe complex systems that link resource development, manufacturing, distribution, and consumption. For example, food chains, when linked vertically, own and operate the farms, processing plants, and distribution systems, and provide food to their customer base in a variety of forms, including meal service. Their integration may also involve them in energy production for their farms, factories, and transportation systems.

In health care, vertical integration commonly refers to the ability of one provider system (i.e., owner or controlling entity) to provide all levels and intensities of service to patients and health care consumers from a geographically contiguous region when these clients present themselves to that system. Primary, sec-

---

*In health care, vertical integration commonly refers to the ability of one provider system to provide all levels and intensities of service to patients and health care consumers.*

---

ondary, tertiary, rehabilitative, custodial, and other care modalities are available within one system. In contrast, mere ownership of a variety of different service modalities in separate areas of the country should be analyzed as a form of diversification, perhaps, but not as vertical integration of service from a consumer's perspective.

In a system of vertically integrated services, a patient presents himself or herself for primary care and moves from one level to another as is medically appropriate, using the most economical and best service necessary and remaining within the ambit of the same provider. One can argue that the greater the extent that all problems are met by one provider, the greater is the vertical integration of that provider. A fully integrated system is capable of providing all services to all patients who present themselves for care.

In addition, since medical care has long been treated by consumers as a service for which one needs to purchase risk protection, a vertically integrated system will provide financial services, much as General Motors provides financial services such as loans to assist in buying a car so that consumers can use its products. Traditionally Blue Cross/Blue Shield provided such services independently of provider. Now providers are adding financial risk services to their portfolios to augment traditional financial risk services.

### History of vertical integration

Hospitals and hospital chains were first attracted to vertical integration because of economies of scale and increase in market share. Economies of scale (quality, cost, production efficiency, profit potential, access to supply of inputs, and access and control of customer markets) relate to decisions about when to own, operate, control, or make an element or service versus contracting for, entering a joint venture, or buying it in the open market. These decisions are made with due consideration for quality of medical care, access for consumers, and competitive factors in the market.

Motivated by economy of scale issues and competitive concerns, the prudent strategist in previous times operated, merged, networked, or otherwise linked with as many elements of a vertically integrated system of hospitals and services as possible. This same strategist also sought to attract independent primary care physicians, who were often in short supply. The strategist sought to network with these physicians for referrals, education, and the economic opportunity brought about by their endorsement of the brand name (most prestigious, biggest, or best) of the system and its secondary and tertiary services.

### Two-stage process

The strategist developed a two-stage process of vertical integration. In the first stage, he or she took advantage of the many economies of operation for hospitals and related services that were available, especially when there were units in contiguous geographic areas. For example, one top-notch management group with specialists could handle 10 or 20 hospitals rather well. Laundries, mobile diagnostic technology, educational systems, representation to government, access to capital, and the like provided attractive opportunities for systems of hospitals with a scale of approximately $300 million to $900 million in revenues.

The greatest opportunity to achieve economies of scale resided in a second stage of integration—control over medical referral patterns. This second stage depended more heavily on physician market competitive factors than on the known economies of scale in hospital operations. In other words, vertical integration had to overcome the resistance (i.e., the refusal to refer patients) of individual practitioners ready to attack any upstream competitor (hospital or specialist) that threatened their opportunities and their freedom to control their own patients.

Indeed, the experiences of voluntary multihospital systems in the late 1960s and 1970s show that integration of medical referrals is easier to attempt than to accomplish. These hospital systems set out to build regionally integrated cluster-type systems that would offer all levels of medical care: treatment in primary settings by independent practitioners; first-level hospital care; specialist care; and, ultimately, subspecialist care. What they found was that physicians insisted on vertical levels of care at one site, their primary site, and not someone else's primary

base. Few, if any, voluntary systems achieved very good results in trying to influence referrals to the other geographically contiguous hospitals they owned. The system's ownership or management of additional hospitals simply did not overcome traditional physician referral patterns. Thus, voluntary hospital systems were able to achieve some degree of vertical integration of hotel-type support services (e.g., bed and board), management services, and capital economies, but not vertical integration of patient care.

### Investor-owned chains

Investor-owned chains also have a history of showing supply-side gains but no real vertical integration. During the 1970s these chains, with their capital advantage, rushed into the most readily penetrable market areas that appeared to have been abandoned by privately owned hospitals: growth areas needing new capacity and overflow areas with breakaway physicians who, for their own competitive reasons, wanted another hospital.

As growth occurred in such investor-owned, horizontally integrated, single-site, and single-purpose hospitals, management specialization developed around organization building, reimbursement, and regulatory process. Shared purchasing, dedicated suppliers, and proprietary interest in manufacturing and distribution were always potential ways to gain additional revenue, but these options were not used much as long as no pressure existed on the pricing side, which controls utilization. Today, with more consumer sensitivity to the price of services, any savings in supply costs go directly to the bottom line, so the scramble for economies in hotel services makes much more sense. Any savings on cost in a price-oriented system benefit the provider's bottom line directly. Of course, the provider may lower prices, thus passing savings to buyers. Again, these economies of operation do not reflect real vertical integration.

### Multihospital systems

A number of multihospital systems have owned and operated prepaid plans, rehabilitation centers, nursing homes, and home care programs, and have offered many subspecialty medical services at one location or another. Such services offered in diverse locations represent a form of diversification but do not address the issues of integrated services for a defined population. Having such experiences and capabilities does, however, aid in positioning such firms for ultimately bringing their other resources into systems of vertically integrated services.

**Current interest in vertical integration**

Since investor-owned systems historically have ignored the opportunities for integration upward into tertiary services and downward into risk services (e.g., ambulatory care, diagnostics), ventures such as Wesley Medical Center in Wichita, Kansas, Lovelace Clinic in Albuquerque, New Mexico, St. Joseph Hospital in Omaha, Nebraska, Humana's Louisville, Kentucky, operations, and similar deals came as a shock to the voluntary and university communities. Corporations thought to be interested only in the simple primary care hospitals in single-hospital or overflow-hospital markets were suddenly interested in hospitals with the potential for becoming the linchpin in a vertically integrated system. The more skeptical observers, of course, seemed to think that such ventures were merely window dressing engaged in for prestige and for marketing purposes, not serious business ventures with their own merits. Less attention seemed to be given at the time to the inherent potential in aggressively seeking preferred provider status with multiple managed care systems or in building or buying such systems to complement the provider capacity in place.

*Increasing profitability*

This new interest in vertical integration in markets where excess capacity exists is understandable as chains such as HCA, American Medical International (AMI), and others announce lower earnings from operations. Having maximized their economies of operations, these chains are now turning to vertical integration to increase their profitability from underutilized assets.

To achieve this goal, the chains must have a solid base of primary physicians, tertiary capacity, and as many ties as possible with insurance companies and managed care systems. Three tasks comprise the real competitive challenge to the chains and regional systems: (1) backward integration to risk services, (2) joint ventures with physicians, and (3) forward integration into referral services. Unless mastered, these tasks represent the Achilles' heel of the for-profit and not-for-profit regional systems.

*Changing competitors*

Vertical integration may also play an increasing role among some hospitals in areas sparsely populated by chain operations. In fact, some observers have said that these hospitals may drop out of the national voluntary alliances, realizing that their biggest competitive threat stems from the potential vertical integration of other systems in their own regions, not from hospital chains.

Now, with the major move by investor-owned chains and voluntary alliances to join with insurance firms to vertically integrate backward into risk services, and with risk service firms striving to move subscribers into managed care systems in order to meet customer demand for more cost control, the entire range of assumptions about who is competing with whom is open for serious examination.

*Management and governance*

In summary, the traditional development of voluntary regional systems, as well as national chains, is built on management, supply, and related economies, not true vertical integration of medical care. Until last year, the voluntary national alliances followed the pattern of the national chains by buttressing their potential advantages in operating costs and ignoring the development of an integrated system of medical referrals.

Even without full vertical integration, voluntary alliances and investor-owned chains can gain much from rebuilding horizontal, somewhat integrated, systems to take advantage of buying power, regional management system sharing, and intramarket program sharing. The biggest roadblock to this process is the notion of local prerogative and discretion. Hospital administrators, especially those who run the larger voluntary and investor-owned chains, have maintained and reinforced the notion that the local administrator has control and autonomy. But these concepts retard movement toward the greater efficiency that national buying and program (product) development afford.

## ENVIRONMENTAL FACTORS SUPPORTING VERTICAL INTEGRATION

Four key factors tend to support vertical integration. First, the distribution of disease in populations dictates vertical integration. Most illnesses are common problems that can be treated by primary practitioners. Because of the relative frequency of these illnesses, primary practitioners can be supported by a relatively small population base. Secondary and tertiary practitioners deal with less frequent problems and thus need a population catchment area of much greater size. A population base in excess of a million may be required for some subspecialty practices; while a family physician can fill a practice in an area that has a few thousand families.

Secondary and tertiary practitioners must depend on the vigilance of the primary care physician to identify those problems requiring specialized care and then to refer the patient to a specialist when more complex diagnostic and therapeutic services are needed. Thus, it is the nature of complicated diseases and complex, expensive technology and specialized treatment to require some form of regionalization or, as has happened most often, a network of referral relationships that move patients to the specialist and then back to the primary practitioner.

---

*Secondary and tertiary practitioners must depend on the vigilance of the primary care physician to identify those problems requiring specialized care and to refer the patient to a specialist.*

---

Second, quality of care by secondary and tertiary practitioners can be ensured only when these physicians continue to develop their skills by serving large population groups. This is a quality of scale issue. It is also an economic value issue, since offering a service without maintaining quality will ultimately cost the practitioner business from sophisticated buyer groups.

Third, there is an efficiency issue involved. Volume helps decrease production cost (at least over some theoretical range of size), and in medical specialties it also increases quality (again, over some theoretical range of activity). Superior value can be produced if there exist the scale and market share to support those specialty services that work efficiently. A comprehensive system has the potential to attract a large volume of patients, thereby lowering the unit cost of services and specialized technology.

Fourth, there is an inherent appeal to the idea that wherever a person comes in contact with a system of care, there exists an incentive within that system that

encourages quality performance and economic treatment, smooth and timely movement among services, and easy communication among caregivers. A good example of this is the perceived quality image of the Kaiser Permanente system.

## ENVIRONMENTAL FACTORS INHIBITING VERTICAL INTEGRATION

There are several key reasons the health care field has not moved toward the concepts of regional and vertical integration.

### Physician autonomy

First, physicians enjoy their independence as economic and medical practitioners. Physicians have always had a keen sense of the potential for hospitals to influence their practice patterns. This potential power and a potential counterweight to it are well known to any physician soon after he or she enters the profession. The question is how to control big, strong, financially well-heeled hospitals. Such hospitals can be controlled by keeping two hospitals viable and using both for patients and referrals. Patient referrals and hospital use patterns are potent tools of control, especially for the primary care physicians who are at the entry level of the medical system. Therefore, some physician groups would resist any movement by hospitals toward scale and increased leverage.

Of the many potential threats to physician autonomy, a hospital's dominance over specialty practices is the oldest and greatest. Physicians truly fear the potential of a dominant institution that fully controls their access to hospital and related services. Regional or vertically integrated systems greatly increase the potential for institutions to control physicians through their ability to shift referrals among competing physician specialists and among competing hospitals. If any geopolitical region had only one vertically integrated set of services, physician power to shift referrals and maintain power or leverage over hospitals would be lost or at least severely diminished. Whether the system is government owned, voluntary, or investor owned makes little difference.

Physicians appear to like the notion of vertical integration of their practices, within their practices, and for their practices where opportunities exist to achieve revenue, profit, quality, and efficiency. In theory, all the ideas that make vertical integration attractive to hospitals (and increasingly attractive to insurance companies) make vertical integration attractive to the practitioner, as long as it is under his or her control.

When there were not enough specialty physicians, there was no incentive for specialists to vertically integrate in order to pressure the primary care physicians for referrals. They did not need more patients. As long as this traditional referral pattern existed, specialists kept their autonomy and so did primary physicians. Perhaps even more important, any moves by secondary and tertiary physicians to invade the primary territory were, and still are, punished by the primary physicians whose referrals control the system of secondary and, especially, tertiary medicine. However, with the current surplus of specialists, increased vertical integration becomes an option.

### Pluralistic system

The second, and supporting, set of reasons for the lack of any serious movement toward regionalization or vertical integration involves the history and underlying motives for societal support for a system of private and public hospitals. For many reasons, the United States has developed a pluralistic system (a variety of owners) of hospitals. This approach is supported by underlying beliefs about religion, ethnicity, and politics. It also suits the intensely competitive nature of medical practice. In the past, competing physicians could almost always find a religious group, a public body, or more recently an investor group to build a hospital for their use, as long as there was some assurance of getting a sufficient number of patients to fill the hospital, carry the debt burden, and secure profits for the equity investment required.

In the past, hospital owners took advantage of the cost-plus reimbursement system. When physicians wanted their own shop to free themselves from outside restrictions or the weight of colleagues more senior or more in control in existing institutions, hospitals made it easy for them to move. When growth occurred, all benefited. One could put a service in place and charge what one needed for a good return, so both physicians and hospitals profited.

### Support of status quo

Another reason for the lack of vertical integration is the fact that the prepayment systems (basically Blue Cross and Blue Shield) were constructed to reinforce those existing arrangements, not undercut them. Insurance was cost, place, physician, and hospital neu-

tral. More recently, with the advent of managed care programs, physicians and hospitals are under intense pressure to sign up with plans that force them to share economic risk for the care of patient groups.

### Support of multiple delivery sites

A fourth reason is that cost-based reimbursement, with its neutral stance toward organization and integration of services, basically supported the development of multiple delivery sites, various degrees of aggregation desired by the provider of service, and competition among all arrangements for the patronage of the individual patient. Under the cost-based system, professional desires regarding technology, place, and service configuration were paramount decision factors. There was no incentive to integrate services.

Now this approach faces rapid obsolescence because of buyer pressure, competitive prices for services, strict utilization review, increasingly fearful insurers who want to get ahead of the game in cost-effective managed care systems, and a real glut of hospitals, beds, services, and physicians. Faced with this obsolescence, many groups are now considering vertical integration.

## IMPLEMENTING VERTICAL INTEGRATION

What are the options for hospitals and multihospital systems to improve performance in multifacility markets, in areas with substantial concentration, and in thinly serviced markets? Before moving to find answers to this question, one should consider how justified the new-found and widely spread belief in vertically integrated systems really is. After all, vertical systems consistently have failed to materialize almost every time they have been attempted in this century.

### Access to physicians who control referrals

The first factor in achieving a measured level of vertical integration is access to the full range of physicians who control referrals. This acknowledges that the vast majority of people are not in managed care programs. Thus, as utilization rates go down, physicians will seek to move their patients to the hospital most likely to offer the broadest service array for their patients. They will enter joint ventures for economic gain, but not if such ventures threaten to tie them up with organizations that lack services their patients may need, i.e., those systems that are not vertically integrated.

For example, in Houston, Texas, both HCA and AMI need access to the kinds of services available at tertiary hospitals like the Texas Medical Center, a large biomedical complex with multiple tertiary facilities. By contrast, in Wichita and in Denver, Colorado, those firms can provide internally almost all the care patients might require in a managed care system. Humana has a similar capacity in Louisville.

### Availability of managed care programs

The second factor in achieving a measured level of vertical integration is preferred access to and availability of health maintenance organizations (HMOs), preferred provider organizations (PPOs), traditional insurance, and other more directly managed care programs. The chains and voluntary alliances are moving to cover this area. Both have made attempts to enter the risk services business.

Any major move by VHA, HCA, or Humana into the full range of risk service products makes that organization's members major competitors with all other systems—hospitals, networks, and insurance. Up to this point, these organizations have been primarily competitors in the market for hospital services. By vertically integrating, they may become formidable in all levels of care and a real competitive threat to any providers that are not vertically integrated. As many of these systems form local alliances, they force others to form counterweight alliances to compete with them. Many older coalitions and status quo arrangements crumble under this pressure.

---

*With alliances and chains bringing the kind of capital needed to capture managed care opportunities, all providers will begin to understand the ultimate power of a new strategy of vertical integration.*

---

With alliances and chains bringing the kind of capital needed to capture managed care opportunities, all providers will begin to understand the ultimate power of a new strategy of vertical integration.

Patients are the coin of the realm for physicians. Hospitals need them. Universities need them. Tertiary care systems need them. By vertically integrating, chains and alliances can have a stake in every market, and they will discover that having a stake in bringing patients to providers makes all other economic joint ventures with physicians seem insignificant by comparison.

## VERTICAL INTEGRATION IN DIFFERENT ENVIRONMENTS

Actually achieving economic advantages of scale in a horizontally integrated firm makes it possible to add all savings to the bottom line in a product priced or managed care environment. Thus shared and centralized services should be developed within cluster and concentrated markets, to the extent that they make economic sense. Even selective backward integration into supply areas, where the firm could benefit from any excess profits being generated by suppliers, can be lucrative in some areas.

Many economies of operation can be achieved by consolidating and centralizing business service functions of existing units. Ensuing economies of scale on purchasing, supplies, standardization of equipment, and the like can and should be done as soon as possible, after a thorough analysis of gain, line by line, area by area. Moves of this type are already under way by most alliances and firms. For each product, the unit of analysis may be as large as the company or as small as two units. For some lines of business, the proper unit for economies and competitive advantage may be larger than the parent firm itself. Risk service may well fall here. In essence, vertical integration takes on the persona of the environment in which it is developed. Several examples follow.

### Concentrated markets with tertiary capacity

In concentrated markets the major gain, beyond shared service economies, stems from the potential for moving patients among programs through physician referral. This is the key to vertical integration. Most approaches to influencing physician referral patterns have involved buying or entering joint ventures with primary care hospitals, or entering joint ventures for diagnostics, ambulatory care centers, managed care programs, PPOs, and other such risk products that can be used to direct patients. But for the near term (three to five years, and possibly longer), winning primary physician loyalty to referral physicians and referral hospitals is the key to achieving vertical integration of medical care capacity in markets where firms own or operate tertiary capacity. In such markets additional equity investments in all levels of services that can utilize existing assets (space and services) also may be attractive.

These concentrated markets should be organized around such concepts as medical care markets and major trade areas, areas within which the population normally seeks and receives 80 to 90 percent of its medical care. Management for the entire market should be under one manager. Such managers might report to a strategic business unit that has overall regional responsibilities for marketing, strategic analysis, investment, and general management of all company activity in the region.

**Markets in which firms have several primary hospitals**

In markets with limited tertiary capacity within the owned and managed system, it will be necessary for primary hospitals to create substantial joint ventures to link with tertiary programs. Only in this way can an organization gain the greatest returns from the care needed by patients who are initially attracted to primary care physicians and primary care treatment in dispersed hospital systems.

This is true for several reasons. First, any managed care, PPO, or HMO insurer wants to contract with the most complete network of providers. If significant types of referral care are not in one's own facilities, then the next best option is to enter a joint venture, network, or independently build and offer such services. In this way, hospitals can become attractive to managed care programs.

Second, under contracting market conditions that necessitate a choice of which hospital to save, physicians typically abandon the overflow or primary care facility in favor of the full-service facility or system. Physicians consider full-service facilities as the best alternative for serving their patients. Not coincidentally, these systems also help physicians maintain their own practice viability. Ironically, when one does not have major referrals for tertiary services, it is not as necessary to seek physician loyalty on referrals. Unlike the markets with tertiary care programs, in primary care markets there is less likelihood that physicians will want or need to move their patients

from one hospital to another. However, as managed care continues to gain ground, those hospitals without the more complex tertiary abilities will lose business as physicians choose to save the more complex facilities needed for their patients. Thus, hospitals must band together with tertiary care systems in order to survive. Fortunately for those with primary care facilities, tertiary facilities are also in oversupply and need alliances for referrals, just as primary hospitals need their referral backup to make their linkage with managed care firms effective.

Third, the supplier with the greatest control over referrals will have the most capital available to offer the next level of technology for medical care and the most advanced systems will become more attractive to upscale consumers, a lucrative target market. For these three reasons, it is essential that primary hospitals link with one or more tertiary care facilities.

**Independent hospitals in markets with several hospitals**

The solo hospital in a market with several hospitals will need to pursue a niche strategy designed to hold what business it can while fending off competitors seeking additional patient days.

Several basic approaches can be developed to support a solo strategy. First, the hospital can link or network with a referral center and try to maintain utilization of primary care services. Second, it can seek to become a primary provider for all managed care plans as they develop. Under this scenario, the hospital must try to keep one plan from becoming dominant in the marketplace. Third, the hospital can try to become the primary provider for at least one managed care plan. When possible, securing an equity position in one or more managed care plans will aid in keeping the directed patient flow from becoming too narrow, or, if it does become narrow, this position will help the hospital to benefit from that flow.

Specialty hospitals will need to find ways to secure the specialty business from all managed care plans or link closely with the general provider most likely to deliver the largest part of the specialty referral market segment to them. Many specialty hospitals depend heavily on the routine work they receive to maintain their more esoteric services, so any strategy that cuts heavily into their overall business may threaten their ability to maintain these referral services.

## Teaching hospitals

Teaching hospitals basically fall into two categories: (1) the major university health science centers where much of the basic health science research is conducted. These centers have a teaching mission, with the hospitals devoted principally to research and education, and (2) the teaching hospitals that offer three or more major residency programs. These hospitals put more focus on patient service, with teaching and research being less primary activities.

### Health science centers

The health science center is likely to have substantial financial support for both its research and its educational role, in addition to the support that is derived from providing patient services. To the extent that these outside support systems can be maintained and enhanced, the health science center will need and be able to compete in the marketplace for referrals from the sophisticated managed care programs. This assumes, however, that the health science centers can and do control their service cost and maintain relatively unique program offerings. Having a research base will continue to make such institutions attractive for the more difficult cases; managed care systems such as Kaiser Permanente, Health America, Maxicare, and others will always need help with their more complex cases. For such firms to try to keep their patients out of these centers of excellence will ultimately test their credibility as major suppliers. Barring a large market share for one firm, they will need to contract for such services for the foreseeable future. This represents a major opportunity for tertiary care suppliers. In fact, health science centers and teaching hospitals might aggressively seek contracts to take on the management of the more complex cases before the insurance programs of such managed care companies decide to take responsibility for them.

Competitors for the more complex and specialized cases will come not from the managed care companies but from those tertiary and teaching centers that do not have major investment in and responsibility for research and teaching of medical students. Additional competition will come from those regional hospital systems and national hospital management companies that have strong regional networks and can offer tertiary services from within their systems.

At this time, it would appear that health science centers can compete effectively, provided they aggressively manage their costs (seek efficiencies) and are careful to seek the role of tertiary supplier for managed care systems early in their development. In other words, the game is just beginning. Many options remain open to those who see change coming, are open to meeting the challenge, and are aggressively examining their markets to determine when to join others, contract, or remain outside the competitive arena when appropriate.

### Other institutions

Those teaching institutions that depend heavily on patient revenues to support their teaching role are at greatest risk of losing some of their preeminence and their roles as centers of excellence. They are faced with the difficult situation of using price discounts to get volume, while simultaneously finding it increasingly difficult to support the residency programs that make it possible to maintain their center of excellence strategy. Ultimately, those who deal with this issue should survive. But they, unlike the academic health science center, will need to network with a large number of providers, managed care firms, and national alliances to secure aggregate volumes of patients necessary for their tertiary programs to maintain quality while performing efficiently.

Since state and federal supporters of academic health science centers are likely to aid their clients in maintaining their viability over the intermediate term of competitive developments, most teaching hospitals will not receive such support. For this reason, some will undoubtedly fail as major tertiary centers of excellence for some services. Maintaining costly specialized programs can be an unbearable burden in a price-sensitive market, especially when buyers seek lower cost.

It is likely that the teaching and tertiary care centers outside of health science complexes will have the greatest need to build regional networks, to link formally and informally with all possible referral sources, and to build as many managed care connections as possible. This expectation seems to be borne out by the large numbers of such institutions that have made up the initial membership of VHA, AHS, and Sun Alliance. Teaching hospitals also seem natural partners for investor-owned firms and managed care firms. The number of joint ventures between these hospitals and investor-owned firms indicates that teaching hospitals are aware that they have a stronger need for multiple alliances than do academic health science centers.

### Alliances between health science centers and management chains

The alliance strategy is relatively new and none of the major linkages to date seem to preclude new initiatives to form alliances between the stronger academic health science centers and hospital management chains. Managed care companies also seem to want strong alliances with primary care providers and referral agreements with those tertiary care providers who wish to maintain their research and teaching capacity but who do not need to subsidize teaching and research programs. In other words, while teaching and tertiary hospitals would like to play a major role in primary care, both hospital chains and managed care companies want to retain this role for their own operations. Thus, it is likely that chains and managed care programs will be selective in seeking out tertiary referral lines with the major academic health science centers. They will reserve the primary and secondary care roles for themselves. In the process, they will bypass their close competitor, the teaching hospital, which has more limited tertiary capacity.

### Managed care companies

Managed care companies are in the business of providing or negotiating for the provision of health care services purchased by employers or other groups. They are required to provide such services within the limits of a contract they make with these employers and groups. At one extreme is the owned and operated health service, such as Kaiser Permanente, which packages physician, hospital, and risk management services within its own family of companies. At the other end of the spectrum is the insurance firm, which contracts for risk and limits liability by specifying the range within which it will cover services or the amount of total payment. In other cases, employers may manage their own risk, specify eligible providers, contract for administration, and use excess insurance coverage to avoid large losses.

---

*Competition among managed care firms is increasing, putting pressure on premium price and thus pushing all suppliers in the direction of more tightly managed utilization and cost controls.*

---

### Increased competition

Competition among managed care firms is increasing, putting pressure on premium price and thus pushing all suppliers in the direction of more tightly managed utilization and cost controls. As these firms compete for the buyers' attention, they will need to control utilization more and more and seek low prices from suppliers of services not offered directly by the managed care firm itself.

Probably the lowest-cost producers of primary care are family physicians. Some of the early HMO service suppliers sought out family physicians, general internists, and similar primary care providers as the core of their original network. Low-cost or low-price hospital providers and willing specialists have been secondary priorities. As patient volume has grown, specialists have been asked to take greater risks and hospitals have been asked to offer greater discounts in order to get the volume business offered by managed care firms that can select the provider for their clients.

Under conditions such as these, physician and hospital providers are under tremendous pressure to take the risk and start their own managed care firms. But in doing so, they must delicately balance their own risk management offerings so that they can gain market share while maintaining business and referrals from competing managed care firms.

Put another way, as providers develop their abilities to offer managed care services directly to employers and groups, they must do so in a fashion that does not simultaneously drive away business from other managed care firms (now competing firms) and from referring physicians whose practices are tied more directly to other managed care firms and hospitals.

If hospital and physician provider groups initiate their own risk services and managed care programs, they may lose referrals from these competing groups.

On the other hand, if they have not positioned themselves to be the provider of choice in such groups, they run the risk of eventually being left out of more tightly managed groups.

### Role of insurance companies

Managed care firms are, with a few exceptions, relatively new. Some have developed with little regard for utilization control and have depended heavily on the lack of tightly managed control for their profitability. As competition builds for the managed care premium dollar, the more loosely managed firms will lose out to more tightly managed groups. But as managed care firms succeed as a sector of the health care industry, it becomes more important than ever for any insurance firm wishing to compete for the full service benefit dollar to offer managed care. Therefore, health care managers now see, and can expect to see, many more insurance firms seeking managed care business, buying up established managed care firms, merging traditional benefit companies into managed care firms, and entering joint ventures between big benefits firms and provider networks and firms.

In short, the strategies of insurance and benefits Firms are so new in their adoption and so tentative in their execution that it seems safe to conclude that the industry is only beginning to discover and answer many of the questions posed and implied here. Few of the strategies that have unfolded so far appear to be clear-cut winners. Few of the players seem secure in the belief that they have the answers. The only thing that seems certain is that change is here. For those who like the excitement of a game in its early stages, this is a great opportunity to participate in the definition of a new health care provider. For those who see only insurmountable problems, retiring to the sidelines or merging with someone more comfortable with the risk seems a more likely strategy.

For those who think that vertical integration is the right way to go, there is plenty of room to maneuver. They can mold the health care system into a more efficient and probably more vertically integrated mode of care. Who will do this is an open question. Where it can be done is similarly open. But since vertical integration runs counter to so many interests, it will remain a high-risk strategy, however it is implemented.

## ASSESSMENT OF FORCES IN THE HEALTH CARE FIELD

Powerful forces are active in the health care field. Voluntary hospital alliances are flourishing as providers seek refuge in networks that will allow independent hospitals and independent physicians to retain control over their destinies in the face of impending radical changes in reimbursement that favor competitive pricing and full-service arrays.

### Assumptions underlying the fears of independent hospitals and physicians

Several assumptions are currently causing great anxiety among independent institutions and practitioners. One assumption is that the powerful hospital chains will use their ability to get market equity to buy up the good business opportunities to the exclusion of the voluntary hospitals. Just how such chains could come up with the new equity to perform this miracle is unclear. (It would probably require in the neighborhood of $50 billion in equity and a similar amount of debt to accomplish this feat.) Given the beating the chains have taken recently in the stock market, this scenario seems improbable. Therefore, the implication that the powerful companies will take over the field seems to be basically a fear tactic to encourage the forging of more horizontal and vertical voluntary alliances.

Another fear is that the powerful insurance and managed care systems will take over control of patients and usurp the role of providers in the system. This argument also assumes that only a few firms will dominate the industry. For this to happen, hundreds of benefits insurers would need to abandon the field; the full-service firms (HMOs) would have to become the sole, or at least dominant, model of delivery; and traditional providers would need to insist on high utilization under traditional methods of payment. Just the opposite seems to be occurring. Utilization is decreasing dramatically. Employers are managing their own care and benefits in a much more effective manner. Traditional providers are adjusting to this new approach, cost is coming down, and providers are accepting PPOs and other price-sensitive approaches fairly well. Also, more and more benefits companies are developing a wide range of approaches to ensure their survival in the marketplace. The world may be changing but it appears that many traditional owners (hospitals and physicians) are responding well to market forces. As a result, they are not losing their control over their hospitals and practices.

A third assumption is that businesses and personal consumers are ready and willing to make changes in how they consume health care services in order to secure a better price and value relationship. This assumption appears to be true. It is unlikely that the industry has fully explored consumers' willingness to change. However, this change is occurring incrementally. Many of the firms that moved first and fastest have experienced difficulty with their model approaches. As consumer groups move inexorably toward tighter controls of their own utilization, providers increasingly respond, albeit reluctantly.

Just how much of the market share will go to tightly managed care firms before traditional suppliers offer equally attractive utilization rates and prices, with greater freedom for consumers to choose physicians? Surely a 5 percent or 10 percent shift to HMOs is too little; but at 20 percent or 30 percent penetration, can traditional suppliers fail to respond? When the responses come, should there not be counter responses? The game has begun, but surely it is not yet decided.

### Current situation

As these fundamental changes occur, providers are indeed finding that circumstances can make for strange bedfellows. Disbelief that change will come has given way to fear that all is lost, only to be replaced by confidence in all-purpose alliances to fight the change. As the battle lines are drawn and readiness to do battle pervades, tenable options emerge with new lines of alliance, vertical and horizontal integration occur, and new partnerships begin to develop.

### New alliances

Vertical integration itself is beginning to emerge as an idea whose time has come. In the early stages many parties saw themselves at the core of such a system. They began the process hoping to solidify this coveted position. Some weaker, more timid players immediately threw in the towel and merged with the stronger partners. Others hedged and joined alliances to wait, see, and sample. A lot of money has been invested in these exercises but for the most part

they were exercises, not the consummation of a vertical system.

Perhaps it is in these alliances that some of the potential for building vertical systems exists. Given the many different services offered for the total health care dollar, it may be that any given provider not only will be a strong part of one alliance, but will play an important role in many alliances. The United States is, after all, a pluralistic society. Many vendors, physicians, and hospitals are interdependent on the unique economies of specialized sectors of the health care economy.

### Significance of new delivery systems

The HMO represents a particular subset of integration. The shared purchasing program represents another subset, and it is unlike the first, though important for its own merit. Maybe the health care industry is moving toward many different types of vertical integration. If new delivery systems do represent subsets of vertical integration, perhaps what is beginning will lead to a more vertically integrated system of services. But it is unlikely to lead to one or two or even a hundred or more super systems. It is more likely that the traditional mode of physician and medical care in general will evolve toward more efficient patterns. Pattern is the key term. In a pattern or set of relationships, more vertically related activities can evolve if and when they provide efficiency or provide a competitive or marketing opportunity for gains in terms of economy, medical care, or access.

Positive economic and medical care gains from joint ventures, networks, and diversification may occur without the parties involved giving up their control in these new negotiated relationships. Gains for consumers can occur without providers totally abandoning their traditional roles and missions. However, these roles will need to be redefined and renegotiated within the context of the larger societal goal of efficiency and access.

### Total integration unlikely

It is unlikely, however, that health care will ever become fully integrated. It is possible, if not probable, that a totally owned and operated vertically integrated system would look and act much like a state owned and operated system, with all the barriers to innovation and change that this might represent. That is, the traditional notion of vertical integration

*It is unlikely that health care will ever become fully integrated.*

may well be a bigger blunder in design than going along with the old cost-plus system despite that system's history of duplication and overuse.

If this is the case, total integration, vertical or horizontal, is undesirable. What is needed are the creativity and innovation that come from highly pluralistic approaches and the energy that comes from competitive behaviors within a pluralistic system that forces change, growth, or failure.

### Rational approach to vertical integration

As today's strategist explores vertical integration, he or she must look for an underlying rationale at each step. Is it for medical quality, efficiency, consumer acceptance, competitive advantage, or some related criterion? In analyzing the alternatives, issues of vertical integration and horizontal integration, corporate restructuring, diversification, merger, and alliance are great starting points, but as goals they fall short. They should be viewed as means or mechanisms for progress, not as goals or outcome measures. Indeed, there is a move toward greater vertical integration not because it represents an unalloyed virtue but because more general risk taking by larger groups of providers stimulates most cost-effective methods of care.

Totally owned and operated vertically integrated systems are not likely to occur as a result of market competitive forces unless all programs, resource requirements, and abilities can be brought to operate at the optimal level of utility simultaneously. This type of situation has never existed in any kind of organization. It certainly does not exist in medical care as it currently operates. Lumping everything into one organization would create a lump, not a set of orderly programs in harmony with one another and collectively meeting consumer needs.

• • •

Health care managers can and probably will network, enter joint ventures, and build and operate in a much more rational fashion—meaning more vertical

and horizontal relationships. But these efforts will not result in a neat textbook example of what a vertical system might represent. The system will be pluralistic. It will meld together and it will break apart whenever the parts do not fit. It will have control and coordination between individuals, groups, and corporations with many voices being heard. The 1990s will not look like the 1970s, but many of the same owners and physicians will be doing many of the things they did in the 1970s with greater efficiency and sound value to consumers, and in competition with others seeking to serve similar markets. In addition, they will be doing things with more and different partners than would have been envisioned in the last decade, or even today.

## REFERENCES

1. *Hospital Literature Index* 40 (1984): 207–8.
2. United Kingdom. Parliament. Consultative Council on Medical and Allied Services, Ministry of Health of Great Britain. *Interim Report on the Future Provision of Medical and Allied Services.* Cmd. 693. 1920.
3. Committee on the Cost of Medical Care. *Medical Care for the American People: The Final Report of the Committee.* Committee Pub. No. 28. Chicago: University of Chicago Press, November 1932.
4. Rosenfeld, L.S., and Makover, H.B. *The Rochester Regional Hospital Council.* Cambridge, Mass.: Harvard University Press, 1956.
5. Clark, H.T. "The Challenge of the Regional Medical Programs Legislation." *Journal of Medical Education* 41 (1966): 71–74.
6. American Hospital Association Special Committee on the Provision of Health Services. *Ameriplan: A Proposal for the Delivery and Financing of Health Services in the United States: Report of the Special Committee on Health Service.* Chicago: AHA, 1970.
7. Brown, M., and Money, W.H. "Promise of Multihospital Management." *Hospital Progress* 56, no. 8 (1975): 36–42
8. Brown, M., et al. "Trends in Multihospital Systems: A Multiyear Comparison." *Health Care Management Review* 5, no. 4 (Fall 1980): 9–22.
9. Brown, M. "Multihospital Systems in the 80s–The New Shape of the Health Care Industry." *Hospitals* 56 (March 1, 1982): 344–61.
10. Brown, M. "Community Hospitals: Caring, Curing, Commerce. Systems Commerce and the Caring Tradition." *Hospital Progress* 64 (May 1983): 37–44, 62.

# The economic transformation of American health insurance: implications for the hospital industry

C. Wayne Higgins
and
Eugene D. Meyers

*The economics of cost containment, growing competition, and the introduction of new technology are forcing major changes on the health insurance industry. This transformation will impact the hospital industry in significant ways, hastening its evolution from a cottage industry to a modern corporate structure.*

*Health Care Manage Rev, 1986, 11(4), 21–27*
© 1986 Aspen Publishers, Inc.

**Pressure from employers** demanding cost containment is transforming the health insurance industry from a passive risk-sharing system into a service industry competing on the basis of cost and utilization controls. At the same time, the development of new products and potential economies of scale resulting from electronic billing promise to drastically reshape the market structure of the health insurance industry. This will force out small insurers and compel larger companies to consolidate with providers in vertically integrated health care systems. As insurers assume the roles of purchasing agents and information and utilization managers for employers and service providers, their power over hospitals will dramatically increase. This article reviews current trends in the health insurance industry and discusses the probable impact on hospitals.

## SELF-INSURANCE

In the United States, health insurance developed largely as a passive risk-sharing system based on the casualty model of insurance.[1] The problem of moral hazard was recognized early, but was addressed, ineffectively, through deductibles and coinsurance rates aimed at the subscriber. Over the years, health insurance came to incorporate a number of inflationary features, such as free choice of provider, cost- and charge-based reimbursement, fee-for-service payment, and differential subsidies favoring inpatient hospital care, which contributed significantly to rising medical costs.[2,3] These cost increases translated into higher insurance premiums; however, federal tax laws exempting employer-paid health insurance premiums from the tax base caused consumers and employers to be less price sensitive. With the passage of Medicare and Medicaid legislation, the public treasury was exposed to health care cost inflation and the government responded with largely ineffective command and control regulations.[4-6]

During the 1970s, high inflation, low productivity gains, and international competition combined to

**C. Wayne Higgins,** *Ph.D., is Associate Professor of Public Health and Health Care Administration, Department of Health and Safety, Western Kentucky University, Bowling Green, Kentucky.*

**Eugene D. Meyers,** *Ph.D., is Coordinator and Assistant Professor, Health Care Administration, Department of Health and Safety, Western Kentucky University, Bowling Green.*

force business and industry to reexamine their passive attitude toward health benefit costs. The 1974 passage of the Employee Retirement Income Security Act (ERISA) provided a means for large corporations to reduce the administration costs of health benefits through self-insurance. Under the provisions of ERISA, self-insured health plans are exempt from state insurance regulations, including reserve requirements and state premium taxes. Total self-insurance is implemented only by large corporations that can efficiently manage in-house billing and can afford the risk of unexpectedly large health care costs. Nonetheless, by 1983 17.5 percent of the private health insurance market was accounted for by self-insured health plans.[7]

Faced with the loss of their largest accounts, insurers sought to recapture this business by offering actuarial support and claims processing through administrative services only (ASO) contracts. Under these arrangements, insurance companies estimate future costs and pay medical bills for self-insured companies but assume no risk for claims costs. Later, insurers offered reinsurance against unexpectedly high costs through minimum premium plans (MPPs). This allowed medium-sized employers to partially self-insure and accounted for 14.3 percent of the market in 1983.[8] Today, alternative financing arrangements, mostly ASO contracts and MPPs, account for roughly half of the private health insurance market.[9]

As the market for insurance services developed, new competitors entered the field in the form of third-party administrators, data companies, and firms specializing in utilization review and claims auditing. These companies provide employers with claims processing, provider-specific cost and quality information, various utilization control services, and review of employee medical bills. Insurers offered these services as well, along with benefits restructuring to control costs, which in effect makes them purchasing agents for the business community.

As insurers become purchasing agents they become the private regulators of the hospital industry. Both utilization controls and benefits restructuring are intended to reduce inpatient hospital utilization. Claims auditing focuses heavily on hospital bills, and information services compile provider-specific cost and service intensity data. Employers can then use these data to pressure expensive hospitals and to direct employees to more efficient facilities. The net results of these programs will be declining demand for inpatient hospital services, substitution of outpatient

care for inpatient care, a progressively ill mix of patients as the less ill are treated in outpatient settings, pressure to decrease service intensity and improve outcomes, and pressure to retire excess capacity and inefficient services. These effects will be reinforced by the incentives of the Medicare prospective payment system and the activities of peer review organizations.[10]

## ELECTRONIC BILLING

Substantial economies of scale in claims processing can be realized through electronic claims submission, editing, and processing.[11] Electronic billing avoids labor-intensive paper claims processing and is already in use by some large firms, such as Electronic Data Systems a subsidiary of General Motors, and National Electronic Information Corporation. To maximize the potential of electronic billing, providers and claims processors must be linked through computer networks. The capital costs of installing such systems will be prohibitive for insurers commanding small market shares. It may also prove impractical for individual providers to be linked to several billing systems simultaneously.

As electronic billing systems grow, many insurance companies are likely to withdraw from the business. Companies that have a small percentage of their total business in health insurance are unlikely to make the investments necessary to develop electronic billing networks. Over time, a large percentage of commercial insurance companies may withdraw from the health insurance business because they lack the market share to justify large new investments. In many large states, 300 or more health insurance companies compete for business and, with the exception of Blue Cross and Blue Shield, few have even a five percent market share.[12] Such a low market share also impedes the efforts of insurers to negotiate discounts and enter into preferred provider organizations (PPOs) and other contractual arrangements with providers.

As a shakeout occurs in the health insurance industry, hospitals will be confronted with fewer but more powerful and better informed payers. Insurers will use data to select cost-effective providers for insurer-provider networks, PPOs, and health maintenance organizations (HMOs). Insurers will have both the information to identify winners among hospitals and the clout to force contractual concessions. Historically, the fragmented third-party payment system and the implicit price competition between payers

*As a shakeout occurs in the health insurance industry, hospitals will be confronted with fewer but more powerful and better informed payers.*

worked to the advantage of providers because cost-containment efforts by any one payer placed its subscribers and beneficiaries at a disadvantage in obtaining services.[13,14] However, the unanimous efforts by payers to contain costs and the consolidation of the health insurance industry will weaken the position of providers relative to that of payers. Hospitals will find their destiny increasingly controlled by third party payers, and the growing demand of payers for efficiency will conflict with medical staff demands for autonomy of practice and control of resource allocations.

## HMOs and PPOs

HMOs have existed in various forms, although not by that name, since the turn of the century.[15] In the last few years, support from employers, unions, and the federal government has greatly accelerated their growth. By early 1985, there were 350 HMOs enrolling more than 15 million people nationwide, and enrollment was growing at approximately 12 percent per year.[16] Growth among multistate for-profit HMOs has been more rapid as hundreds of millions of dollars in private capital are invested in these organizations. Sustained HMO growth is expected, with total revenues for the industry projected to reach $35 billion by 1990.[17]

The growth of HMOs challenges both hospitals and insurers. Hospitals face declining occupancy because group model HMOs utilize fewer inpatient services than traditionally insured systems.[18,19] Hospitals are also pressured to compete for HMO contracts by offering discounts. Insurers face the prospect of declining market share as HMOs offer employers more favorable benefit and premium packages. To compete, insurers and providers are developing competitive, at risk products, such as independent practice associations (IPAs).[20] Like group model HMOs, these organizations embody incentives for reduced inpatient utilization and employ increased managerial control.

PPOs, like IPAs and group model HMOs, are presently undergoing rapid development. A recent survey by Thomas Rice and colleagues found that almost six million people are eligible to use PPOs, a fourfold increase in less than one year (from late 1984 to mid-1985). The study also revealed that utilization review, aimed at reducing inpatient hospital utilization, is now almost universal among PPOs.[21] PPOs facilitate competition among both providers and insurers. For insurers they provide new products, featuring discounts and utilization controls, that can compete with HMOs, IPAs, and conventional insurance. Hospitals and physicians view the PPO as a mechanism for protecting and expanding market share.

While PPOs have been developed by hospitals, physician groups, insurers, and entrepreneurs, the insurance industry and hospital organizations are now the leaders in expanding PPO networks. As insurers negotiate PPO contracts with hospitals, the demand for discounts and utilization controls can cause considerable friction. The conflict between Blue Cross and the hospital industry over the insurer's rapidly growing PPO system reflects the divergence of interests between insurers and providers.[22]

## VERTICALLY INTEGRATED SYSTEMS

Along with the growth of HMOs and PPOs has come the development of vertically integrated health care systems that offer both medical services and health insurance products. These systems are being developed by hospital corporations to protect market share and by insurance companies to gain greater control over utilization and efficiency. Current examples of vertically integrated health care systems include Humana Care Plus, which controls, through ownership or affiliation, about five percent of the nation's hospital beds,[23] and Partners National Health Plans, a joint venture between Aetna Life and Casualty and Voluntary Hospitals of America, a group of 550 nonprofit hospitals. The integration of health care plans and service delivery creates opportunities for lower priced, more cost-effective benefit packages than does traditional indemnity or service-benefit plans. Partnerships also facilitate the development of HMO and PPO products. More cost-effective benefit packages will allow integrated systems to expand market share at the expense of traditional insurance, effectively forcing some insurers out of the health insurance business and causing others to create integrated systems in order to compete. Current estimates project rapid growth for integrated systems. Some forecasts predict that 70 percent of the privately insured population will be enrolled in such plans by 1990.[24] Because only the largest and strongest insurance plans will be desirable partners in integrated systems, the growth of these arrangements will promote consolidation in the health insurance industry.

If the integrated health care systems of today evolve into vertically and horizontally integrated health care corporations offering a full range of medical services and health insurance products, hospitals will face a loss of autonomy as they are forced to affiliate with these corporations in order to survive. Furthermore, while some of today's partnerships are mechanisms for retaining and expanding market share for hospital corporations, tomorrow's health care corporations are unlikely to be dominated by hospitals. Indeed, hospitals are more likely to be cost centers than profit centers and it is unlikely that health care corporations will tolerate excess capacity in their most costly component. Thus, a private sector solution to the problem of excess hospital capacity could unfold as large corporations sell and convert hospital assets and independent hospitals are forced out of business.

## IMPACT OF CHANGES ON HOSPITALS

### Declining demand

Hospitals are already experiencing declining demand. The American Hospital Association reports a decline in admissions of 6 percent during the first quarter of 1985; this followed a 2.8 percent drop from 1983 to 1984.[25,26] The trend toward declining admissions should continue and accelerate as all third party payers seek to minimize inpatient hospital care. In addition to aggravating the excess capacity problem, these measures will leave hospitals with patients who are more ill and more costly to treat. During the first quarter of 1984, average cost per case for hospital inpatients increased at an annual rate of 8.2 percent. By the first quarter of 1985, the rate of increase jumped to 9.1 percent,[27] reflecting a more costly mix of patients. As the full potential of outpatient care is exploited, hospitals can expect to admit an even more ill patient mix. This will result in higher production costs while pressure to reduce inpatient expenditures

increases. It may also aggravate the problem of malpractice insurance costs since more adverse outcomes can be expected with more severely ill patient populations.

### Pressure to integrate

The hospital industry has already experienced considerable horizontal integration with the growth of proprietary hospital corporations in the 1970s and the growth of voluntary chains in the 1980s. Vertical integration is rapidly occurring as hospitals and multihospital chains acquire ambulatory clinics and long-term care facilities. The development of insurer–provider networks is but the latest stage in the hospital's evolution from a cottage industry to the modern corporation. Competition from HMOs, the demand for cost containment, and the intense competitive pressure in both the hospital industry and the health insurance industry will increasingly force these sectors to merge the functions of risk sharing and service delivery in a single corporate entity. Today's partnerships are likely to evolve into unified corporations as competition among insurer–provider networks requires greater managerial control and organizational complexity.

For hospitals, integration will mean a loss of autonomy and demands to subordinate the needs of the institution to the needs of the corporation. It will also mean progressive growth in the power of management, relative to clinicians, and a broadening of the managerial purview as a single management entity becomes responsible for both clinical services and insurance products. This growth in administration is already in evidence and will likely continue.[28]

### Excess capacity

For hospitals, the pressure for integration arises from the need to protect market share and access investment capital. In the long run, however, integration is likely to exacerbate the problem of excess hospital capacity and force a contraction of the hospital industry.

Regarding patient volume, integrated systems face pressures similar to those of HMOs, i.e., minimize the cost of health plans by controlling inpatient hospital utilization and substituting outpatient care for inpatient care. Since hospitals will be the major cost centers for the integrated systems, competition will force health care corporations to sell or convert excess hospital assets. However, if this occurs on a large scale, several problems will arise. First, from an architectural perspective, hospitals do not lend themselves to conversion. Second, the market for used hospital equipment is weak. Third, as health care corporations move to sell surplus facilities the market value of hospital assets will fall, thereby reducing the borrowing capacity of independent hospitals and creating greater pressures to integrate. Corporations will also be affected as the value of their hospital assets declines. This will hasten their efforts to diversify into outpatient services, insurance products, and other investments while reducing capital investments in hospitals. Consequently, over the long term, moves to integrate will solve neither the problem of declining demand nor the problem of access to investment capital. Many analysts estimate that up to one-third of all hospital beds will close during the next decade.[29] The integration of hospitals into health care corporations should facilitate that process.

### Increased managerial control

As hospitals are incorporated into integrated systems and are forced to compete on the basis of costs and outcomes, their management will exercise greater control and their administrative structure will grow more complex. Historically, hospitals have experienced dual lines of authority whereby managers focused on day-to-day operations and maximizing efficiency for nonreimbursable services while physicians largely controlled the revenue-producing clinical services. As the entire hospital becomes the major cost center of a larger organization, management must focus on efficiency in clinical services as well. This will cause friction as managers begin to assert authority in ways that affect physician practice and autonomy. However, the balance of power is shifting in favor of administration because hospitals are increasingly at financial risk, and because the physician surplus is making physicians replaceable.[30]

Management will also expand control through the use of management information systems that integrate cost and clinical data. Known as financial and production data in most industries, this information will allow managers to compare costs and revenues across services, diagnostic groups, and physicians. Management will have strong incentives to cut costs by reducing or eliminating unprofitable services, avoiding unprofitable patients, and dropping costly physicians from medical staffs. Concern has already

been expressed that the Medicare prospective payment system will bias treatment decisions and service offerings.[31-33] Hospitals participating in private at-risk contracts or integrated systems will face similar incentives. Likewise, the topic of closed medical staffs has been raised and procedures for granting and withdrawing practicing privileges is currently under review in many hospitals.[34] In the future, information systems will also incorporate quality assurance variables, such as treatment outcome, infection rate, and accident rate by service and physician. This will allow administrators to provide enhanced risk management programs in response to rising malpractice costs. It is possible that tomorrow's health care corporations may provide corporate malpractice coverage for their physicians, making risk management and quality control major administrative responsibilities.

### Control of medical practice

It is widely recognized that the utilization of medical services varies substantially among geographical regions and these variations are primarily attributed to differences in style of physician practice.[35-38] In addition, there is little evidence that more care results in observable improvements in health status and treatment outcome.[39,40] In the absence of evidence that more is better, pressures for cost containment will almost certainly dictate that less is good enough. Ultimately, hospitals and health care corporations can control cost only by encouraging conservative practice patterns on the part of their physicians. The use of standardized treatment protocols and monitoring of physician practice will enable management to influence clinical practice to an unprecedented degree. This will undoubtedly be seen by some physicians as an infringement on their autonomy. However, the growing power of insurers and corporations, along with pressure to practice normative medicine as a defense against malpractice claims, will facilitate increased administrative control. In a related trend, physicians are unlikely to influence hospital capital spending in the future to the extent that they have in the past. Efficiency and cost-containment needs will require that major capital outlays will be governed more by cost–benefit studies than by physician relations.

In the short term, hospital management can realize savings by exerting greater control over scheduling decisions. Many facilities can reduce staffing and

*The structural changes now occurring in health care financing will cause a progressive transfer of authority and control from physicians to managers.*

save resources by scheduling admissions and procedures, especially the use of operating rooms and expensive diagnostic services, to maximize hospital efficiency rather than physician convenience. Again, this reflects increased managerial control at the expense of physician prerogatives. Overall, the structural changes now occurring in health care financing will, if continued, cause a progressive transfer of authority and control from physicians to managers. How physicians will adapt to an inferior role remains to be seen but the physician glut, the growing power of management, and the bureaucratization of the health care industry suggest few alternatives.

•   •   •

The economic transformation of the health insurance industry is in its infancy, but already significant trends are observable that will, if continued, radically alter the relationships between insurers and providers. Hospitals, because of their importance, their costs, and their role as the major arena in which payers' demands for efficiency will clash with the professional sovereignty of physicians, will be drastically affected.

Today, health insurers are rapidly becoming the purchasing agents and information sources for American business. In this role, they have become private regulators intent on minimizing inpatient utilization and length of stay while maximizing efficiency. The traditional roles of hospital as physician workshop and physician as independent contractor will be obsolete in this environment. To survive, hospitals will have to expand administrative control of clinical practice and exert tighter control over medical staff membership.

In the future, there will be fewer health insurers, but survivors will have larger market shares, bill electronically, offer a full range of products including capitation plans, and tightly control price and utilization through contractual arrangements or direct affiliation with providers. This phase will be characterized by declining hospital autonomy, pressure to integrate, and increased management purview and control. The power of management will grow as managers assume responsibility for both insurance products and service delivery in a variety of settings. In most metropolitan areas, physicians will be seen as replaceable and will be increasingly subordinate to management.

During the final phase of the transformation, competition among insurer–provider partnerships will result in consolidation of the health care industry into a few large vertically and horizontally integrated corporations intent on enhancing and protecting capital by minimizing costs. If current policies and economic trends continue, it is likely that capitation health plans will be their principal insurance product. These corporations will complete the integration of both hospital and physician into a modern organizational structure. They will seek to minimize costs by eliminating excess hospital capacity and tightly controlling utilization. In doing so, they are likely to be more successful than government regulations. As recent experience in the transportation industry suggests, the public is far more tolerant of private sector solutions.

## REFERENCES

1. Starr, P. *The Social Transformation of American Medicine.* New York: Basic Books, 1982.
2. Feldstein, P. *Health Care Economics.* 2d ed. New York: Wiley, 1983.
3. Enthoven, A. *Health Plan.* Reading, Mass.: Addison-Wesley, 1981.
4. Ibid., 93–110.
5. Higgins, C., and Bruhn J. "Health Care Regulations and the Economics of Federal Health Care Policies." *Health Care Management Review* 6 (Fall 1981): 41–47.
6. Salkever, D., and Bice, J. *Hospital Certificate of Need Controls.* Washington, D.C.: American Enterprise Institute, 1979.
7. Ibid.
8. Arnett, R., and Trapnell, G. "Private Insurances: New Measures of a Complex and Changing Industry." *Health Care Financing Review* 6 (Winter 1984): 31–42.
9. Etheredge, L. "The World of Insurance: What Will the Future Bring?" *Business and Health* 3 (January-February 1986): 5–9.
10. Arnett, R., et al. "Health Spending Trends in the 1980's: Adjusting to Financial Incentives." *Health Care Financing Review* 6 (Spring 1985): 1–26.
11. Etheredge, "The World of Insurance."

12. Ibid.

13. Paringler, L. *The Medicare Assignment of Rates of Physicians: Their Responses to Changes in Reimbursement Policy.* Washington, D.C.: Health Care Financing Administration, 1979.

14. Greenspan, N., and Vogel, R. "Taxation and Its Effect upon Public and Private Insurance and Medical Demand." *Health Care Financing Review* 1 (Spring 1980): 39–45.

15. Mayer, T., and Mayer, G. "HMO's: Origins and Development." *New England Journal of Medicine* 312 (1985): 590–94.

16. *The HMO Industry Ten Year Report.* Minneapolis, Minn.: InterStudy, 1985.

17. Masso, A. "HMO's in Transition: What the Future Holds." *Business and Health* 2 (1985): 21–29.

18. Manning, W., et al. "A Controlled Trial of the Effects of a Prepaid Group Practice on Use of Services." *New England Journal of Medicine* 310 (1984): 1505–10.

19. Enthoven, A. "The Rand Experiment and Economical Health Care." *New England Journal of Medicine* 311 (1984): 1528–30.

20. Iglehart, J. "The Twin Cities' Medical Marketplace." *New England Journal of Medicine* 311 (1984): 343–48.

21. Rice, T., et al. "The State of PPO's: Results From a National Survey." *Health Affairs* 4 (Winter 1985): 25–40.

22. Powills, S. "Blue Program Divides Hospitals." *Hospitals* 59 (1985): 20.

23. Etheredge, "The World of Insurance."

24. Ripps, J., and Werronen, H., "Insurer–Provider Networks: A Marketplace Response." *Business and Health* 3 (January–February 1986): 20–22.

25. American Hospital Association. *Hospital Statistics 1985.* Chicago: AHA, 1985.

26. American Hospital Association. *Economic Trends.* Chicago: AHA, Summer 1985.

27. Ibid.

28. Himmelstein, D., and Woolhandler, S. "Cost Without Benefit: Administration Waste in U.S. Health Care." *New England Journal of Medicine* 314 (1986): 441–45.

29. Blendon, R. "Health Policy Choices of the 1990s." *Issues in Science and Technology* 2 (1986): 65–73.

30. Ginsberg, E., and Ostow, M. *The Coming Physician Surplus.* Totowa, N.J.: Rowman & Allheld, 1984.

31. Omenn, G., and Conrad, D. "Implications of DRG's for Clinicians." *New England Journal of Medicine* 311 (1984): 1314–17.

32. Relman, A. "Cost Control, Doctor's Ethics and Patient Care." *Issues in Science and Technology* 1 (1985): 103–11.

33. Jencks, S., et al. "Evaluating and Improving the Measure of Hospital Case-Mix." *Health Care Financing Review* supplement (November 1984): 1–11.

34. Keenan, C. "Closed Medical Staffs not Inevitable." *Hospitals* 59 (1985): 28.

35. Bunker, J. "Surgical Manpower: A Comparison of Operations and Surgeons in the United States and in England and Wales." *New England Journal of Medicine* 290 (1970): 1051–55.

36. Wennberg, J., and Gittelson, A. "Small Area Variations in Health Care Delivery." *Science* 180 (1973): 1102–8.

37. LoGerfo, J. "Variations in Surgical Rates: Fact or Fantasy." *New England Journal of Medicine* 297 (1977): 38789.

38. Chassin, M., et al. "Variations in the Use of Medical and Surgical Services by the Medicare Population." *New England Journal of Medicine* 314 (1986): 285–90.

39. Bunker, J., and Wennberg, J. "Operation Rates, Mortality Statistics and the Quality of Life." *New England Journal of Medicine* 289 (1973): 1249–51.

40. Chassin, M. "Variations in Hospital Length of Stay: Their Relationship to Health Outcomes." HCFA Pub. No. OTA-HC5-24. Washington, D.C.: Government Printing Office, 1983.

# Health maintenance organizations: improvements in the regulatory environment

H. Glenn Boggs

*Health maintenance organizations (HMOs) can help slow rising health care costs. State regulatory statutes are needed that will protect critical interests of HMO members while freeing HMOs from needless statutory requirements. A model HMO regulatory law is designed to strike a balance between protection of members and freedom for HMOs to deliver programs that can reduce health care costs.*

Health care costs comprise a major element of the U.S. national economy today. In previous years these costs have escalated rapidly. For example, from 1970 to the early 1980s, the U.S. GNP increased by more than 200 percent, but health care costs increased by more than 300 percent.[1]

Although various initiatives are now being tried that may moderate this trend, undoubtedly a complex problem of this magnitude will not be solved with any single bold solution. More likely, a combination of innovations, market forces, governmental influence, and much hard work by individuals will be necessary to bring rising health care costs under control and move Americans closer to the goal of effective and affordable health care for all citizens.

One new device, designed to control spiraling health care costs, which has emerged with a widening impact on the health care scene in recent years, is the health maintenance organization (HMO). Health care administrators, consumers, and regulators alike have a stake in the HMO regulatory environment—all should be sensitive to developments and concepts that can improve this environment. After briefly tracing the history of the HMO concept, a proposed model for state regulation of the HMO is presented. A narrative outline discussion of both desirable and undesirable regulation is followed by a detailed model statute—the statute is attached in appendix form for those readers who wish to refer to that level of detail.

For the sake of clarity in this discussion, the term HMO is defined rather broadly to include any entity that meets the following two-part test: (1) fixed payments by members for an agreed time period and (2) provision of specified, comprehensive medical services by the entity without further charge to the member (or covered dependent) on an as-needed basis. The HMO can be profit or not-for-profit and can use physicians on its staff or physicians under contract. Members can join individually or pursuant to a collective bargaining agreement.

Conceptually, it is readily apparent that there should be inherent incentives in the HMO design to maximize good medical care while at the same time

**H. Glenn Boggs,** *J. D., is an Assistant Professor at the Florida State University College of Business, where he teaches law-related courses. He is a member of The Florida Bar and an honors graduate of the Florida State University College of Law.*

*Health Care Manage Rev, 1986, 11(2), 45–59*
© 1986 Aspen Publishers, Inc.

minimizing costs. This is the case since the HMO's income is predetermined and fixed and therefore its economic advantage lies in delivering the required medical services at the least possible cost. HMO members are protected from an organization's temptation to cut corners to save money because the HMO remains responsible for the member's medical care for better or worse. Accordingly, if a member's health worsens, the HMO will still have to care for that member with the attendant resulting costs. Strictly from a financial viewpoint, then, the HMO profits by keeping its members as healthy as possible and avoiding expensive, time-consuming medical problems for its members.

## HMO DEVELOPMENT TRACED

If an HMO has these virtues, one might legitimately wonder why there have not been more of them around, sooner. Accordingly, a brief review of the history of HMO development is in order.

Group medical practice organizations with characteristics similar to HMOs began forming as industrialization marched into the American West around the beginning of the twentieth century. Railroads, mines, lumber, and other interests sought to provide medical care for workers using various group arrangements since workers were frequently far removed from the traditional fee-for-service medical system established in the East.[2] In 1887 Dr. W.W. Mayo and his sons started their now world-famous practice in Rochester, Minnesota, on a group practice basis,[3] and in 1929 Drs. Donald E. Ross and H. Clifford Loos began a group practice in Los Angeles, called the Ross-Loos Medical Clinic, which is accorded the distinction by some researchers of being the first HMO-type entity.[4] Other clinics and group practices were formed in following years, including the prominent Kaiser-Permanente Medical Care Program in 1945.[5] However, by 1970 there were still only 33 HMOs with about 3 million members throughout the country.[6]

Any observer of HMO development would have to consider 1973 to be a watershed year since after much debate and wrangling Congress passed the Health Maintenance Organization Act of 1973. Critics of the new statute were numerous, especially within the HMO industry, and in 1976 several amendments were adopted that accorded the HMO industry most of the changes it wanted.[7] The federal law, as amended, does not require an HMO to qualify under it since both before and after the act, HMOs could qualify under the appropriate laws and regulations of their respective states without any necessity to meet federal requirements. However, one important aspect of the federal enactment was that it prohibited any state from maintaining certain artificial legal roadblocks inhibiting the formation and development of HMOs under state law. For example, 42 U.S.C. §300e-10 provides that for HMOs qualified under the federal statute, no state may stop such an HMO from doing business by requiring: (1) that approval of the HMO by a medical society be obtained, (2) that physicians constitute all or some specified portion of the governing body of the HMO, (3) that all physicians or a specified portion of physicians in the HMO's area be allowed to provide services for the HMO, or (4) that the HMO meet requirements for insurers of health care services regarding capitalization and financial reserves against insolvency. In addition, all states are precluded from prohibiting HMOs qualified under 42 U.S.C. §300e-10 from advertising for members by describing "services, charges or other nonprofessional aspects of its operation." Thus, consistent with the concept of federalism and the autonomy of the states, while an HMO must satisfy the legal requirements of its particular state before engaging in business, an HMO that elects to qualify under the federal act can avoid the aforementioned state requirements that Congress has determined to be unduly restrictive and that would tend to frustrate the national policy to encourage the development and creation of HMOs.

As an additional incentive to form HMOs under the federal act, from 1973 to 1981 Congress provided approximately $364 million in either grants or loans to federally qualified HMOs to stimulate their formation and success.[8] To indicate the success of this device and for comparative purposes, Figure 1 illustrates how membership in HMOs has increased.[9]

In addition to the various legal and procedural impediments that sometimes confounded HMO development under state laws (previously discussed) at least one knowledgeable commentator has suggested that one possible reason for the relatively slow pace of HMO development heretofore has simply been the sheer difficulty of building and maintaining an organizationally complex entity like an HMO.[10] This notwithstanding, since the federal grant and loan program was curtailed in 1981, HMOs have increasingly turned to the nation's public equity and bond mar-

## FIGURE 1

### MILLIONS OF MEMBERS IN ALL HMOs

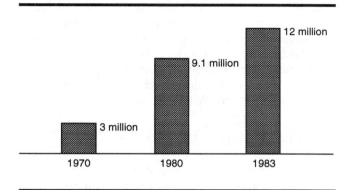

## A PROPOSED MODEL LAW FOR STATE REGULATION

At the heart of the HMO concept consumers make financial payments to a business entity in return for a promise of specified medical care if and when they need it. Arrangements of this type, which shift the risk of providing needed medical care from the individual to a group entity, might well be viewed as a form of insurance that would traditionally be subject to regulation—often fairly substantial regulation—by a state insurance department. Given that a public policy choice to enhance the development of HMOs to assist in the effort to contain rising medical care costs is appropriate, it is logical to relieve HMOs from unnecessarily burdensome regulations. Indeed

*Given that a public policy choice to enhance the development of HMOs to assist in the effort to contain rising medical care costs is appropriate, it is logical to relieve HMOs from unnecessarily burdensome regulations.*

kets to obtain the capital needed for expansion and growth and have, in turn, been well received by those markets.[11]

Recent HMO growth has also been achieved by multistate HMO firms that have perhaps mastered the organizational and management techniques needed to successfully operate and that are now applying their knowledge in one locale after another. Of the approximately 14 major "chains" or multistate HMOs, some expanded their operations as much as 100 percent in 1982. Data available at mid-1983 showed that about 73 percent of all enrolled HMO members belonged to multistate HMOs.[12]

At this point, before discussing state regulation, a brief summary to focus on several key facts is necessary: (1) The concept of the HMO appears to have intrinsic incentives to help control rising medical costs; (2) federal policy as expressed through the HMO Act of 1973, as amended, is designed to encourage the growth and development of HMOs; (3) states, by their inherent police power to legislate for the promotion of the public health, safety, and welfare, have the authority to regulate HMOs within their jurisdictions; (4) HMOs of one form or another are in place throughout the country and currently serve more than 12 million members; and (5) it is reasonable to assume that HMOs will grow and serve still more members in the foreseeable future.

it will be recalled that the federal HMO statute expressly prohibits the states from mandating that federally qualified HMOs meet the capitalization and financial reserve requirements of health care services insurers. Accordingly, the public interest would appear to be best served by exempting all HMOs from state insurance regulation and by adopting a special statute specifically designed to accommodate the HMO entity.

This, of course, has occurred on a fairly broad scale throughout the country. For example, in 1972 the National Association of Insurance Commissioners (NAIC) prepared and promulgated a proposed model HMO act. Its influence has been widely felt and by early 1982, after several amendments, the model or substantial portions of it had been adopted in 27 states.[13] In spite of the influence of the NAIC model act, even a cursory review of HMO legislation on the various state statute books reveals a wide variety in regulatory approach and scope. Questions naturally arise regarding the quantity of necessary regulation. How much is absolutely required and how much is too much?

## RESEARCH

In order to shed light on this area two separate and independent research initiatives were undertaken during the summer of 1984. First, the regulators themselves were polled in a mail questionnaire. Officials responsible for administration of HMO statutes in all states were queried concerning formation of HMOs, insolvency of HMOs, and administrative discipline of HMOs in their respective states. Replies were received from 41 states and also from both the Virgin Islands and Washington, D.C., resulting in a response rate of over 80 percent. Data obtained from this survey are reproduced in Tables 1, 2, and 3, and will be referred to subsequently in discussion of appropriate specific regulatory initiatives.

In addition to the survey, legal research was conducted to locate any reported judicial decision that construed either the federal HMO statute or any state HMO regulatory statute. The process to conduct this search involved first identifying each state HMO statute (if one was on the books) and then checking to see if there were any reported judicial decisions construing the statute. After obtaining the citation to a case, it was reviewed and catalogued relative to its application to regulatory law. Perhaps surprisingly, this tedious process of legal research yielded fewer than 25 case decisions construing either the federal statute or one of the state HMO laws. What emerges from a review of the litigation in this area is a picture of a *relatively* tranquil regulatory environment in which the parties have resorted to litigation on a generally infrequent basis.

In light of the data both collected and available in the literature a substantive critique of HMO regulation should contemplate the regulatory goals to be achieved and the means to achieve them. First, as has already been postulated, the HMO concept should be encouraged and provided a favorable regulatory climate in which to germinate and, hopefully, flourish. Second, the members of HMOs, who make financial payments in advance in exchange for future medical services if needed, should be protected regarding their receipt of the medical services. Often there will be a tension between these two objectives and the task is to strike as harmonious a balance as possible when such tensions arise.

To facilitate consideration of specific statutory language that could accomplish the desired regulation reference will be made in the proposed model law (see the Appendix) to certain sections of the Florida HMO statute that has been on the books since 1972 and amended on several subsequent occasions, including 1984. In terms of population, Florida is one of the larger states, and its HMO law is relatively comprehensive so examples made with Florida statutory language should have a general application throughout the country. Obviously, many, if not most, states have their own individual peculiarities and consequently will modify suggested statutory provisions to meet specific individual needs.

## REGULATORY ISSUES

Following is a narrative outline of regulatory issues, with annotations to the proposed Model Law in the Appendix.

### I. Licensing applications

To begin an HMO regulatory statute it is conventional to have a title section, announce the legislature's objective, and define terms. In the proposed model law Sections 1, 2, and 3 accomplish those tasks. In Section 2 outlining the legislature's objectives, the policy choices are announced that remove HMOs from regulation under the state's ordinary insurance laws and remove artificial legal barriers to HMO development and growth. Since definitions of terms can have a critical bearing on the ultimate interpretation of statutes, particular attention should be paid to the definition of terms such as the HMO itself, the health maintenance contract, and comprehensive health care services as contained in Section 3 of the proposed model law.

One fairly simple and relatively effective method of protecting HMO members from fraud is to compel HMO organizers, owners, and operators to disclose their identity and to require regulators to substantiate their backgrounds for veracity and honesty. This can be accomplished by requiring each HMO to have a certificate to operate that, in turn, will not be issued until specified documents and information are submitted to regulators for review. Each bit of data required should have a rational connection to ensuring that the HMO will be run fairly by honest persons. If that connection cannot be made, the data should not be required. Regulators should be given reasonable statutory deadlines within which to process the application to avoid unnecessary delay.

| **TABLE 1** | | | | | | |
|---|---|---|---|---|---|---|
| HMOs FORMED BETWEEN 1973 AND 1984 | | | | | | |
| State | 1983 | 1982 | 1981 | 1980 | 1979 | Total 1973–date* |
| Alabama | 1 | 0 | 0 | 0 | 0 | 3 |
| Arizona | 1 | 1 | 1 | 0 | 0 | 8 |
| Alaska | 0 | 0 | 0 | 0 | 0 | 0 |
| Colorado | 0 | 0 | 0 | 1 | 2 | 8 |
| Delaware | 1 | 0 | 0 | 0 | 0 | 1 |
| Florida | 4 | 1 | 2 | 2 | 0 | 21 |
| Georgia | 0 | 0 | 3 | 1 | 1 | 5 |
| Idaho | 0 | 0 | 0 | 0 | 0 | 2 |
| Illinois | 1 | 2 | 1 | 2 | 3 | 21 |
| Indiana | 2 | 3 | 0 | 2 | 0 | 7 |
| Iowa | 1 | 2 | 0 | 1 | 0 | 4 |
| Kansas | 1 | 0 | 1 | 0 | 0 | 6 |
| Kentucky | 1 | 0 | 0 | 0 | 0 | 3 |
| Louisiana | 0 | 0 | 1 | 1 | 0 | 2 |
| Maine | 0 | 0 | 0 | 0 | 0 | 1 |
| Maryland | 1 | 0 | 2 | 4 | 6 | 15 |
| Massachusetts | 0 | 0 | 2 | 4 | 2 | 17 |
| Michigan | 3 | 3 | 2 | 0 | 3 | 20 |
| Minnesota | 3 | 0 | 0 | 0 | 1 | 5 |
| Mississippi | 0 | 0 | 0 | 0 | 0 | 0 |
| Missouri | 0 | 2 | 0 | 0 | 0 | 6 |
| Nebraska | 0 | 0 | 0 | 0 | 0 | 1 |
| New Hampshire | 0 | 0 | 0 | 0 | 1 | 1 |
| New Jersey | 1 | 1 | 1 | 1 | 0 | 12 |
| New York | 3 | 0 | 0 | 1 | 1 | 15 |
| North Carolina | 0 | 0 | 2 | 0 | 0 | 4 |
| North Dakota | 2 | 0 | 0 | 0 | 0 | 3 |
| Ohio | 5 | 2 | 3 | 0 | 2 | 19 |
| Oklahoma | 3 | 0 | 1 | 0 | 0 | 6 |
| Oregon | 1 | 0 | 0 | 0 | 1 | 6 |
| Pennsylvania | 0 | 2 | 0 | 0 | 0 | 10 |
| Rhode Island | 0 | 0 | 0 | 0 | 1 | 1 |
| South Carolina | 0 | 0 | 0 | 0 | 0 | 4 |
| South Dakota | 0 | 0 | 0 | 0 | 0 | 0 |
| Tennessee | 0 | 0 | 0 | 2 | 0 | 2 |
| Texas | 0 | 4 | 2 | 1 | 3 | 17 |
| Vermont | 0 | 0 | 1 | 0 | 0 | 1 |
| Virginia | 2 | 1 | 0 | 0 | 1 | 6 |
| Virgin Islands | 0 | 0 | 0 | 0 | 0 | 0 |
| Washington | 2 | 0 | 2 | 1 | 0 | 13 |
| Washington, D.C. | 0 | 0 | 0 | 0 | 0 | 0 |
| West Virginia | 0 | 0 | 0 | 1 | 2 | 4 |
| Wisconsin | 4 | 2 | 0 | 3 | 0 | 17 |
| Total | 43 | 26 | 27 | 28 | 30 | 297 |

*Data collected in late spring and summer 1984.

| **TABLE 2** | | | | | | |
|---|---|---|---|---|---|---|
| INSOLVENT HMOs FROM 1973 TO 1984 | | | | | | |
| State | 1983 | 1982 | 1981 | 1980 | 1979 | Total 1973–date* |
| Alabama | 0 | 0 | 0 | 0 | 0 | 0 |
| Arizona | 0 | 0 | 0 | 0 | 0 | 1 |
| Alaska | 0 | 0 | 0 | 0 | 0 | 0 |
| Colorado | 0 | 0 | 0 | 1 | 0 | 1 |
| Delaware | 0 | 0 | 0 | 0 | 0 | 0 |
| Florida | 1 | 0 | 1 | 0 | 1 | 4 |
| Georgia | 0 | 0 | 0 | 0 | 0 | 0 |
| Idaho | 0 | 0 | 1 | 0 | 1 | 2 |
| Illinois | 0 | 0 | 2 | 0 | 1 | 3 |
| Indiana | 0 | 0 | 0 | 0 | 0 | 0 |
| Iowa | 0 | 0 | 0 | 0 | 0 | 1 |
| Kansas | 0 | 0 | 0 | 0 | 0 | 0 |
| Kentucky | 0 | 0 | 0 | 0 | 0 | 0 |
| Louisiana | 0 | 0 | 1 | 1 | 0 | 2 |
| Maine | 0 | 0 | 0 | 0 | 0 | 0 |
| Maryland | 1 | 0 | 2 | 0 | 0 | 3 |
| Massachusetts | 0 | 0 | 0 | 0 | 0 | 0 |
| Michigan | 0 | 1 | 1 | 0 | 0 | 2 |
| Minnesota | 0 | 0 | 0 | 0 | 0 | 0 |
| Mississippi | 0 | 0 | 0 | 0 | 0 | 0 |
| Missouri | 0 | 0 | 1 | 0 | 0 | 2 |
| Nebraska | 0 | 0 | 0 | 0 | 0 | 0 |
| New Hampshire | 0 | 0 | 0 | 0 | 0 | 0 |
| New Jersey | 0 | 0 | 0 | 0 | 2 | 2 |
| New York | 0 | 0 | 2 | 0 | 0 | 2 |
| North Carolina | 0 | 0 | 0 | 0 | 0 | 0 |
| North Dakota | 0 | 0 | 0 | 0 | 0 | 0 |
| Ohio | 0 | 0 | 0 | 1 | 0 | 1 |
| Oklahoma | 0 | 0 | 0 | 0 | 0 | 0 |
| Oregon | 0 | 0 | 1 | 0 | 0 | 1 |
| Pennsylvania | 0 | 0 | 2 | 0 | 0 | 2 |
| Rhode Island | 0 | 0 | 0 | 0 | 0 | 0 |
| South Carolina | 0 | 0 | 0 | 0 | 0 | 0 |
| South Dakota | 0 | 0 | 0 | 0 | 0 | 0 |
| Tennessee | 0 | 0 | 0 | 0 | 0 | 0 |
| Texas | 1 | 0 | 1 | 1 | 0 | 3 |
| Vermont | 0 | 0 | 0 | 0 | 0 | 0 |
| Virginia | 0 | 0 | 0 | 0 | 0 | 0 |
| Virgin Islands | 0 | 0 | 0 | 0 | 0 | 0 |
| Washington | 0 | 1 | 1 | 2 | 2 | 6 |
| Washington, D.C. | 0 | 0 | 0 | 0 | 0 | 0 |
| West Virginia | 1 | 0 | 1 | 0 | 0 | 2 |
| Wisconsin | 0 | 0 | 0 | 0 | 0 | 0 |
| Total | 4 | 2 | 17 | 6 | 7 | 40 |

*Data collected in late spring and summer 1984.

**TABLE 3**

ADMINISTRATIVE OR DISCIPLINARY ACTIONS TAKEN AGAINST HMOs FROM 1973 TO 1984

| State | 1983 | 1982 | 1981 | 1980 | 1979 | Total 1973–date* | State | 1983 | 1982 | 1981 | 1980 | 1979 | Total 1973–date* |
|---|---|---|---|---|---|---|---|---|---|---|---|---|---|
| Alabama | 0 | 0 | 0 | 0 | 0 | 0 | New Hampshire | 0 | 0 | 0 | 0 | 0 | 0 |
| Arizona | 0 | 0 | 0 | 0 | 0 | 0 | New Jersey | 0 | 0 | 0 | 1 | 2 | 3 |
| Alaska | 0 | 0 | 0 | 0 | 0 | 0 | New York | 10 | 10 | 11 | 10 | 6 | 47 |
| Colorado | 0 | 0 | 0 | 0 | 0 | 0 | North Carolina | 0 | 0 | 0 | 0 | 0 | 0 |
| Delaware | 0 | 0 | 0 | 0 | 0 | 0 | North Dakota | 0 | 0 | 0 | 0 | 0 | 0 |
| Florida | 1 | 0 | 0 | 0 | 0 | 1 | Ohio | 0 | 0 | 0 | 0 | 0 | 0 |
| Georgia | 0 | 1 | 1 | 0 | 0 | 2 | Oklahoma | 0 | 0 | 0 | 0 | 0 | 0 |
| Idaho | 0 | 0 | 0 | 0 | 0 | 0 | Oregon | 0 | 0 | 0 | 0 | 0 | 0 |
| Illinois | 0 | 0 | 0 | 0 | 0 | 0 | Pennsylvania | 0 | 0 | 0 | 0 | 0 | 0 |
| Indiana | 0 | 0 | 0 | 0 | 0 | 0 | Rhode Island | 0 | 0 | 0 | 0 | 0 | 0 |
| Iowa | 0 | 0 | 0 | 0 | 0 | 0 | South Carolina | 0 | 0 | 0 | 0 | 0 | 0 |
| Kansas | 0 | 0 | 0 | 0 | 0 | 0 | South Dakota | 0 | 0 | 0 | 0 | 0 | 0 |
| Kentucky | 0 | 0 | 0 | 0 | 0 | 0 | Tennessee | 0 | 0 | 0 | 0 | 0 | 0 |
| Louisiana | 0 | 0 | 1 | 0 | 0 | 1 | Texas | 0 | 0 | 1 | 0 | 0 | 1 |
| Maine | 0 | 0 | 0 | 0 | 0 | 0 | Vermont | 1 | 0 | 0 | 0 | 0 | 1 |
| Maryland | 6 | 0 | 0 | 0 | 0 | 6 | Virginia | 0 | 0 | 0 | 0 | 0 | 0 |
| Massachusetts | 0 | 0 | 0 | 0 | 0 | 0 | Virgin Islands | 0 | 0 | 0 | 0 | 0 | 0 |
| Michigan | 0 | 1 | 1 | 1 | 1 | 4 | Washington | 0 | 1 | 1 | 1 | 2 | 6 |
| Minnesota | 4 | 0 | 0 | 0 | 0 | 7 | Washington, D.C. | 0 | 0 | 0 | 0 | 0 | 0 |
| Mississippi | 0 | 0 | 0 | 0 | 0 | 0 | West Virginia | 0 | 0 | 0 | 0 | 0 | 0 |
| Missouri | 0 | 0 | 0 | 0 | 0 | 0 | Wisconsin | 0 | 0 | 0 | 0 | 0 | 0 |
| Nebraska | 0 | 0 | 0 | 0 | 0 | 0 | Total | 22 | 13 | 16 | 13 | 11 | 80 |

*Data collected in late spring and summer 1984.

Regulators with expertise in public health and medicine should have the duty to examine an HMO's capability to deliver competent medical care. The proposed model law calls for HMO applications to be initially filed with a state's insurance department that has the primary responsibility for licensing, but the model also provides that the responsibility for passing on an applicant's ability to deliver medical services be placed with a state's department of health or its equivalent.

## II. Rate making

The Florida HMO statute, as well as similar statutes in other states, provides that one of the regulator's responsibilities is to pass on the actuarial soundness of an applicant's proposed rates. The proposed model omits this requirement entirely. The rationale for this omission is that the marketplace itself will serve as a better barometer of pricing than regulatory planning. If the HMO's rates are too high, members are unlikely to join, and if the rates are too low, the HMO will experience financial difficulty and be forced to adjust within its contractual limits. Ultimately, this process should produce the lowest rates possible, which is the chief reason for promoting the development of HMOs.

If a particular HMO is unable to make the necessary financial adjustments and fails, its members will nevertheless be protected in their expectation to receive future medical services by a reinsurance contract that HMOs will, under the proposed model law, be required to obtain prior to being licensed. The reinsurance contract contemplated here is an agreement between the HMO and a carrier with a track record acceptable to regulators that obligates the carrier to underwrite the delivery of medical services promised to members if, for any reason, the HMO fails to render them. A simple requirement of this nature leaves it to HMO organizers to obtain reinsurance in the market, eliminating a substantial number of regulatory provisions aimed at reaching determinations regarding the financial viability of a proposed HMO. If the reinsurance is commercially unavailable, the department has the statutory authority in the model to waive the requirement and substitute a satisfactory bond or deposit. Data that appear to support this approach are available in Tables 1 and 2, which reveal a relatively low rate of HMO insolvency compared with the number of HMOs in existence.

### III. Malpractice liability protection

In addition to reinsurance to cover delivery of promised services, a proposed HMO should provide evidence of professional liability insurance to protect it from claims arising out of the delivery of medical services to members. In cases discovered in the litigation research such as *Pulvers v. Kaiser Foundation Health Plan*, 99 C.A. 3d 560 (1979), the courts have upheld liability attached to the HMO for acts or omissions of its agents. Consequently, this type of insurance protection or adequate self-insurance should be mandated by state regulatory authority.

To help ensure fair treatment to members and prospective members, the model law requires the HMO to implement a complaint system for member grievances and requires that member solicitation documents be submitted to and reviewed by the department for clarity and accuracy. A cooling off period during which members may cancel a contract is also provided. Sections 4 and 5 of the model law deal with these issues.

### IV. Contracts

The chief point of intersection between the HMO as an entity and the member is the contract, which is discussed in Section 6 of the model. Regulatory statutes should require that the contract be in writing and that the language used be written clearly in understandable English. As long as the contractual provisions do not violate any statutory requirements, the HMO should be free to structure its program as it sees fit. One or two exceptions to this general approach seem warranted from legal research. If an HMO member is a victim of a tortious act for which a third party is liable, the model would permit the HMO to recover its costs for treatment from the member, but only to the extent that the member has actually recovered funds from the third party who was at fault. This approach seems appropriate since otherwise the member would reap a windfall at the expense of the HMO. The member's interest is safeguarded since the HMO cannot recover from the member unless the member has actually recovered from the tortfeasor.

Member protections are also built into the model law that: (1) prohibit the HMO from summarily dropping a member, (2) allow a member to continue with the HMO if he or she leaves the group in which he or she initially gained membership, (3) clarify coverage for newborn and handicapped children, and (4) require that providers of services and materials look only to the HMO and not to members for their compensation.

Sections 7, 8, and 9 of the model control routine regulation of HMOs by requiring an annual report, mandating that HMOs invest extra funds in the same manner as life insurance companies, and prohibiting certain specified practices, respectively.

### V. License revocations

Since the model incorporates the concept of state licensing of HMOs before they are permitted to operate, it must follow that what the state gives, it can take away. Accordingly, Sections 10 and 11 give state regulators power to conduct inspections of licensed HMOs and specify the conditions under which regulators have authority to initiate revocation or suspension procedures. In addition to the normal suspension or revocation sanctions against an HMO's license, the model also provides that civil administrative fines may be levied. A policy choice is made in the model unlike some states, to delete misdemeanor criminal penalties from the arsenal of HMO regulatory authority. An HMO engaging in serious misconduct such as criminal fraud, for example, will almost certainly be liable to prosecution under criminal statutes already on state law books. Thus the model HMO regulatory law avoids duplication and is likely to be more clearly and fairly administered procedurally if confined to the civil administrative area.

Sections 12 and 13 are straightforward provisions that set fees for filing specified documents and give the departments authority to promulgate rules. To minimize confusion, both the Department of Insurance and the Department of Health are required to cooperate in rule making.

Since HMO promoters are investigated for integrity prior to licensure it follows that the identity and trustworthiness of HMO ownership transferees be examined. Section 14 provides for this eventuality.

Sections 15, 16, and 17 tie up such loose ends as: (1) regulation of third party contracts with the HMO to ensure that members are not liable thereunder, (2) provisions for the confidentiality of member medical records, and (3) a requirement that the HMOs give their members an annual report on the status of the organization.

## VI. Dual choice

The federal HMO statute and the HMO laws of a number of states currently include the so-called "dual choice" concept. These provisions allow an HMO that meets prescribed statutory criteria to legally compel employers (who also meet the statutory criteria) to offer the HMO program to their employees. This is an unusually strong marketing tool for HMOs, and it should be carefully analyzed on its merits. Recent data gathered by the U.S. Office of Health Maintenance Organizations in a national survey of employer attitudes indicate that only 6 percent of employers experienced HMO access demands through dual choice.[14] Since HMOs do not appear to be making extensive use of this coercive tool the model law proposed herein deletes this device.

•   •   •

The HMO appears to have some intrinsic qualities that will work to slow rising health care costs. Indeed, a recent survey indicates

that HMOs, with their unique system for financing and delivering care, are able to better control the rising costs of health care. HMOs are able to provide a more comprehensive benefit package at the same, if not lower, cost of the indemnity plan. HMOs do this while keeping their premiums from increasing as rapidly as the indemnity plans. Based on current trends, the HMO premium costs will be lower than the indemnity plan premiums in all regions within the next one to three years. This should have a very positive effect on HMO enrollment growth nationwide.[15]

This expected growth can best be managed by state regulatory statutes that are designed to protect critical interests of HMO members while at the same time freeing HMO entities from needless statutory requirements. The proposed model HMO regulatory law is designed to strike this delicate balance between protection of members on one hand and freedom for HMOs to innovate and deliver programs that actually succeed in reducing rising health care costs on the other. The HMO, in this environment, should play a significant part in reaching the goal of adequate health care for all Americans at a reasonable cost.

## REFERENCES

1. National Industry Council for HMO Development. "The Health Maintenance Organization Industry Ten Year Report 1973–1983." National Industry Council for HMO Development, 1983, p. 15.
2. Shouldice, R.G., and Shouldice, K.H. *Medical Group Practice and Health Maintenance Organizations.* Washington, D.C.: Information Resources Press, 1978, p. 20.
3. Ibid., 20, 21.
4. Ibid., 21.
5. "The Health Maintenance Organization Industry Ten Year Report," 5.
6. Ibid.
7. Brown, L.D. *Politics and Health Care Organizations: HMOs as Federal Policy.* Washington, D.C.: Brookings Institution, 1983, pp. 404–405.
8. "The Health Maintenance Organization Industry Ten Year Report," 5–6.
9. Ibid., 4–5.
10. Brown, *Politics and Health Care Organizations,* 31.
11. "The Health Maintenance Organization Industry Ten Year Report," 5, 21, 22, 23.
12. Ibid., 21.
13. NAIC Model Health Maintenance Organization Act. Model Regulation Service, National Association of Insurance Commissioners, May 1982, p. 4.
14. U.S. Office of Health Maintenance Organizations. "Employer Attitudes Toward Health Maintenance Organizations." Division of Private Sector Initiatives Pub. No. HRS-M-HM 83-2. Washington, D.C.: Government Printing Office, August 1983, p. 50.
15. Ibid., 64.

## APPENDIX

## MODEL HEALTH MAINTENANCE ORGANIZATION STATUTE

SECTION 1:
Short Title.—This Act shall be referred to as the Health Maintenance Organization Act.

SECTION 2:
Legislative Objective and Public Policy.—It shall be the policy of this state to:
(a) Eliminate legal barriers to the organization, promotion, and expansion of health maintenance organizations;
(b) Recognize that health maintenance organizations shall be exempt from operation of the insurance laws of this state except in the manner and to the extent set forth in this part; and
(c) To permit insurance companies or combinations of insurance companies to create health maintenance organizations.

SECTION 3:
Definitions.—As used in this Act, the following terms are defined to mean:
(1) *Comprehensive health care services* means services, medical equipment, and supplies furnished by a provider which may include, but which are not limited to, medical, surgical, and dental care; psychological, optometric, optic, chiropractic, podiatric, nursing, physical therapy, and pharmaceutical services; health education, preventive medical, rehabilitative, and home health services; inpatient and outpatient hospital services; extended care; nursing home care; convalescent institutional care; laboratory and ambulance services; appliances, drugs, medicines, and supplies; and any other care, service, or treatment of disease, the correction of defects, or the maintenance of the physical and mental well-being of human beings.
(2) *Department* means the Department of Insurance.
(3) *Entity* means any legal entity with continuing existence, including, but not limited to, a corporation, association, trust, or partnership.
(4) *Guaranteeing organization is* an organization which is domiciled in the United States; which has authorized service of process against it; and which has appointed the Insurance Commissioner as its agent for service of process issuing upon any cause of action arising in this state, based upon any guarantee entered into under this part.
(5) *Health maintenance contract* means any contract entered into by a health maintenance organization with a member or group of members to provide comprehensive health care services in exchange for a prepaid per capita or prepaid aggregate fixed sum.
(6) *Health maintenance organization* means any organization authorized under this part which:
(a) provides, either directly or through arrangements with other persons, health care services to persons enrolled with such organization, on a prepaid per capita or prepaid aggregate fixed-sum basis; and
(b) provides, either directly or through arrangements with other persons, those member services which members reasonably require to maintain good health specified in paragraph (9) herein; and
(c) provides physician services either directly through physicians who are either employees or partners of such organization or under arrangements with a physician or any group of physicians.
(7) *Insolvent* or *insolvency* means the inability of the health maintenance organization to discharge its liabilities as they become due in the normal course of business.
(8) *Member* means an individual who has contracted, or on whose behalf a contract has been entered into, with a health maintenance organization for health care services.
(9) *Minimum services* includes, but is not limited to, emergency care, inpatient hospital, and physician care, ambulatory diagnostic treatment, and preventive health care services.

(10) *Provider* means any physician, hospital, or other institution, organization, or person that furnishes health care services and is licensed or otherwise authorized to practice in the state.

SECTION 4:    Issuance of Certificate.—Before any entity may operate a health maintenance organization, it shall obtain a certificate of authority from the department. Each application for a certificate shall be on such a form as the department shall prescribe and shall be verified by an officer or authorized representative of the applicant and shall be accompanied by the following:

(1) A copy of the basic organizational document of the applicant, if any, such as the articles of incorporation, articles of association, partnership agreement, trust agreement, or other applicable document, and all amendments hereto;

(2) A copy of the bylaws, rules and regulations, or similar form of document, if any, regulating the conduct of the affairs of the applicant;

(3) A list of the names, addresses, and official capacities with the organization of the persons who are to be responsible for the conduct of the affairs of the health maintenance organization, including all members of the governing body, the officers and directors in the case of a corporation, and the partners or associates in the case of a partnership or association. Such persons shall fully disclose to the department and the governing body of the health maintenance organization the extent and nature of any contracts or arrangements between them and the health maintenance organization, including any possible conflicts of interest;

(4) A statement generally describing the health maintenance organization, its operations, the manner in which comprehensive health care services will be regularly available, the location of the facilities at which comprehensive health care services will be regularly available to members, the type of health care personnel engaged to provide the comprehensive health care services and the quantity of personnel of each type;

(5) Forms of all health maintenance contracts the applicant proposes to offer the members, showing the benefits to which they are entitled, together with a table of the rates charged, or proposed to be charged, for each form of such contract;

(6) A statement describing with reasonable certainty the geographic area or areas to be serviced by the health maintenance organization;

(7) A financial statement prepared on the basis of generally accepted accounting principles;

(8) A description of the procedures to be used for members to file complaints which includes a provision requiring copies of all complaints and responses to be forwarded to the department; and

(9) Copies of all the solicitation documents which shall contain all information necessary to enable a consumer lacking special knowledge of health maintenance organizations to make an informed, rational choice as to whether or not to enroll in the organization. Such information shall include a specific description of the comprehensive health care services to be available and a general description both of the times and locations at which the services will be rendered and the approximate number and type of full-time equivalent medical practitioners. Such information shall be presented in the solicitation document in a manner which is clear, concise, and intelligible to prospective members. Any changes in the health maintenance organization's solicitation document shall be filed with the Department of Insurance. At any time the department may, upon at least ninety days written notice to an organization, disapprove any solicitation documents, or amendment thereto, on any of the grounds stated in this Act. Every potential member whose subscription is solicited shall receive, at or before the time of such solicitation, the solicitation document approved of in this section. Any person obligated for any part of a prepayment in connection with an enrollment agreement, in addition to any right otherwise available to revoke an offer, may cancel such agreement within seventy-two hours after he has signed an agreement or offer to enroll. Cancellation occurs when written notice of cancellation is given to the health maintenance organization, its agents or representatives.

SECTION 5:  Issuance of Certificate of Authority.—The department shall issue a certificate of authority within 60 days of the filing of a properly completed application to any entity filing a completed application upon payment of the prescribed fees and upon the department's being satisfied that:

(1)  The entity proposes to establish and operate a bona fide health maintenance organization having the capability to provide comprehensive health care services in the geographic area proposed, as certified by the Department of Health as a condition precedent to the issuance of any certificate,

(2)  The health maintenance organization shall have a written guarantee insuring the payment of covered member claims which guarantee is provided by a guaranteeing organization which must be acceptable to and approved by the Department of Insurance. This contract shall protect members' contractual rights to services if the health maintenance organization fails to deliver such services for any reason. If the health maintenance organization can demonstrate that such a contractual guarantee is commercially unavailable on any reasonable basis, then the department may permit the substitution of either a deposit or bond or combination thereof in amounts acceptable to the department to satisfy this requirement in lieu of such guarantee,

(3)  The health maintenance organization has made acceptable arrangements to provide all comprehensive health care services offered,

(4)  The terms of the contracts such entity proposes to offer to members will, in fact, assure that the comprehensive health care services required by such members will be rendered under reasonable standards of quality of care, as certified by the Department of Health. The Department of Health shall have 45 days from the receipt of the health maintenance organization's application to advise the Department of Insurance whether or not the applicant satisfies this requirement,

(5)  The entity has provided, through contract or otherwise, for periodic review of its medical facilities and services,

(6)  The entity furnishes evidence of adequate insurance coverage or an adequate plan for self-insurance to respond to claims for injuries arising out of the furnishing of comprehensive health care services,

(7)  The ownership, control, or management of the entity is competent and trustworthy and possesses managerial experience that would make the proposed health maintenance organization operation beneficial to the members. The department shall not grant or continue authority to transact the business of a health maintenance organization in this state at any time during which it has good reason to believe that the ownership, control, or management of the organization is under the control of any person whose business operations are or have been marked by business practices, or conduct that is to the detriment of the public, stockholders, investors, or creditors; by the improper manipulation of assets or of accounts; or by bad faith,

(8)  The entity has a blanket fidelity bond in the amount of $100,000 issued by a licensed insurance carrier in this state, that will reimburse the entity in the event that anyone handling the funds of the entity either misappropriates or absconds with such funds,

(9)  This section shall not prohibit reasonable underwriting classifications for the purposes of establishing contract rates, nor shall it prohibit experience rating, and

(10)  A copy of the contract the entity proposes to offer to its members which meets the requirements of this Act shall be attached and reviewed by the department as a part of the application process.

SECTION 6:  Health Maintenance Organization Contracts

(1)  Any entity issued a certificate and otherwise in compliance with this part may enter into contracts in this state to provide an agreed upon set of comprehensive health care services to members in exchange for a prepaid sum. Every member shall receive a copy of the contract, but no contract shall be delivered to any member until it is first filed with and approved by the Department of Insurance.

(2)  Every health maintenance contract must clearly state all of the services to which a member is entitled under the contract and must include a clear and understandable

statement of any limitations on the services or kinds of services to be provided, including any copayment, deductible, or waiting period feature required by the contract or by any insurer or entity which is underwriting any of the services offered by the health maintenance organization. The contract shall also state where and in what manner the comprehensive health care services may be obtained and how member complaints shall be handled.

(3) Every member shall receive a clear and understandable description of the health maintenance organization's method for resolving member grievances.

(4) The total payments for a health maintenance contract shall be a part of the contract and shall be stated in individual contracts issued to members.

(5) Any amendments or changes to the contract shall be approved by the department before they are effective or provided to members.

(6) A health maintenance organization providing medical benefits or payments to a member who suffers injury, disease, or illness by virtue of the negligent act or omission of a third party is entitled to reimbursement from the member, on a fee-for-service basis, for the reasonable value of the benefits or payments provided. However, the health maintenance organization is not entitled to reimbursement for expenses rendered in excess of the member's monetary recovery from the third party.

(7) Persons or entities providing services or products to the health maintenance organization shall look only to it for payment and shall have no legal rights to hold members liable for such payments.

(8) All health maintenance contracts which provide coverage, benefits, or services for a member of the family of the member shall, as to such family member's coverage, benefits or services, also provide that the coverage, benefits, or services applicable for children shall be provided with respect to a newborn child of the member, or covered family member of the member, from the moment of birth. The coverage, benefits, or services for newborn children shall consist of coverage for injury or sickness, including the necessary care or treatment of medically diagnosed congenital defects, birth abnormalities, or prematurity, and transportation costs of the newborn to and from the nearest appropriate facility appropriately staffed and equipped to treat the newborn's condition, when such transportation is certified by the attending physician as medically necessary to protect the health and safety of the newborn child.

(9) No contract may be cancelled or otherwise terminated or not renewed without giving the member at least 30 days notice in writing of the cancellation, termination or nonrenewal of the contract. The written notice shall state the reason or reasons for the cancellation, termination or nonrenewal. All contracts shall contain a clause which requires that this notice be given.

(10) Any contract which is issued, delivered or renewed in this state and provides that coverage of an unmarried dependent child will terminate upon attainment of the limiting age for dependent children specified in the contract shall also provide in substance that attainment of such limiting age shall not operate to terminate the coverage of such child if the child is and continues to be both:

(a) incapable of self-sustaining employment by reason of mental retardation or physical handicap;

(b) primarily dependent upon the member for support and maintenance.

Proof of such incapacity and dependence shall be furnished to the health maintenance organization within thirty-one days of the child's attainment of the limiting age. Upon request, but not more frequently than annually after a two-year period following the child's attainment of the limiting age, the organization may require proof satisfactory to it of the continuance of such incapacity and dependency.

(11) Every group contract issued by a health maintenance organization shall provide an option for conversion to a direct payment basis to any member covered by the group contract who terminates employment or membership in the group.

(12) No health maintenance organization may cancel or fail to renew the coverage of a member because of his health status or his requirements for health care services.

SECTION 7:              Annual Report
                      (1) Every health maintenance organization shall, annually on or before April 1, or within
3 months of the end of the fiscal year for a health maintenance organization operating
under a valid certificate of authority, or within such extension of time therefore as the
department, for good cause, may grant, on forms prescribed by the department, file a
report with the department, verified by the oath of two persons who are principal
managing directors of the affairs of the organization, showing its condition on the last
day of the preceding calendar year. Such report shall include the information requested by the department on its forms.
    (2) Any health maintenance organization which neglects to file the annual report in the
form and within the time required by this section shall forfeit $100 for each day
during which the neglect continues; and, upon notice by the department to that effect,
its authority to do the business in this state shall cease while such default continues.

SECTION 8:              Investment of Funds.—The funds of any health maintenance organization shall be invested
only in securities permitted by the law of this state for the investment of assets of life or
property and casualty insurance companies.

SECTION 9:              Prohibited Practices
    (1) No health maintenance organization shall permit the use of advertising which is
untrue or misleading, solicitation which is untrue or misleading, or any form of evidence of coverage which is deceptive.
    (2) No entity certificated as a health maintenance organization, other than a licensed
insurer insofar as its name is concerned, shall use in its name, contracts, or literature
any of the words "insurance," "casualty," "surety," "mutual," or any words descriptive of the insurance, casualty, or surety business or descriptively similar to the name
or description of any insurance or surety corporation doing business in the state.
    (3) No person, entity, or health care plan not certificated under the provisions of this part
shall use in its name, logo, contracts, or literature the phrase "health maintenance
organization" or the initials "HMO"; imply, directly or indirectly, that it is a health
maintenance organization; or hold itself out to be a health maintenance organization.

SECTION 10:             Examinations.—The department shall examine the affairs, transactions, accounts, business
records and assets of any health maintenance organization as often as it deems it expedient
for the protection of the people of this state, but not less frequently than once every three
years. The Department of Health may conduct periodic examinations regarding the quality
of comprehensive health care services being provided by the organization. Every health
maintenance organization shall submit its books and records and take other appropriate
action as may be necessary to facilitate an examination. For the purpose of examinations, the
respective departments may administer oaths to and examine the officers and agents of a
health maintenance organization concerning its business and affairs. The expenses of examination of each health maintenance organization by the departments shall be paid by the
organization. In no event shall expenses of all examinations exceed a maximum of $15,000
per year. Any rehabilitation, liquidation, conservation, or dissolution of a health maintenance organization shall be conducted under the supervision of the department, which shall
have all power with respect thereto granted to it under the laws governing the rehabilitation, liquidation, conservation, or dissolution of life insurance companies.

SECTION 11:             Regulatory Powers
    (a) The department may revoke or suspend any certificate issued to a health maintenance
organization, or order compliance within 60 days, if it finds that any of the following
conditions exist:
        (1) The organization is not operating in compliance with this Act;
        (2) The organization is in substantial violation of its health maintenance contracts, as
certified by the Department of Health;

(3) The organization is unable to fulfill its obligations under outstanding health maintenance contracts entered into with its members, as certified by the Department of Health;

(4) The organization has advertised, merchandised, or attempted to merchandise its services in such a manner as to misrepresent its services or capacity for service or has engaged in deceptive, misleading, or unfair practices with respect to advertising and merchandising;

(5) The organization is insolvent; or

(6) The organization knowingly utilizes or has knowingly utilized a provider that is furnishing or has furnished health care services who does not have a license or other authority to practice or furnish health care services in this state.

(b) The Department of Health shall participate in any proceedings under this section involving matters related to the quality and nature of comprehensive health care services being delivered. The recommendations and findings of the Department of Health with respect to such matters shall be conclusive and binding upon the department.

(c) The department may, in lieu of revocation or suspension, levy an administrative penalty in an amount not less than $100 or more than $10,000.

SECTION 12:    Fees.—Every health maintenance organization shall pay to the department the following fees:

(1) For filing a copy of its application for a certificate of authority or amendment thereto, a nonrefundable fee in the amount of $150.

(2) For filing each annual report, $150.

Fees charged under this section shall be distributed as follows: one-third to the Department of Health and two-thirds to the Department of Insurance.

SECTION 13:    Rule Making.—The Department of Insurance, together with the Department of Health, on a joint basis, shall promulgate rules necessary to carry out the provisions of this Act. The approval of both departments is required as a condition to the implementation of any rule governing health maintenance organizations. The department shall collect and make available in a single volume all health maintenance organization rules promulgated by the departments.

SECTION 14:    Transfer of Ownership.—Each health maintenance organization which desires to transfer ownership of more than 10 percent of the stock or ownership interest in the health maintenance organization shall submit to the department an application for approval of the new stockholder or owner. The application shall contain the name and address of the applicant or applicants and such other information as required by the department. The application shall be filed with the department no later than 60 days prior to the effective date of the transfer of ownership.

SECTION 15:    Third Party Contracts.—Whenever a contract exists between a health maintenance organization and a provider of either services or products and the organization fails to meet its obligations to pay fees, the health maintenance organization shall be liable for such fee or fees rather than members; and the contract shall so state.

SECTION 16:    Medical Information, Confidentiality of.—Information pertaining to the health of any member or applicant obtained from any health maintenance organization shall be held in confidence except to the extent that it may be necessary to carry out the purposes of this Act; or upon the express consent of the member or applicant; or pursuant to statute or court order; or in the event of claim or litigation between such person and the health maintenance organization wherein such information is pertinent. A health maintenance organization shall be entitled to claim any statutory privileges against such disclosure which the provider who furnished such information to the health maintenance organization is entitled to claim.

SECTION 17: Annual Statement to Members.—Every health maintenance organization shall annually provide to its members written information including but not limited to a list of the times and locations at which covered health care services will be provided; a description of the structure, facilities, enrollment, and primary providers of the organization; and a statement advising members of their right to refer any complaints respecting quality or appropriateness of care to the organization which has been set up to monitor the quality or appropriateness of provider services. In addition, the organization shall make available upon the request of any member its most recent financial statement.

NOTES

1. States which do not have an existing Administrative Procedures Act or its equivalent should add a section to the Model Act describing administrative procedures to be followed by regulators.

2. Various sections of the foregoing proposed model law were selected from existing statutes of certain states including but not limited to Florida. Modifications, alterations, and reorganizations were made by the author as deemed appropriate.

# Hospital–health care plan affiliations: considerations for strategy design

Richard A. Reid,
Julie H. Fulcher,
and
Howard L. Smith

*Hospital-health care plan affiliations are designed to use idle hospital service capacity while minimizing the resulting financial risks.*

Health care managers have focused with increasing intensity on issues of cost containment and competition. The federal government's concern with the accelerated growth in health care costs under Medicare and Medicaid programs has produced a new approach to financing care. This prospective payment scheme has instituted fixed rates for specified groups of related patient diagnoses regardless of the actual service costs incurred. In the private sector, cost-effective alternatives to traditional hospital care have proliferated in recent years. Day surgery centers, urgent care facilities, home health care programs, and occupational rehabilitation services are representative of lower-cost options available to many patients. Moreover, employers and third party payers are becoming more concerned with overall health care costs. These financial sponsors are demanding more accountability from health care managers, fearing that government limits on payments will increase tendencies toward cost shifting. These environmental changes have yielded an unheralded management challenge to hospital administrators.

## HEALTH CARE PLANS

In order to thrive in this environment, hospitals need to monitor and control service costs while aggressively meeting competitive challenges in the marketplace. One particular managerial strategy that has gained recent popularity is affiliation with a health care plan. These plans are known under a variety of labels, including health maintenance organizations (HMOs), prepaid group practices (PGPs), individual practice associations (IPAs), preferred

**Richard A. Reid,** *Ph. D., is a Professor in the Anderson Schools of Management, University of New Mexico, Albuquerque. He has published over 30 articles in national and international journals. He is coauthor of* Competitive Hospitals: Management Strategies, *published by Aspen Publishers, Inc.*

**Julie H. Fulcher,** *M. B.A., is a financial analyst with Southwest Community Health Services in Albuquerque, New Mexico. She is currently installing a new cost accounting system in a multihospital organization.*

**Howard L. Smith,** *Ph.D., is a Professor in the Anderson Schools of Management, University of New Mexico, Albuquerque. He has published and consulted extensively in the health services administration field. He has recently completed a text,* Competitive Hospitals: Management Strategies, *currently being published by Aspen Publishers, Inc.*

*Health Care Manage Rev, 1986, 11(4), 53–61*
© 1986 Aspen Publishers, Inc.

provider organizations (PPOs), and foundations for medical care (FMCs).

In general, health care plans (HCPs) can be described as organizations that contract with enrolled patients to provide a relatively comprehensive set of health care services in return for a fixed periodic premium. A variety of relationships provides the structure for HCP organizations. For example, there are a growing number of national proprietary chains of HCPs. Other arrangements include joint ventures between community hospitals and their medical staffs. These plans often appear to be developed in response to perceived competitive threats from HCPs sponsored by for-profit chains. In addition, physician groups and third party payers have initiated several different types of HCPs.

Although HCPs have existed since the 1930s, a dramatic increase in the number of plans and enrollments in these plans has occurred during the last couple of years. Two major reasons appear to account for this growth. First, HCPs present an attractive alternative to both cost-conscious employers and their employees. The use of health care services is low compared to alternative fee-for-service programs. Moreover, there are relatively few forms for patients to complete in the care-consumption process. A second and more important reason for the recent increase in HCPs is the significant change in financial incentives available to hospitals. Reduced patient census and decreased inpatient revenues resulting from the establishment of Medicare diagnosis related groups (DRGs) have stimulated interhospital competition for patients. Since HCP members are urged (or even required) to use designated hospitals and physicians, participation in an HCP provides a stable and attractive source of responsible clients. Thus, efforts to contain costs and respond to increased levels of competition have provided the impetus for the development of HCPs into a major alternative health services provider organization.

Hospital managers seeking an effective strategy for prospering in a dynamic marketplace need to consider developing an association with one or more HCPs. The purpose of this article is to analyze and discuss the managerial implications resulting from hospital–HCP affiliations. First, the significance associated with each of five basic HCP structural characteristics will be considered from a hospital administration perspective. Next, some specific considerations for designing a productive relationship with HCPs will be presented. Finally, relevant environmental factors related to successful future hospital–HCP affiliations will be evaluated. Although this analysis considers the hospital and the HCP as separate bargaining entities, many of the same issues are relevant to partnership agreements that could evolve between these two organizations.

## CHARACTERISTICS OF HEALTH CARE PLANS

A wide variety of HCP organizational structures have evolved during the past decade. Although HCPs have adapted their organizations to local environments, five common interrelated attributes have been identified in the design of these plans.[1] The following characteristics appear to be present in all HCPs:

1. A contractual responsibility exists between the HCP and its clients that states that the plan will provide a specified and relatively comprehensive set of health services.
2. The HCP has a defined enrollment that can be accurately identified at any time.
3. Membership in an HCP is voluntary and is the result of a choice between alternatives that include the traditional fee-for-service system.
4. HCP members prepay a fixed periodic fee that does not reflect actual services used.
5. At least one of the three functional components of an HCP (hospital, physician, or administrative) must be responsible for the financial risk associated with the contractual obligation to the clients.

Table 1 summarizes the implications associated with hospital involvement with HCPs relative to each of the five defining characteristics. In the development of a mutually beneficial relationship with an HCP, it is necessary for hospital managers to be aware of the inherent incentives that administrators of HCPs need to capitalize on in order to remain viable competitors in a dynamic health care market.

### Contractual responsibilities

Several implications result from the contractual obligation to provide needed client services. The most significant of these is that the HCP physician has assumed the role of a purchasing agent for the client in the procurement of health services. Because HCPs employ physicians who decide between alternative approaches to patient care, these plans are not third

---

**TABLE 1**

---

FIVE DEFINING CHARACTERISTICS OF HEALTH CARE PLANS

---

| Characteristics | Implications |
|---|---|

---

| | |
|---|---|
| Contractual responsibilities | • HCP physician acts as informed purchasing agent for client, concerned with both the quality and costs of care |
| | • HCP administration addresses policy and financial matters with client |
| | • HCP hospital increases admission and collection efficiencies with potentially reduced bad debt expenses |
| Defined enrollment | • Provides HCP providers with access to prescribed client groups |
| | • Provides demographic characteristics of HCP members |
| Voluntary membership | • Comprehensive product must be offered at a competitive price |
| | • HCP hospital must deliver cost-efficient services and maintain favorable reputation to remain affiliated |
| | • HCP hospital may be actively involved in marketing efforts |
| Fixed periodic payment | • HCP requires minimal enrollments |
| | • HCP administration seeks provider affiliates that minimize health care costs |
| Assumption of risk | • Risks assumed by HCP components reflect respective bargaining strengths |
| | • HCP hospital's risk is manifested in its negotiated payment scheme |

---

party payers in a traditional sense. Instead of negotiating with providers or clients regarding service coverage, HCPs can (through designated physicians) directly affect the selection of cost-efficient diagnostic and treatment modalities. In the fee-for-service system, the typical physician focuses almost exclusively on providing high quality patient care regardless of cost. In contrast, HCP physicians remain concerned with providing quality care, but have a much greater incentive to consider the cost of care being prescribed. Thus, HCP physicians can be viewed as highly informed purchasing agents for the enrolled membership. They are aware of both the level of effectiveness and the cost associated with alternative approaches to caring for their patients. It is significant that many newer HCPs are the result of physician–hospital joint ventures. In light of increasing trends toward fixed payment practices of third party payers, hospitals view these HCP relationships as a positive approach to allying physician interests.[2]

Most cost savings realized by HCPs result from lower inpatient utilization rates.[3] However, upon being hospitalized, HCP members and other patients seem to have little difference in treatment efficiencies.[4] This situation is not unexpected as the major portion of hospital costs results from direct labor and overhead. While physicians may directly affect the rate at which hospital resources are employed for a single patient, they are unable to have direct influence over policies that govern the resource levels that the hospital as a whole provides.

Another implication of the HCP–client contractual relationship is the simplification of patient admission and bill collection procedures. Often the hospital is only directly responsible for collecting small user fees from HCP patients. Fees for hospital services come directly from the HCP administrative component. Moreover, bad debt expenses are nonexistent for patients enrolled in a financially viable HCP.

**Defined enrollment**

In a market that is characterized by uncertainty and increased levels of competition, direct access to a well-defined group of clients represents an extremely attractive opportunity for health care providers. In general, the larger the HCP's enrollment is, the more desirable an affiliation becomes for a provider. Any situation that will increase inpatient census and associated service unit revenues is highly prized by hospital managers. Moreover, demographic data collected on HCP clients provides affiliated hospitals with the ability to forecast service use and related revenues. This ability to reduce levels of future uncertainty through informed planning is highly desired by hospitals.

In future evaluations of HCP opportunities, hospital managers will need to consider both size and demographic characteristics of alternative HCP client groups in ranking their respective attractiveness. Hospitals should seek different types of financial arrangements with HCP administration that reflect the risk being undertaken. For example, hospitals could accept preestablished rates for a group of HCP clients whose rate of resource utilization is predicted to be relatively invariant. Conversely, it appears appropriate for hospitals to demand payment guarantees for HCP clients who are expected to have a high degree of variability in their inpatient lengths of stay and consumption of hospital resources, or who reflect other risky characteristics.

### Voluntary membership

Belonging to a particular HCP remains an option that must be exercised on a periodic basis by all plan members. Thus, HCP viability is ensured only if plan administrators continue to offer a competitive product. Maintaining existing members and attracting new enrollees require the delivery of a comprehensive set of health services at an acceptable price. HCPs must keep their premiums at an appropriate level relative to perceived costs of alternative care modalities including the traditional fee-for-service system. Since goals of comprehensive services and low premium costs conflict, HCP administrators are challenged to creatively resolve this issue. Motivating affiliated providers to incorporate innovative operational efficiencies is one approach to resolving the dilemma and remaining competitive.

In selecting hospitals as potential candidates for affiliation with their plans, HCP administrators appear to focus on the following factors: cost containment performance levels, types of services provided, geographic location relative to HCP membership, reputation with existing clients and HCP physicians, and managerial flexibility.[5] Although current thinking supports the premise that the dominant focus of HCP administrators centers on a hospital's cost-containment profile, the importance of the other factors should not be underestimated. To illustrate, one study[6] concluded that a hospital's reputation was of greater importance than its ability to control costs in influencing selection by an HCP. Notwithstanding the importance of community image and good will, however, it appears that most hospitals will compete for affiliation with HCPs on the basis of unit cost per delivered service. This situation reflects the fact that HCPs will be marketing to clients on the basis of services offered per premium dollar. Thus, hospitals that will be most attractive to HCPs are those having effective cost-control procedures with available capacities to provide needed services at readily accessible locations while remaining adaptable to changing client needs.

An affiliate hospital has a vested interest in the successful development and implementation of a marketing plan for its associate HCP. Increased membership provides opportunities to utilize available and unused service capacity. Moreover, in situations where affiliated hospitals are sharing some of the financial risk, larger client groups can yield surpluses for provider participants.

Closely affiliated HCP hospitals may desire involvement in the determination of which market segments should be aggressively sought. After assisting in the identification of suitable market targets, it is not unusual for HCP hospitals to be asked to provide special assistance in promoting the plan to potential client groups. For example, hospitals may have to provide chest X-rays for employee physicals at discounted rates or provide speakers for health and safety promotion programs to help market the HCP in local business organizations. The extent to which hospital management will be motivated to cooperate with its HCP will depend on the degree to which the hospital perceives a similarity between its interests and those of the HCP administration. This, in turn, will depend on the type of agreement that has been negotiated between the two as well as the working relationships that each has with affiliated HCP physicians.

### Fixed periodic payments

To maintain their HCP membership, plan enrollees are regularly required to submit a fixed, preestablished payment. The HCP then pays providers for all services rendered on behalf of their clients. Since expenses incurred are independent of payments received during any month, sufficient fiscal reserves must be available for an HCP to ensure economic survival. A minimum membership size is required to achieve financial solvency. Analysis indicates that enrolled HCP clients must number between 15,000 and 30,000, depending on premium payments amounts, local health care costs, and the health status of the enrolled membership.[7]

---

*Hospitals considering an affiliation with an HCP need to assess the long-term viability of the plan as well as the receptivity of local businesses to promoting an HCP among their employees.*

---

Hospitals considering an affiliation with an HCP need to assess the long-term viability of the plan as well as the receptivity of local businesses to promoting an HCP among their employees. Many HCPs have failed during the past decade because they did not have sufficient capital reserves to ensure survival during the initial phase of the service life cycle.[8] To help increase the probability of short-term solvency, both proprietary and not-for-profit HCPs are giving serious thought to mergers or other forms of consolidation. A merger provides an opportunity to allocate risk over a larger financial base. Moreover, linkages can yield access to needed managerial expertise, more efficient operational procedures, and greater experience in effectively establishing and maintaining provider relationships. Thus, hospital management needs to thoroughly investigate the structure and commitment of the HCP's administration and sponsorship before becoming affiliated.

Each HCP seeks economic survivability and since fixed revenues must cover generated expense, plan administrators desire provider relationships that will promote the containment of costs and the reduction of resource utilization rates. At the negotiating table, HCP administrators will be seeking prescribed service levels for the least cost. A research study has shown that service payments were based on billed charges by hospitals in over one-half of all hospital–HCP agreements.[9] In almost one in five cases, discounted payments were negotiated while all-inclusive per diem rates were used only in approximately one out of every eight agreements. With increased probability of additional prospective payment programs, it appears likely that many HCP administra-

tors will be seeking more fixed and risk-sharing agreements with hospitals in order to minimize costshifting possibilities. Moreover, HCPs seek committed affiliates who are willing to share the financial risks whenever possible.

**Assumption of risk**

There are three basic methods by which an affiliated hospital can receive payment from an HCP for services rendered to its clients. HCP hospitals that receive payment for billed charges assume minimal risk through their affiliation with a plan. A second type of payment scheme involves a risk-sharing agreement between the plan and an affiliated hospital. This approach implies that a prescribed portion of the HCP's annual surplus or loss is allocated between plan providers and administrators, usually in direct relation to their assumed risk or cost-control responsibilities. The third type of payment plan involves acceptance of a preestablished fixed payment for each HCP client admission. This approach is modeled after the DRG payment program that Medicare has instituted and entails the most risk to hospitals. It should be noted, however, that HMOs are generally adamant about not developing DRG-type reimbursement relationships with hospitals. DRG-type reimbursement may dilute or prevent the basic financial incentives that drive prepaid systems, as shown in the experience of HMOs in New Jersey.[10]

A wide variety of payment arrangements exist in practice. For example, negotiated payment schemes range from the acceptance of fixed payments for certain groups of diagnoses to arrangements where costs for complications due to provider error or nosocomial infections are absorbed by the provider. Another available risk-sharing agreement involves switching from the billed charges approach to a fixed payment scheme after a certain number of HCP clients have been admitted to an affiliated hospital. The allocation of risk through payment schemes reflects the relative bargaining strengths of the plan administrators and associated hospitals.

HCPs can influence hospital efforts in cost containment and operational efficiencies. In particular, if an affiliated hospital is receiving fixed payments for admitted HCP clients, it will be highly motivated to reduce operating expenses. On the other hand, HCP hospitals receiving payment based on billed charges will have little incentive to contain costs because they

---

**FIGURE 1**

---

KEY DETERMINANTS IN NEGOTIATING A HOSPITAL–HCP AFFILIATION AGREEMENT

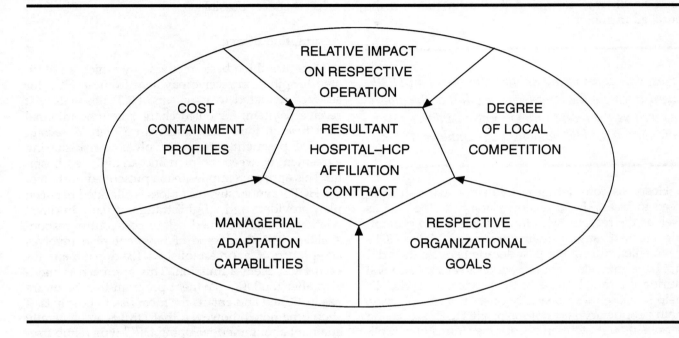

---

are legitimately reimbursed through a negotiated agreement with the plan.

## NEGOTIATING CONSIDERATIONS

The basic goal of a hospital considering affiliation with an HCP is to increase the utilization of idle service capacity while keeping its financial risk at a minimum. In turn, HCP administrators seek to provide appropriate levels of health care for enrolled clients at the lowest total cost. A mutually beneficial agreement between these two organizational entities requires that each have a high perceived probability of meeting its goals. Moreover, the final contract will reflect the relative bargaining strengths of the two negotiating entities. The key determinants associated with the design of a hospital–HCP contractual agreement are shown in Figure 1. Hospital managers need to be aware of their relative negotiating strengths in order to achieve realistic expectations in the design of a harmonious relationship with an HCP.

**Relative impact on operations**

If the enrolled membership of an HCP represents a significant proportion of a negotiating hospital's catchment area residents, then the HCP administration will be able to exercise meaningful leverage in bargaining with the hospital. One study found that HCPs were able to translate this leverage into payment discounts when the percentage of expected revenues generated by plan clients was as low as 3.1% of total hospital receipts.[11]

In regard to mature and larger HCPs, the general trend is toward greater aggressiveness in all aspects of negotiation with providers.[12,13] In some communities with well-established HCPs, affiliated hospitals are trying to reduce their dependence on revenues generated from HCP clients. It is reported, for example, that certain hospitals in the Minneapolis/St. Paul, Minnesota, area are actively seeking patient admissions from outside their immediate communities while other inpatient facilities are broadening their inpatient services to include psychiatric and chemically dependent patients.[14]

Hospitals appear to have their greatest bargaining strength with recently organized HCPs that have relatively few members.[15] This implies that hospitals should actively cultivate association possibilities with newly established HCPs: In designing payment arrangements with affiliated hospitals, first-year HCPs tend to negotiate fewer discounts of smaller magnitude and to rarely require risk sharing.[16] Another reason that hospitals should initiate affiliations with recently formed HCPs is to establish a good working relationship that will have the opportunity to endure during the plan's growth and maturation phases. Mutual dependency and trust grow stronger with time and as personal linkages solidify, it becomes more difficult for HCP administrators to realistically consider switching between major providers.[17]

## Competition

The amount of competition that the hospital and the HCP administration will encounter affects the resultant negotiated arrangement. An HCP would have a difficult time becoming established in a single hospital community if that hospital manager was not cooperative. On the other hand, even relatively small HCPs command respect in multihospital urban areas because of competition between the hospitals for affiliation.

In multi-HCP areas, plans that offer the most attractive payment schemes will be preferred by inpatient providers. In general, it is to the hospital's benefit to affiliate with as many HCPs as possible. The only situation that should be avoided is one in which the costs of treating the clients of an HCP are expected to exceed the preestablished payment levels. As fixed and per diem payment agreements become more common, careful consideration of these options will be necessary to ensure desirable contractual arrangements for associate hospitals. Managerial familiarity with actual service costs will become critical in determining the attractiveness of a particular payment approach.

## Changing HCP orientations

Early HCP founders were often visionaries with strong beliefs concerning the superiority of prepay-

ment and group practice concepts. Most of these pioneering organizations were nonprofit entities that focused on delivering high-quality care and a broad range of cost-efficient health services. In recent years, large and aggressive entrepreneurially oriented firms with a national scope have rapidly established chains of HCPs. Many of these newly constituted, well-financed organizations are using multiple strategies to meet their developmental goals. Market penetration is being achieved through the purchase of locally designed HCPs and through the financial sponsorship of joint ventures between local providers. These newer plans appear to have a more short-run operations focus as illustrated by the establishment of lowcost claims processing systems and a lower degree of tolerance for providers who do not adhere to stricter cost controls. This latter attitude raises some ethical conflicts for service providers who must decide between cost and efficacy in individual patient care situations.

Hospital managers need to examine closely the policies and constraints associated with membership in one of these national HCP chains. Managerial expertise, good financial planning, and sufficient capital reserves are the major attractions of the chains. However, it may be more effective for a hospital to negotiate with a locally oriented physician-initiated HCP. Alternatively, it may be advantageous to both a hospital and its medical staff to form their own joint venture HCP. The ability to respond to local needs and the opportunity to reinvest any surplus funds in community endeavors are benefits that can accrue to a locally owned and developed HCP.

## Additional issues

Initially, hospital–HCP agreements tend to be relatively informal and thus easily adapted to changing marketplace conditions.[18] As financial arrangements grow more complex to reflect evolving managerial concerns associated with improved operational performance, more formal agreements are likely to be required. Since a dynamic health care environment poses potential problems of adaptation to a contractually obligated HCP hospital, it is necessary that management design sufficient flexibility into the HCP agreements to enable appropriate responses to challenges in the marketplace.

Hospitals should consider whether to specify that HCP clients must use hospital ancillary services.

Some plans are providing their own ancillary services in competition with these traditional hospital surplus-generating centers.[19] Additional competition is also being provided by some plans that are contemplating the purchase of their own hospitals or hospital beds.[20]

Another important issue associated with designing a mutually beneficial contract involves the establishment of valid and reliable processes for establishing the true costs of patient care services. The implementation of Medicare's prospective payment plan has forced many hospitals to develop more elaborate cost accounting systems. HCP administrators are particularly interested in how costs are calculated by affiliated hospitals because of the requirements to distribute resulting surpluses under risk sharing arrangements. In joint ventures between physicians and hospitals, cost finding processes will be subjected to ever greater scrutiny. Major interest centers on processes for allocating overhead and bad debt expenses.

Since HCP administrators have sought to market a relatively comprehensive set of health services for a reasonable prepaid premium, population segments that are expected to be heavy service users, such as the elderly, have not been actively recruited. However, counterintuitive results were generated from an experiment that enrolled 5,500 newly eligible Medicare beneficiaries in an HMO.[21] After 12 months of high costs, hospital utilization and claim rates decreased for this group of elderly clients of a western Kaiser-Permanente Medical Care Program. Since that study, a high percentage of eligible HMOs have examined contractual associations with the Health Care Financing Administration for the Medicare population. It is likely that HCPs will continue these trends. Hospital managers realize that there are not any inherent financial disincentives to providing care for this age group. As long as a hospital is receiving adequate payments for inpatient services delivered, it should welcome all patients. Therefore, hospitals should encourage HCPs to design and market financially viable programs that focus on serving the elderly.

•   •   •

It is obvious that the health care industry has been undergoing dramatic changes during the last several years. The dynamics of these evolutionary processes are likely to continue. Both competitive and cost-con-

> *Hospitals should encourage HCPs to design and market financially viable programs that focus on serving the elderly.*

tainment factors in the health services market will persist in stimulating the development of a wide variety of HCPs. The structure of the HCPs necessitates that affiliated physicians act as agents for HCP clients in their consumption of health services. These physicians will exercise their concern for the cost as well as the quality of care primarily through cost-effective decisions on diagnostic and treatment modalities. Although a new structure has evolved to link the hospital and physician, the physician retains the role of gatekeeper for the hospital.

Since HCPs have a well-defined membership, an opportunity to develop meaningful service utilization forecasts exists for the interested hospital manager. Different HCP subscriber characteristics provide distinctive cost and negotiating implications for hospitals. HCPs have operational thresholds related to the number of enrollees required to financially break even. The majority of HCPs are likely to want to negotiate fixed payment or risk-sharing agreements because their limited capital reserves and preestablished revenue streams make them economically vulnerable to sustained durations of heavy service utilization by enrolled clients. Although fixed-payment arrangements provide affiliated hospitals with strong incentives to contain costs, they remain the most financially risky type of arrangement.

It appears to be virtually impossible to analyze one of the five defining characteristics of an HCP without having the discussion naturally unfold into the others. This is evidence of a strong interrelationship existing between these five major attributes. Although the hospital manager may elect to analyze the impact of each characteristic independently, it is important to realize that an effective HCP relationship requires that the implications be considered from an integrated and comprehensive perspective.

In seeking HCP affiliations, hospital managers want to increase the utilization of their idle service capacity while minimizing their susceptibility to adverse financial risk. Reaching an agreement requires an awareness of the HCP administrator's goals and an appreciation of the relative bargaining strengths of each negotiator. Key determinants in the design of a viable hospital–HCP relationship include the impact of an affiliation contract on current operations and the extent of the competition for an affiliated agreement. A hospital manager must be aware of orientation and policy differences between local and national and not-for-profit and proprietary HCPs to make an enlightened affiliation decision.

Unlikely as it seemed just a couple of years ago, HCPs are rapidly becoming a dominant force in the health services market. It is imperative that hospital managers develop effective strategies for interacting with these plans and aggressively seek the establishment of productive relationships with them. Failure to act in a timely manner may erode current market share and provide an unnecessary threat to long-term survivability.

## REFERENCES

1. Luft, H.S. *Health Maintenance Organizations: Dimensions of Performance.* New York: Wiley, 1981.
2. Richards, G. "How Do Joint Ventures Affect Relations with Physicians." *Hospitals* 58, no. 23 (1984): 68–71.
3. Gans, C.R., Cooper, B.S., and Hirschmann, C.G. "Contrast HMO and Fee-for-Service Performance." *Social Security Bulletin* 3, no. 5 (1975): 3–14.
4. Luft, H.S. "Health Maintenance Organizations and the Rationing of Medical Care." *Milbank Memorial Fund Quarterly* 60 (1982): 268–306.
5. Kralewski, J.E., et al. "HMO–Hospital Relationships: An Exploratory Study." *Health Care Management Review* 8, no. 2 (1983): 27–35.
6. Kralewski, J.E., Countryman, D.D., and Pitt, L. "Hospital and Health Maintenance Organization Financial Agreements for Inpatient Services: A Case Study of Minneapolis/St. Paul Area." *Health Care Financing Review* 4, no. 4 (1983): 79–84.
7. Reisler, M. "Business in Richmond Attacks Health Care." *Harvard Business Review* 63, no. 1 (1985): 145–55.
8. Ibid.
9. Morrisey, M.A. "The Nature of Hospital–HMO Affiliations." *Health Care Management Review* 9, no. 2 (1984): 51–60.
10. Coelen, C., and Sullivan, D. "An Analysis of the Effects of Prospective Reimbursement Programs on Hospital Expenditures." *Health Care Financing Review* 5 (1981): 1–40.
11. Morrisey, "The Nature of Hospital–HMO Affiliations," 58.
12. Kralewski, et al., "Hospital and Health Maintenance Organization Financial Agreements for Inpatient Services."
13. Kralewski, et al., "HMO–Hospital Relationships: An Exploratory Study."
14. Appel, G.L., and Aquilina, D. "Hospitals Won't Compete on Price until Spurred by Buyers' Shopping." *Modern Healthcare* 12, no. 11 (1982): 108, 110.
15. Morrisey, "The Nature of Hospital–HMO Affiliations."
16. Kralewski, et al., "HMO–Hospital Relationships: An Exploratory Study."
17. Morrisey, "The Nature of Hospital–HMO Affiliations."
18. Ibid.
19. Christianson, J.B. "The Competitive Approach to Health Care Reform: Implications for Hospital Management." *Health Care Management Review* 6, no. 4 (1981): 7–15.
20. Kralewski, et al., "HMO–Hospital Relationships: An Exploratory Study."
21. Greenlick, M.R., et al. "Kaiser-Permanente's Medicare Plus Project: A Successful Medicare Prospective Payment Demonstration." *Health Care Financing Review* 4, no. 3 (1983): 85–97.

Part III

# CONTRACTUAL NETWORKS: HOSPITALS and MANAGED CARE

# Strategies employed by HMOs to achieve hospital discounts: A case study of seven HMOs

John E. Kralewski,
Roger Feldman,
Bryan Dowd,
and
Janet Shapiro

*This article is a summary of seven health maintenance organization (HMO) case studies focusing on strategies used to obtain favorable prices for inpatient hospital services. All of the HMOs stressed that the effort should be based on the local environment and should accommodate the special circumstances of organization of physicians' practices and hospitals, as well as the structure of the HMO and its strategic plan for growth.*

*Health Care Management Rev,* 1991, 16(1), 9–16
© 1991 Aspen Publishers, Inc.

This article presents a summary of seven health maintenance organization (HMO) case studies that focused on the strategies used to obtain favorable prices for inpatient hospital services. Four communities were included in the study: a mature market area, an intermediate market, and two new market areas. Two HMOs were studied in each community. Because of lack of sufficient data, one HMO in the fourth community dropped out of the study. Where possible, a centralized model (staff or network) and a decentralized independent practice association (IPA) model were studied in each community. Table 1 shows the configuration of the HMOs and the markets studied. Data were collected through site visits and questionnaires distributed to physicians and administrators in each plan. The study was completed in 1987.

## HMO STRATEGIES

The HMOs included in this study presented an interesting mix of strategies designed to obtain accessible, high-quality hospital services at favorable prices.

### Findings from the case studies

One of the most pronounced findings in this regard is that virtually every HMO–new or old, centralized or decentralized, new or mature market–had a well-defined strategy to deal with hospitals. Conversely, in previous hospital studies we found that, except mature HMO markets, hospitals rarely had a strategy for dealing with HMOs.[1]

Clearly, HMOs think and act strategically. This does not mean that all activities are dictated by a long-range plan. The HMOs in this study cleverly maximize short-term opportunities for hospital services but they do not

**John E. Kralewski,** *Ph.D., Professor and Director of the Division of Health Services Research and Policy, holds the William Wallace Chair in Health Services Management at the University of Minnesota.*

**Roger Feldman,** *Ph.D., Director of the Health Care Financing Administration Research Center, is a Professor in the Division of Health Services Research and Policy and the Department of Economics, University of Minnesota.*

**Bryan Dowd,** *Ph.D., is an Associate Professor in the Division of Health Services Research and Policy at the University of Minnesota.*

**Janet Shapiro,** *B.A., is a Research Associate in the Division of Health Services Research and Policy at the University of Minnesota.*

**TABLE 1**

CASE STUDY SITES

| Study site | Health plan | HMO type | Enrollment | Hospitals in enrollment area | Percentage of hospitals used | HMO maturity | Number of HMOs in service area |
|---|---|---|---|---|---|---|---|
| I | A | Staff/network | 198,000 | 71 | 10 | Intermediate | 10 |
|   | B | IPA | 115,000 | 107 | 43 |   |   |
| II | C | Staff/network | 42,000 | 36 | 22 | New | 2 |
|   | D | IPA | 25,000 | 36 | 36 |   |   |
| III | E | Staff/network | 216,000 | 32 | 47 | Mature | 6 |
|   | F | Staff/network | 201,000 | 33 | 25 |   |   |
| IV | G | IPA | 60,000 | 53 | 34 | New | 5 |

let those opportunities dictate their long-term strategies. One HMO, for example, took advantage of the low-cost excess beds available from a second-choice hospital as an interim measure while attempting to gain better financial arrangements with their first-choice hospital.

A second and related dominant characteristic of the HMOs studied is that they are extremely innovative in their ability to leverage what are, at times, relatively low numbers of patients to obtain financial concessions for hospital services. One IPA model HMO, for example, convinced a hospital laboratory that they would obtain fee-for-service (FFS) as well as HMO patients from their generalist physicians as a spillover effect of the HMO designating the lab as a sole provider. Consequently, the HMO obtained very favorable prices for their inpatient and outpatient laboratory services even though they had very few enrollees.

A third important finding is that although HMOs deal quite differently with hospitals than with physicians and in fact often assign responsibility for these two provider groups to different departments, it is clear that the relationships between the HMOs and their physicians often dictate hospital arrangements. To obtain the services of some physicians considered important to an HMO's program because of location, technical competence, or reputation, the HMO may agree to a contract with the hospital where those physicians have privileges even though it gains few concessions. Similarly, the group practice HMOs in our case studies had

totally different bargaining positions with hospitals and employed different strategies than the IPA plans.

A fourth major finding from the case studies relates to the effects of the local environments on the strategies and structures of HMOs. Although there are important characteristics, such as a strong sense of entrepreneurship, across all of the HMOs included in this study, they each have unique structural patterns and strategies to deal with their providers. These patterns are largely determined by the characteristics of the local environment. Three environmental factors, in particular, appear to have a major influence on the structure and function of HMOs.

### Environmental influences

The first environmental factor is the structure of the health insurance market in the HMO's service area. A pattern of extensive coverage and few utilization controls provides a favorable economic environment for HMOs, but dictates a competitive strategy focused on price and access to service. The group model HMO in this environment was required to offer a plan with coverage comparable to or better than the FFS plans at a significantly lower price in order to offset consumer access concerns. If this cannot be achieved, group practice HMOs in these environments tend to adopt network models or wraparound service plans to improve their competitive position. Conversely, in a market characterized by lower levels of health insurance coverage, HMOs can often compete on the basis of their spectrum of services rather than price and access.

The other two market factors which are important are the structure of the physicians' practices and the hospitals in the community. A community characterized by concentrated providers presents a more difficult environment for negotiations but conversely provides organizational entities with which the HMO can negotiate. HMOs in the community with a large number of physicians in group practices and hospitals consolidated into multi-institutional systems pursued strategies that are less controlling and are more organizationally sophisticated. Negotiations were elevated to the organizational level rather than with individual physicians, and utilization controls were often delegated to the physicians and their organization. Contracts with hospitals in these communities were negotiated at the corporate systems level and included several hospitals. These contracts were often more complex than single hospital agreements with multiple levels of services, volume guarantees, and financial risk-sharing provisions. When the HMOs must negotiate with individual physicians or small three- or four-physician group practices and individual hospitals, the contracts are typically simpler and focused on prices, with controls on physician utilization of services usually centralized at the HMO level.

## HOSPITAL NEGOTIATIONS

The HMOs included in this study have developed unique and extremely effective techniques to obtain hospital discounts, often while maintaining access to a wide range of institutions. As noted previously, physician relationships are key to these strategies. The successful HMOs in this regard are those that are able to develop organizational mechanisms that create a willingness among physicians to use the desired hospitals. In some cases this is achieved by close organizational

*The HMOs included in this study have developed unique and extremely effective techniques to obtain hospital discounts, often while maintaining access to a wide range of institutions.*

ties between the HMO and the physicians wherein they act as one organization. This approach is indicative of HMOs that are established and run by a medical group practice or the staff/network model HMOs.

### Staff/network HMO negotiating strategy

The physicians in staff/network HMOs identify very closely with the plan and are more willing to change hospital allegiances to protect the HMO's economic base. In two of the HMOs studied these organizational relationships linked at least part of the physician's income to the financial performance of the HMO. Even in these cases, however, physician compliance is not automatic. As noted by Ottensmeyer, even physicians in group practice HMOs feel that their professional prerogatives are eroded as their HMOs begin to dictate hospital choice.[2]

The HMOs in this study that have been the most successful in obtaining physician commitment to selected hospitals are those that have been able to create an ownership culture among their physicians. In one case this was accomplished by employing the physicians on a salary basis with bonuses tied to the financial performance of the HMO.

In another case, a group practice model, an ownership culture was achieved by encouraging a strong collegial/professional cultural environment among the physicians and then appealing to them as rational decision makers to limit their choice of hospitals to one prestigious, high-quality institution. By guaranteeing a certain volume of patients, the HMO was then able to obtain a significant discount for hospital services.

Obtaining discounts from prestigious teaching hospitals is difficult in any setting and was particularly difficult in the setting described here, since the institution in question was operating at a high occupancy level. The HMO management was largely successful in this case because it approached the hospital in a friendly rather than an adversarial manner. Over time, it was able to convince the hospital management that HMOs were going to be a dominant factor in the community, that hospital utilization was going to decline (and it already was starting to decline), and that the hospital would be protecting its long-run market share by selling some beds at reduced cost to the HMO in return for a guaranteed volume of patients. The result was an extremely satisfactory agreement in which the HMO obtained substantial discounts for hospital services (up to 30 percent for some services), gained prestige from the hospital's stature in the community, and enhanced the professional image of its physicians. Consequently, the physicians were more than willing to cooperate.

This approach also had a down side, however, in that it inadvertently created professional–organizational conflict regarding practice styles. The physicians in this HMO began to assume a resource-intense practice style consistent with that of other physicians at this prestigious teaching hospital. In addition, some of the HMO's physicians were recruited from the hospital medical staff and they brought their practice culture to the HMO. The resultant conflict over resource use caused these physicians to be significantly more dissatisfied with the quality of care and the administrative structure of the HMO than were those in the other group model plans included in the study.[3]

### IPA model HMO negotiating strategy

The IPA model HMOs in the study dealt with the hospital issue in a totally different manner. While they have attempted to develop close relationships with their physicians and to use that commitment to deal with hospitals, they largely have been unsuccessful in doing so. Consequently, they have deteriorated to an adversarial relationship.

While the three plans studied differ somewhat in the methods used to gain organizational control over their physicians, all relied heavily on centralized decision making and rules and regulations. Contracts are developed with hospitals, and physicians are then coerced into hospitalizing their patients in those institutions. In most negotiations the physicians were consulted during this process but the decision clearly was made by the HMO and was based on a combination of quality perceptions, location, and price. In each case this did not result in the degree of concentration of patients achieved by staff/network HMOs. However, they achieve at least some concentration by shifting physicians who have appointments at competing hospitals to one institution and by selecting physicians who are willing to change hospital appointments or are new to the community and are still developing their hospital affiliations.

The IPA HMOs studied also tended to deal with other physician practice-style issues in a similar manner. Physicians, for example, must clear all nonemergency hospitalizations with the HMO before admission, and referrals are carefully controlled. To employ this controlling strategy successfully, an IPA must be in a position to withstand a physician boycott. Therefore,

this strategy can only be employed in communities where there is a surplus of physicians or where there are a relatively large number of physicians who, for one reason or another, are finding it difficult to develop or maintain a satisfactory patient workload. Clearly, this is a less-than-optimal strategy, since it creates a great deal of anxiety among physicians and undoubtedly has an effect on patient care. However, the strategy is effective under certain conditions and should not be discredited. In our interviews with IPA executives they expressed the belief that they cannot gain control over costs any other way, given the conditions in their communities. This is especially true for new HMOs that must control physicians' resource use quickly in order to survive. A controlling strategy therefore appears to be a less-than-optimal but effective approach under some environmental conditions.

It is important to note, however, that this approach may be effective only as a short-term strategy. These HMO executives acknowledge that in the long term their adversarial relationships must mature into relationships built on trust and respect. If this transition does not occur, the conflict inherent in this approach will ultimately adversely affect the efficiency and effectiveness of the organization and the HMO will fail.

This adversarial approach to physicians is mirrored in hospital negotiations. The IPAs identify strategic hospitals and negotiate very hard upfront for discounts, threatening to shift their patients to different institutions if the hospital does not cooperate. Unlike the staff/network HMOs, price is the main issue, and IPAs bargain especially hard for price discounts if there is an alternate hospital nearby. Threats to boycott a hospital are not uncommon. The IPAs in our study had target figures in mind during the negotiations and only agreed to a contract if a price was achieved that was close to that target.

The sophistication of the HMO management in this regard is impressive. They clearly do their homework and in some cases appear to know more about the hospital's cost picture than the hospital management. They, therefore, enter negotiations with an important advantage. In most cases the HMO management obtains the cost data from published hospital and rate review documents augmented by rather low-key industrial espionage.

The IPA HMOs also use hospitals' physicians to gain hospital cooperation. For example, one of the IPAs had sufficient enrollment to influence the market for hospital services in the community. Consequently, it unilaterally set a price for services and notified the hospital about its decision. If a hospital did not want to accept that price it had to notify its physicians that they could no longer hospitalize those HMO patients at that hospital. Most hospitals, although violently opposed to these techniques, reluctantly cooperate. Two factors are at work. First, if the IPA's admissions account for a large proportion of the hospital's patient load, it often cannot afford to lose them. On the other hand, if the IPA's patients represent only a small proportion of the hospital's workload, the financial implications of the discount are too small to risk offending the physicians who provide services for the HMO. This is especially true if those physicians are providing services for other patients as well and might move all of their patients to another hospital if a conflict developed.

## FINANCIAL RISK SHARING WITH PHYSICIANS

Recognizing that in the long run they must develop collaborative rather than adversarial relationships with their physicians, the IPAs are attempting to capture physician loyalty by experimenting with programs that involve them in the financial structure of the plan. The basic approach common to this strategy is some form of capitation rate for the physicians providing services for the plan. Since these HMOs use generalist physicians as gatekeepers for services, this strategy often focuses on those providers first and then progresses to other physicians. Hospitals are also included in this strategy, but the main focus is on physicians. As noted by one HMO chief executive officer, hospitals can hardly be expected to engage in any real financial risk sharing when HMO physicians determine their costs.

In order to implement this strategy the IPA HMOs must form their physicians into some type of organization which can be capitated. This, of course, presents a major problem in that by definition these physicians are independent practitioners with little or no organizational structure. Even when it is possible to organize small groups of physicians into viable risk-sharing units they often are too small and have too few HMO patients to form effective risk pools. This strategy, therefore, has two dimensions.

The first dimension focuses on the formation of relatively small organizations made up of logically related primary care physicians. This includes a wide variety of organizational approaches ranging from the generalist physicians practicing in a certain office building to loose federations of family practitioners or general internists. After identifying the physicians, an umbrella organization is formed to represent their interests. Al-

though these units resemble IPAs, in general they are smaller, are usually limited to one specialty, deal with physician services only, and are much more cohesive. Consequently, the physicians are able to develop reasonably close collegial relationships and they use that structure to control resource utilization.

The second dimension of this strategy focuses on the development of effective risk pools for (or with) these physicians' organizations. Again, there is a wide variety of approaches, depending on the nature of the physicians' organization, the size of its HMO population, and the physicians' willingness to assume more financial risk in return for greater potential profit. Common dimensions of these IPA-inspired physician organizations are as follows:

- The physicians are at risk for primary care.
- A stop-gap reinsurance program is offered to the physicians at low cost by the HMO.
- Specialty services are paid for by the HMO through separate contracts or risk-sharing agreements with specialists or specialty groups.
- Hospital services are paid for by the HMO in a manner similar to specialty services.
- The HMO establishes a pool of funds for specialty services and hospital services and the generalist physicians share in any savings in that fund at the end of the year.
- The HMO limits hospital and specialty physician use to those with contracts; the HMO negotiates these contracts for the generalist physician organization, and the generalists benefit from any discounts through increased end-of-the-year sharing in the hospital/specialty pools.

All of the HMOs included in this study viewed capitation of all providers as a potentially useful strategy. Capitation of physicians and selected hospitals was well underway in some plans. However, extending this concept to other providers such as pharmacies, laboratories, home health agencies, etc., presents major problems. Even the physician capitation program is undergoing considerable change in most HMOs and some are reconsidering the viability of hospital capitation given the lack of control hospitals have over resource utilization.

---

*All of the HMOs included in this study viewed capitation of all providers as a potentially useful strategy.*

The problem centers on the economic relationships between capitated physicians and their use of services not included in the capitation rate. Although hospitals and pharmacists often can improve the efficiency of their organizations and thus provide services at lower costs and practice effectively within the constraints of capitation payment, they are still largely at the mercy of the HMO physicians in terms of overall utilization and costs. Linking physician incentives to their use of resources in these other capitated organizations is therefore a high-level priority.

## HOSPITAL DISCOUNTS

The discounts obtained for hospital services varied considerably depending on the type of service and type of HMO. Group practice HMOs with a highly integrated medical staff were able to obtain discounts up to 29 percent for obstetrics services and 25.7 percent for medical/surgical inpatient services. Conversely, the two IPAs with widely dispersed physicians were only able to obtain discounts in the 5 percent to 10 percent range. Both types of HMOs obtained better discounts for specialized services such as mental health or chemical dependency than they did for general hospital services. Group practice HMOs tended to favor contracts based on per diem rates while the IPAs favor discounts off billed charges. (For a more detailed discussion of the type and amount of discounts see Kralewski, et al.[1])

While all of the HMOs included in this study have obtained discounts for services from at least their main hospitals, it is clear that those who are the most effective in this regard have developed long-range strategies that recognize both hospital and HMO needs and attempt to build a trust relationship that will result in high-quality, accessible hospital services at a favorable price. Short-run opportunities to obtain favorable financial arrangements for inpatient services clearly exist and while the well-run HMOs take advantage of these opportunities, they do not do so at the expense of long-run strategies. The one HMO that pursued a short-run opportunistic strategy found that they alienated their physicians, hospitals, and enrollees for the sake of some rather minimal short-term gains.

On the other hand, it is clear that HMOs do not obtain favorable price concessions from hospitals unless they aggressively seek to do so by maximizing every opportunity. Thus while long-range strategies are fundamental, the successful HMOs appear to be able to stay flexible enough to maximize short-run opportunities. The following eight factors appear to be key to successful negotiations with hospitals by the HMOs included in these case studies:

1. Hospitals are first of all recognized as fundamental organizational units in the health care system. The importance of high-quality, accessible physician services (both inpatient and outpatient) is stressed as essential to the success of the HMO, and the hospital is considered a unit which can be dealt with *organizationally*. This is an important distinction in that it recognizes that, unlike most other health care providers, hospitals are driven by many of the same factors as HMOs and can respond organizationally to external opportunities provided by the HMOs.

2. The strategies used to deal with hospitals are driven by the environment and the structure of the HMO. The organization of the HMO's physicians and the organizational and economic relationships between the HMO and its physicians often dictate hospital strategies.

3. Hospitals are respected as influential actors in the field and the community but are considered businesses which must be dealt with on a business-like basis. It is, therefore, not considered unprofessional or antisocial to challenge every element of a hospital's pricing structure and to refuse to allow the costs of extraneous services to be included in prices simply because the hospital and the community has found it expedient to do so.

*The HMO knows as much (and often more) about the target hospital's cost structure as the hospital's management.*

4. The HMO knows as much (and often more) about the target hospital's cost structure as the hospital's management. The strategy is simply to know where concessions can be gained and to prevent deceptive pricing. For example, it is becoming more and more difficult to determine the price on which discounts are based. Hospitals may offer a 20 percent discount but raise prices substantially to offset the discount, especially if few are actually paying billed charges. Well-run HMOs consider accurate information regarding hospital costs in the community and the costs of providing services in the target hospitals as essential to a sound long-range strategy for hospital services. Often much of this information is obtained from public documents such as the Medicare costs reports. Some, however, is also obtained from the hospitals as a

condition for being included in the HMO's long-run strategy.

5. The HMO recognizes that hospitals are economic units that must maintain favorable financial performance in order to remain viable. The HMO also recognizes that strategically located hospitals must remain viable or they (the HMO) will need to establish their own inpatient services. Most successful midsized HMOs do not want to own and operate their own hospitals, preferring to pursue a long-run strategy that will obtain the best prices possible for those services while maintaining the economic viability of the hospital as a separate unit. As part of this strategy HMOs often help their hospitals reduce costs by supporting efforts to improve efficiency. Unlike the FFS medical staff, HMOs often provide the support of their physicians when one of the hospitals in their strategic plan faces tough cost/benefit issues such as staffing, adding new equipment, etc.

6. The HMO identifies strategically positioned hospitals and attempts to develop a long-term relationship with them. Price is generally not a major consideration in the first stages of this strategy. The quality of the hospital as measured by reputation in the community, the quality of the medical staff, and the assessment of HMO physicians is paramount. Location and range of services is a close second-level consideration. This goes hand in hand with the HMO's strategic plan for growth. Once a geographic area is identified as a market area, the hospitals in or close to that area are profiled and considered as candidates for a long-term relationship. Depending on the geographic distribution of the potential enrollees and the location and the range of services offered by the hospitals, one or two institutions are selected as target hospitals. Other hospitals may be used during the initial phases of the implementation of this strategy but all effort is devoted to strengthening the relationship with the target hospitals and obtaining favorable prices from those institutions. If after a reasonable time it proves impossible to obtain favorable prices, a target hospital will be replaced. However, most HMOs that have developed successful long-range strategies for inpatient services appear to be reluctant to change a target hospital unless they absolutely must do so.

7. While the successful HMOs appear to be tough negotiators for hospital prices they attempt to give the hospital something in return whenever possible. Patient volume is one of the most important bargaining chips, especially when hospital demand in the community is declining. Indeed some HMOs have been able to help a hospital improve its net revenue while obtaining substantial discounts by increasing hospital admissions and achieving favorable economies of scale.

8. Successful HMOs attempt to mesh their strategic plans for growth with their target hospital's strategic plans so that they can accommodate their expanded needs for inpatient services while maintaining favorable prices. These HMOs recognize that there is a delicate balance of power between the HMO and the hospital and that changes in the availability of hospital beds or HMO patients can shift the power balance. They also recognize that it is very disruptive to change hospitals or even phase down the use of one hospital in favor of another. They are, therefore, very realistic about their power at any given time, and the successful HMOs never overstep their power bounds. Consequently, a close organizational working relationship between the HMO and hospital is a fundamental element in the HMO's long-range strategy for hospital inpatient services.

The above is by no means an exhaustive list of factors which appear to be important in HMO negotiations for hospital services. However, they represent the main elements around which the HMOs in this study organized the nuances dictated by the local environment into successful strategies. All of the HMOs stressed that while there are key elements common to a long-run strategy for hospital services, it is fundamental that the effort be based on local conditions and accommodate the special circumstances described by the organization of physicians' practices and hospitals, as well as the structure of the HMO and its strategic plan for growth.

• • •

These case studies focus on seven HMOs in four communities. Therefore, while important insights have been gained about the strategies used by these HMOs to obtain favorable hospital prices, the limited number of observations must be kept in mind. The local environment clearly plays a major role in shaping these strategies and consequently many variations on the themes identified in this study can be expected to exist.

Given these conditions, the population ecology conceptual perspective of organizations articulated by Hannan and Freeman may provide a particularly fruitful framework for the analysis of the strategies and structures of HMOs.[4] This perspective emphasizes the environment as a major factor determining the common form of populations of related organizations through an evolutionary process. It is, therefore, argued that the strategies, structures, and performance of individual organizations can be best understood by focusing on the characteristics of the population to which the organization belongs and the process by which it evolved to that stage.

All but one of the HMOs included in this study recently restructured their organizations to meet changing conditions in their environments. In a previous study we found that similar changes in a highly competitive community blurred the traditional structural differences between HMOs.[5] In that community the entire "population" of HMOs shifted their strategies to a more balanced emphasis on access as well as price even though they were operating in a highly price-competitive setting. As a consequence, their organizational structures became very similar. The relative influence of various environmental conditions, the effectiveness of alternate strategies in different settings, and the relationships of both to the structure and life cycle of the HMO organization are important areas for future research.

## REFERENCES

1. Kralewski, J.E., et al. "An Analysis of Investor-Owned and Not-for-Profit Multi-Institutional Hospital Systems." Division of Health Services Research and Policy and Division of Health Services Administration, University of Minnesota, 1987.
2. Ottensmeyer, D.J., and Smith, H.L. "Patterns of Medical Practice in an Era of Change." Frontiers of Health Services Management 3 no. 1 (1986): 3–28.
3. Kralewski, J.E., Feldman, R., and Dowd, B. "Organizational and Economic Relations between Hospitals and HMOs: The Creation of Competitive Markets for Hospital Services." Final report to the U.S. Department of Health and Human Services, January 20, 1988.
4. Hannan, M., and Freeman, J. "The Population Ecology of Organizations." American Journal of Sociology 82 (1977): 929–64.
5. Feldman, R., Kralewski, J., and Dowd, B. "Health Maintenance Organizations: The Beginning of the End?" Health Services Research 24 (1989): 191–211.

# The growth and effects of hospital selective contracting

Glenn A. Melnick,
Jack Zwanziger,
and
Alicia Verity-Guerra

*Since the passage of California's ground-breaking PPO legislation in 1982, enrollment in managed-care systems has risen dramatically in California and throughout the United States. This article charts the growth of selective contracting and presents data on the effects of these programs on hospital costs.*

Selective contracting with hospitals by third party payers has grown rapidly in recent years. This article charts the growth of selective contracting throughout the country and in California, which leads the nation in the adoption of selective contracting. Hospital cost data comparing California with the rest of the United States show that hospitals are being significantly affected by selective contracting programs. The rapid and widespread growth of hospital selective contracting requires that hospital managers develop strategies and management systems in order to operate effectively in the new managed-care environment.

## BACKGROUND

The introduction of selective contracting to stimulate competition among health care providers on the basis of price is an important policy initiative in the widely heralded new competitive environment of the health care market. Selective contracting is a policy option that enables third party payers to negotiate prices with providers for health service delivery. An important development is that many states have enacted selective contracting legislation that reduces the threat of antitrust prosecution for third party payers who exclude providers from their participating provider list. The ability to exclude "high-cost" providers, coupled with the introduction of price competition among providers, reduces a third party payer's expenditures. Selective contracting has been used both by Medicaid programs and by private third party payers such as Blue Cross and commercial insurance companies.

**Glenn A. Melnick,** *Ph.D., is an assistant professor at the School of Public Health, University of California at Los Angeles and a Resident Consultant with the RAND Corporation in Santa Monica, California. Dr. Melnick has worked and written extensively in the area of health care competition and the hospital reimbursement systems.*

**Jack Zwanziger,** *Ph.D., is a Resident Consultant with the RAND Corporation. Dr. Zwanziger has worked extensively in the area of health care competition and in the application of DRGs to the CHAMPUS system.*

**Alicia Verity-Guerra,** *M.S.P.H., is currently manager of marketing services for MetLife Healthcare Network of Denver, Colorado. She has worked in the area of health care competition and hospital selective contracting over the past several years.*

This study was supported in part by a grant from the Robert Wood Johnson Foundation and in part by a grant from the Office of the Assistant Secretary for Planning and Evaluation, U.S. Department of Health and Human Services.

*Health Care Manage Rev,* 1989, 14(3), 57–64

A central objective of selective contracting is to foster price competition among health care providers by encouraging the formation of preferred provider organizations (PPOs). PPOs, sometimes referred to as preferred provider arrangements (PPAs), are contractual arrangements between a panel of health care providers (physicians and hospitals) and a purchaser of health care services (insurers and self-insured employers). PPOs provide subscribers with financial incentives (usually the sharing of decreased costs) to encourage the use of specific providers who, in turn, offer discounts from charges or accept fixed payment rates, such as a per diem or per discharge, negotiated in advance. Additionally, many PPOs require providers to agree to utilization review procedures such as preadmission certification. Hospitals and physicians located in areas with many competitors or substantial excess capacity are likely to agree to accept lower fees and increased utilization oversight in return for the promise of a continued or increased flow of patients. Providers who do not sign contracts with PPOs in their areas run the risk of being "locked out" of a substantial portion of the market.

In addition to PPOs, selective contracting is carried out by some health maintenance organizations (HMOs). An HMO is an organized plan that guarantees the delivery of comprehensive health care services to a voluntarily enrolled population at a prepaid fixed premium. HMOs exert a large degree of control over costs by channeling subscribers into a closed provider panel. HMOs that do not own hospitals must contract with hospitals to provide services to their enrollees. Although HMOs can reimburse hospitals by a variety of mechanisms, most arrangements impose a substantial amount of financial risk on hospitals and/or physicians.

---

*"PPOs seem to have provided the health industry with a mechanism to facilitate competition among both providers and insurers."*

---

HMOs and PPOs have grown due to their promise to control costs. HMOs control costs through the use of primary physician "gatekeepers" to keep tight control over hospital admissions, through utilization review procedures, and through financial incentives for decreased utilization of services. PPOs control costs by contracting with low-cost providers, by establishing reimbursement methods that realize savings (e.g., discounts or fixed payments that provide incentives for reduced utilization), and by enforcing such utilization review procedures as mandatory second opinions, preadmission certification, concurrent review, and retrospective review.

## THE GROWTH OF PPOs IN THE UNITED STATES

In the spring of 1985, Gabel and Ermann published an article that presented a very bleak future for PPOs.[1] They noted that only 1.3 million Americans (less than 0.5% of the U.S. population) were eligible to use PPO plans and that these plans placed only limited emphasis on utilization review. Synthesizing over 200 articles on the subject and interviews with 20 plan administrators, the authors concluded that PPOs would not be a meaningful competitive force in the health care marketplace and that provider-sponsored PPOs were "little more than a marketing tool."

A few months later, Rice et al. reported a dramatically different picture of the PPO and its future in the health care marketplace.[2] They conducted 134 telephone interviews of operating PPOs over a five-month period. Eligibility had increased to 5.4 million. The majority of plans reimbursed hospitals on the basis of fixed per diem rates or discounted charges. Importantly, employers were inducing employees to use preferred providers through positive incentives in the form of lower co-insurance, lower deductibles, and services such as well baby care. The report concluded that "PPOs seem to have provided the health industry with a mechanism to facilitate competition among both providers and insurers."[3]

Gabel et al. evaluated a 1986 study by the Health Insurance Association of America (HIAA) that examined the characteristics and geographic distribution of PPOs. The HIAA used the results of a screening questionnaire to divide its 198 insurer/members into four groups: (1) operating PPOs, (2) planning PPOs, (3) not operating or planning PPOs, and (4) nonrespondents. All of the insurers then operating a PPO were interviewed, and one-half of the insurers within each of the remaining groups were chosen for interviews, resulting in a sample of 121 insurers.[4] From this information, Gabel et al. concluded that most PPOs target major metropolitan areas rather than rural areas and small towns. The typical insurer-sponsored PPO was active

## TABLE 1

PPO PLANS AND SUBSCRIBERS IN THE UNITED STATES, 1983–1988

| Category | 1983 | 1984 | 1985 | 1986 | 1987* | 1988 |
|---|---|---|---|---|---|---|
| Number of plans | 73 | 143 | 325 | 369 | 674 | 575 |
| Number of subscribers (millions) | N/A | 1.3 | 5.5 | 17 | 32 | 35 |
| % of non-Medicare population | N/A | .62 | 2.63 | 8.10 | 15.14 | 16.56 |

*These numbers may be inflated due to double counting.

Sources: American Association of PPOs; American Medical Care Review Association; Health Care Financing Administration, Department of Statistics; U.S. Department of Commerce, Bureau of the Census.

in five states, with 43% of the survey respondents indicating California as their major market and 73% citing location as an important influence on the selection of providers. Employees of self-insured employers constituted 46% of those eligible for the surveyed PPO plans.[5]

Table 1 summarizes the dramatic growth of PPOs nationwide. The number of plans increased from 73 in 1983 to a high of 674 in 1987, then declined in 1988 to 575. The decline in the number of PPOs may be the result of consolidation as PPOs take advantage of economies of scale. Additionally, duplicate counting occurred in the past but was reduced if not eliminated in the more recent figures. The number of people having a PPO option rapidly increased from fewer than a million in 1983 to over 35 million in 1988. This represents a jump from less than 1% of the non-Medicare population in 1984 to over 16.5%. Industry officials believe that while the number of plans may stabilize, the number of subscribers will continue to increase.

According to Gabel et al., the HIAA study shows that one of every three health insurance companies offers a variation of a PPO arrangement. In 1986 the typical insurer-sponsored PPO served 62,400 eligibles and signed contracts with 75 employers, 80 hospitals, and 6,500 physicians. (The 62,400 eligibles represent those individuals who may elect to act on their privilege to use a preferred provider within the PPO network.[6])

## THE GROWTH OF HMOs IN THE UNITED STATES

HMOs agree to provide a defined set of services for a given period of time at a rate that is fixed in advance. They are at risk if the expenses of providing services exceed payments. HMOs experienced a period of steady growth in the late 1970s and early 1980s. However, competition and selective contracting have inspired new interest in this alternative delivery system. Table 2 illustrates the growth of HMO plans and enrollment in the United States. In 1987 there were an estimated 662 HMO plans nationally that covered 28.6 million enrollees, representing over 11% of the U.S. population.[7]

InterStudy reported in December of 1986 the existence of 22 open-ended HMOs with a total enrollment of 343,163.[8] Open-ended HMOs allow enrollees to use a physician outside of the closed panel, in which case the plan switches to an indemnity plan that holds the enrollee responsible for copayments and deductibles. In addition, insurance companies are beginning to market insurance products that imitate HMOs. Prudential has such a product, with 360,000 enrollees. The emergence of these hybrids is blurring the distinction between traditional HMOs and indemnity plans.

Another new development among HMOs is the single benefit organization (SBO). SBOs provide specialized service benefits, such as dental care, vision care, and physical therapy, on a capitated basis using a closed provider panel. Nationally there are more than 45 SBOs, of which 40 are in California.[9]

## TABLE 2

HMO PLANS AND ENROLLEES IN THE UNITED STATES FOR SELECTED YEARS, 1977–1987

| Category | 1977 | 1980 | 1984 | 1985 | 1986 | 1987 |
|---|---|---|---|---|---|---|
| Number of plans | 165 | 236 | 306 | 480 | 626 | 662 |
| Number of enrollees (millions) | 6.3 | 9.1 | 15.1 | 21.0 | 25.8 | 28.6 |
| % of total population | 2.86 | 4.0 | 6.37 | 8.79 | 10.70 | 11.74 |

Sources: InterStudy; Health Care Financing Administration, Department of Statistics; U.S. Department of Commerce, Bureau of the Census.

In summary, PPOs and HMOs have grown dramatically in the United States in recent years. In 1984, HMOs and PPOs together covered less than 7% of the total U.S. population. By 1987 these managed care plans covered almost 25% of the population. As PPOs and HMOs that contract for hospital services expand their market share, hospitals located in markets with heavy PPO and HMO penetration are likely to experience increasing competitive pressure as a result of these organizations. Hospitals must compete for these contracts, with price in addition to quality being an important component, in order to provide inpatient services to HMO enrollees.

## METHODS OF REIMBURSEMENT UNDER SELECTIVE CONTRACTING

Selective contracting uses many reimbursement schemes, including payment of full and discounted charges, fixed rates per diagnosis related group (DRG) and capitation fees with a risk pool. The predominant payment methods used are discounts from charges and fixed per diems. Hospitals report granting up to a 40% discount from charges, but average discounts range between 10% and 20%.[10] According to Rahn and Traska, a recent survey by the American Hospital Association (AHA) found that per diems, multiple per diems, capitated fees, and fixed rates per DRG are more frequent in facilities with more than 100 beds than in smaller facilities.[11]

## TABLE 3

### PPO PLANS, SUBSCRIBERS, AND CONTRACTS, CALIFORNIA, 1983–1987

| Category | 1983 | 1984 | 1985 | 1986 | 1987 |
|---|---|---|---|---|---|
| Number of plans | 25 | 37 | 60 | 66 | 70 |
| Number of subscribers (millions)* | .23 | .43 | 4.0 | 8.7 | 12 |
| % of non-Medicare population | 1.03 | 1.89 | 17.15 | 36.65 | 49.57 |
| Number of hospital contracts | 490 | 876 | 2,000 | 3,300 | 4,891 |

* Estimates of PPO subscribers are based on the number of people with PPOs as a health insurance option. The actual number of people selecting this option is likely to be lower.

Sources: *Insights* 11, no. 15 (1987) (California Association of Hospitals and Health Systems); Health Care Financing Administration, Department of Statistics; U.S. Department of Commerce, Bureau of Census.

According to the AHA survey, facilities in the East South Central region are most likely to receive full charges. The Middle Atlantic, Mountain, and Pacific regions have higher frequencies of per diem rates for HMO agreements. This is probably a reflection of the higher HMO penetration and/or greater market competition in these regions.

The market power of the HMO or PPO is very important in determining the preferred reimbursement method. "Although the prevalence of certain payment mechanisms could be linked to HMO penetration or market sophistication, it also can be influenced by an HMO's ability (or inability) to deliver patient volume to a hospital in exchange for competitive pricing of hospital services."[12] In communities where the population base is large and where HMOs or PPOs have significant market penetration, reimbursement of a hospital's full charges is rare.

## THE GROWTH AND CONSEQUENCES OF SELECTIVE CONTRACTING IN CALIFORNIA

California leads the nation in the use of hospital selective contracting by PPOs and HMOs. While the full effects of selective contracting in California have not yet been felt, some initial effects can be observed. This section details the growth of PPOs and HMOs in California and some of the early effects of selective contracting on hospitals in California. It presents recent data comparing trends in hospital costs in California with those in the rest of the United States to show that the enactment of selective contracting legislation has had significant effects on California hospitals.

California first introduced selective contracting as a response to a Medicaid-driven budget crisis. The legislation permitted both the state Medicaid program and private third party payers to contract with selected hospital and physician providers. This law was to encourage the formation of PPOs as a means of fostering price competition among health care providers.

The growth of PPO enrollment in California is summarized in Table 3. Precise PPO enrollment data are not available. Potential enrollment (i.e., employees who have a PPO as a benefit option) in PPOs had grown from 230,000 in 1983 to over 12 million by July 1987.[13] In 1983, PPO insurance plans were available to only 1% of California's non-Medicare population; by 1987 they were available to nearly 50% of the state's non-Medicare population. Another indicator of the growth of contracting PPOs is the number of different contracts that each hospital has with different PPOs. The number

## TABLE 4

### HMO PLANS AND ENROLLEES IN CALIFORNIA, 1977–1987

| Category | 1977 | 1980 | 1984 | 1985 | 1986 | 1987 |
|---|---|---|---|---|---|---|
| Number of plans | 30 | 32 | 30 | 40 | 49 | 49 |
| Number of enrollees (millions) | 3.1 | 4.0 | 5.3 | 6.2 | 6.7 | 7.1 |
| % of total population | N/A | 16.90 | 20.69 | 23.80 | 25.30 | 26.38 |
| % of non-Kaiser plans | N/A | 19.0 | N/A | 39.0 | N/A | 45.0 |

Sources: *Insights* 11, no. 12 (1987) (California Association of Hospital and Health Systems); Health Care Financing Administration, Department of Statistics; U.S. Department of Commerce, Bureau of the Census.

of separate hospital PPO contracts has grown dramatically, from 490 in 1983 to almost 5,000 by mid-1987, or an average of more than 10 different contracts per hospital in California.

California has historically been an area of strength for HMOs, as Table 4 shows. From 1977 until the end of 1987, HMOs increased their enrollment in California from 3.1 million to 7.1 million members, representing 26.4% of the population of California.[14] California has in excess of 5 million more enrollees than any other state in the nation. (The closest state is New York, with a total of 2 million enrollees.) Much of the recent growth in enrollment in California has occurred in HMOs that do not own or operate hospitals (i.e., non-Kaiser HMOs) and so must contract with hospitals to serve their members. The percentage of the HMO market served by non-Kaiser HMOs grew from 19% in 1980 to 45% by 1987, an increase of over 130%.

Hospitals are now operating in an environment in which a substantial portion of their business is enrolled in managed-care insurance programs. Over 50% of California's population is covered by a managed-care plan, and the proportion is even higher if one looks only at the insured population (21.6% of California's population was uninsured in 1986). Hospitals that do not meet the market price face an increasing risk of not being awarded contracts to serve a growing share of their markets. If they cannot successfully compete for contracts, they will eventually be "locked out" of the market.

## CONSEQUENCES OF SELECTIVE CONTRACTING IN CALIFORNIA

The 1983 introduction of the prospective payment system (PPS) for hospitals under Medicare changed hospitals' incentives across the nation. Suddenly hospitals had an incentive to reduce their costs. The event that makes California unique occurred prior to the implementation of Medicare's PPS: enactment of the selective contracting law.

Selective contracting has spread more rapidly in California than in the rest of the nation. This section presents data that show some of the effects of increased competitive pressures. All expense data are adjusted for inflation (base year = 1974), using the Health Care Financing Administration's hospital market-basket input price index. Consequently, all changes in expense variables are in real terms.

Hospital costs are the largest component of medical costs and have been increasing at the fastest rate. The reasons most often cited for this are the limited direct payment by patients for hospital care, the lack of insurance coverage for less costly substitutes, and the growth of high-cost technology. As third party payers focus their efforts on reducing medical care costs, hospital costs are the first component that must be controlled. Unless their cost-containment strategies reduce the rate of increase in hospital expenses, third party payers will be unlikely to achieve much of a reduction in the overall rate of increase in health care costs.

---

*Hospitals that do not meet the market price face an increasing risk of not being awarded contracts to serve a growing share of their markets.*

---

As admissions decline, the less costly admissions are being treated on an outpatient basis. For this reason alone, we would expect expense per admission to increase. However, as Figure 1 shows, trends in expense per admission reveal that other factors constrain the growth in expenses. In the period 1975–1982, California hospitals generally had larger percentage increases in their expense per admission than did hospitals in the rest of the nation. In 1982 this changed, and the percentage increase in expense per admission was greater in the rest of the nation than in California. While both the United States and California were subject to PPS in late

## FIGURE 1

PERCENTAGE OF CHANGE IN EXPENSE PER
ADMISSION: CALIFORNIA VERSUS UNITED
STATES

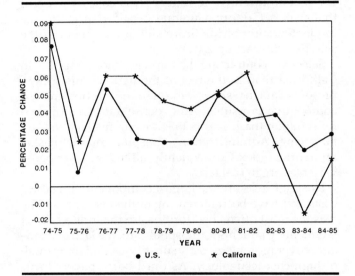

## FIGURE 2

PERCENTAGE OF CHANGE IN EXPENSE PER
INPATIENT DAY: CALIFORNIA VERSUS UNITED
STATES

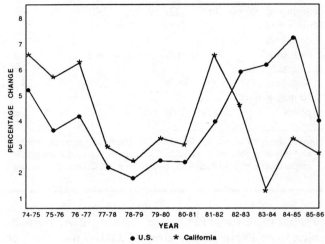

1983, the decline in expense per admission in California hospitals started before PPS and was greater than in the rest of the country. Selective contracting provided California hospitals with an additional incentive to reduce the rate at which their expenses were escalating.

The rapid growth of HMOs without their own facilities in the early 1980s led to an increase in contracting by these HMOs even before the implementation of California's selective contracting law in 1982. Consequently, the rate of increase in hospital expenses per admission in California began to slow during 1981–1982, with the decline accelerating through 1983–1984.

Expense per inpatient day is a second measure that can demonstrate the effect of selective contracting on California hospitals. As is shown in Figure 2, after having been consistently greater than in the rest of the United States, annual percentage increases in expense per inpatient day were lower in California after the advent of selective contracting. The cost per day accelerated for the rest of the nation, while California's rate declined beginning in 1982.

Perhaps the best measure of the effect of market competition and incentives by third party payers to reduce health care costs is the effect of such pressures on the portion of per capita income spent on hospital services. This measure summarizes the effects of

changes in hospital-related expenditures as well as changes in the total population and in the population's ability to pay for hospital care. If income is rising along with the increase in total population, then it is reasonable to expect that total spending for hospital services will increase more than if the income level were declining or relatively stable.

As Figure 3 shows, the percentage of per capita income spent on hospital services in California and the rest of the United States started at the same level in 1974, 2.71%, and followed a similar pattern of increase for the period 1974 through 1982. The percentage peaked in California in 1982, when Californians spent 3.80% of their per capita income on hospital services. The rest of the nation spent 3.96% of its per capita income on hospital services during 1982 and reached a peak in the following year at 4.19%. In 1983, with the advent of PPS, the portion of per capita income devoted to hospital services in the remainder of the United States began to decline, but the level for the United States still exceeded that for California. In 1986 the share of per capita income spent on hospital services in California declined slightly to 3.56%, while in the rest of the nation it actually reversed and began to climb, reaching 4.03% that year. The decline in hospital-related spending as a percentage of national per capita income during the

## FIGURE 3

HOSPITAL EXPENSE AS A PERCENTAGE OF PER CAPITA INCOME: CALIFORNIA VERSUS UNITED STATES

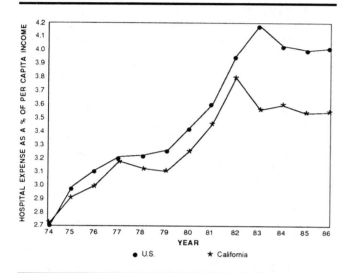

early years of PPS may have been due to hospitals' anticipating the ensuing effects of PPS. By 1985 these effects may have become depleted, and the prior trend of increasing hospital expenditures may have returned. In California, the continuing pressure of selective contracting has kept spending for hospital services, as a percentage of per capita income, in check.

## MANAGEMENT IMPLICATIONS OF SELECTIVE CONTRACTING

The United States, and California in particular, has experienced a dramatic increase in the enrollment of managed-care systems. The data on the growth of such systems that have been presented indicate consumers' willingness to accept restricted freedom of choice in exchange for reduced costs. Moreover, the recent emergence of open-ended HMOs, SBOs, and other hybrid organizations is blurring the traditional distinctions between HMOs, PPOs, and managed fee-for-service plans.[15] Although such organizations are difficult to classify, they give employers a greater range of flexibility with respect to health care benefits to their employees. Recent estimates are that 25% of the private pay population in the United States are covered by managed-care insurance programs, and that proportion is expected to reach 70% by the year 2000.[16]

Selective contracting, a cornerstone of PPOs and other managed-care systems, has had a significant impact on hospital cost behavior in California. The three measures of expense just presented indicate a change in hospital behavior after the 1982 advent of selective contracting in California. The rate of increase in hospital-related spending fell substantially in California compared to the rest of the nation.

Prior to the era of prospective reimbursement and selective contracting, hospitals competed largely on the basis of nonprice factors. To be successful, hospitals tried to attract physicians, who in turn brought in patients. Often the means by which hospitals attracted physicians—for example, acquisition of new technologies and improvement of service amenities—resulted in cost increases. Because most hospital reimbursement resulted from fee-for-service, cost-based methods, hospitals were able to recover the costs of providing additional amenities through higher charges to third party payers. Studies have shown that during this era hospitals in more competitive markets had higher costs than hospitals in less competitive markets, providing evidence of nonprice competition.[17,18] However, with the shift from cost-based to prospective, fixed-price methods of reimbursement, hospitals are beginning to compete on the basis of price. To compete effectively, hospital managers must learn to operate with fewer resources than in the past and must now promote greater efficiency within their organizations.

*With the shift from cost-based to prospective, fixed-price methods of reimbursement, hospitals are beginning to compete on the basis of price.*

Health care managers must keep abreast of emerging delivery systems and develop strategies for competing in this new environment. By joining HMO and PPO networks, hospitals can substantially improve their competitive position in the market. However, they must avoid the pitfall of treating all contracts identically. PPOs and HMOs are quite different in terms of their economic structure and risk apportionment and in terms of the magnitude of risk that they represent for the provider. For example, some HMOs require that hospitals bear the financial risk of out-of-plan use by HMO enrollees. Thus hospitals must have adequate information systems to monitor and control out-of-plan use—something that many HMOs have been unable to do very effectively.

Successful management in a contracting environment requires several measures, including aggressive case management, payment monitoring, and cost accounting. From a strategic point of view, managers must know their costs. Inaccurate or incomplete knowledge of their costs means that they cannot know the real profit margin. Under these circumstances negotiating contracts is imprecise and can have devastating consequences. In addition, without accurate cost information, managers cannot identify the product lines that are profitable for their particular facilities.

Good information systems are vital to a successful management process. The information system should offer, at a minimum, a cost-accounting system integrated with a case mix management system; the ability to inventory and monitor all contracts in order to determine contractual allowances accurately; the capability of screening admissions in terms of contract requirements; retrospective analysis capabilities; and software with which to measure quality of care for contracted patients.[19]

The landscape of the health care industry is evolving rapidly. Hospital managers must be aware of the changing environment in which they operate. Successful hospital managers understand the incentive structure of different payment systems, and they market and manage their operations with this conceptual understanding as a guide. An essential component of any successful management program is a thorough understanding of how evolving payments systems are affecting the hospital's medical staff and how the hospital can improve its competitive position in the market by working with its medical staff. The establishment of common goals by management and the medical staff ensures mutual success in contracting.

## REFERENCES

1. Gabel, J., and Ermann, D. "Preferred Provider Organizations: Performance, Problems, and Promise." *Health Affairs* 4, no. 1 (1985): 25–40.
2. Rice, T., et al. "The State of PPOs: Results from a National Survey." *Health Affairs* 4, no. 4 (1985): 25–40.
3. Ibid., 38.
4. Gabel, J., et al. "The Commercial Health Insurance Industry in Transition." *Health Affairs* 6, no. 3 (1987): 40–60.
5. Ibid.
6. Ibid.
7. InterStudy. *InterStudy Edge*. Excelsior, Minn.: InterStudy, Summer 1988.
8. Ibid.
9. American Medical Care and Review Association, *HMO Trends Report*.
10. Johns, L., Derzon, R., and Anderson, M. "Selective Contracting in California: Early Effects and Policy Implications." *Inquiry* 22, no. 1 (1985) 24–32.
11. Rahn, G., and Traska, M.R. "Formal Hospital/HMO Contracts Increase: Survey." *Hospitals* 61, no. 14 (1987): 47–50.
12. Ibid, 48.
13. Arstein-Kerslake, C. "PPOs Continue to Grow." *Insights* 11, no. 12 (1987): 1–8.
14. Arstein-Kerslake, C. "HMOs Flourishing in California." *Insights* 11, no. 15 (1987): 1–8.
15. Boland, P. "The Evolving Market for Preferred Provider Contracting." *Journal of Ambulatory Care Management* 10, no. 2 (1986): 13–21.
16. Matherlee, T. "HNLA Symposium on Managed Care, Change and Diversification." *Health Lawyers News Report* 16, no. 1 (1988): 1–8.
17. Farley, D.E. *Competition Among Hospitals; Market Structure and its Relation to Utilization, Cost and Financial Position*. Hospital Studies Program, National Center for Health Services Research and Health Care Technology Assessment, 1985.
18. Robinson, J.C., and Luft, H.S. "the Impact of Market Structure on Patient Volume, Average Length of Stay, and the Cost of Care." *Journal of Health Economics* 4 (1985): 83–94.
19. Green, L. "Managing Contractual Allowances: The New Profitability Imperative." *Foresight* 3, no. 1 (1988): 1–10.

# Contracts between hospitals and health maintenance organizations

Roger Feldman,
John Kralewski,
Janet Shapiro,
and
Hung-Ching Chan

*This article describes the contractual relations that are emerging between health maintenance organizations (HMOs) and hospitals. Six HMOs in four large metropolitan areas provided information on 102 hospital contracts. The authors found that the HMOs are becoming more aggressive in placing hospitals in competition with each other for HMO patients. Staff and network HMOs are able to obtain a higher concentration of patients and substantially larger discounts for inpatient services than are individual practice association (IPA) plans in this study.*

*Health Care Manage Rev*, 1990, 15(1), 47–60
© 1990 Aspen Publishers, Inc.

This article presents an analysis of the contractual relationships between health maintenance organizations (HMOs) and hospitals in four communities. The data are from a larger research project that the authors conducted for the U.S. Department of Health and Human Services. The study was designed to determine the degree to which HMOs create competitive markets for hospital services and to document the strategies used to achieve those ends. It had three parts: a qualitative assessment of HMO strategies for obtaining favorable price concessions from hospitals, a descriptive analysis of the resulting contracts, and an economic analysis of patient concentration and price differentials for hospitalized HMO patients. This article presents the results of the descriptive analysis of HMO–hospital contracts.

Since hospital costs constitute a large share of the typical HMO's budget, it is not surprising that HMOs have concentrated considerable effort on reducing hospital utilization rates and prices. Efforts to reduce utilization apparently pay off in lower admission rates[1] and shorter length of stay[2] than is usual for traditional fee-for-service health plans. It is not clear, however, that HMOs have been able to reduce the unit prices of hospital services.

In previous studies by the authors of the Minneapolis-St. Paul metropolitan area, a rapid increase was found in the number of formal contracts between HMOs and hospitals from 1977 to 1980, but little evidence was found of competitive bidding for those contracts.[3,4] Many of the contracts, in fact, were initiated by hospitals rather than HMOs. In some cases a hospital collaborated with a medical group practice to develop an HMO and retained close organizational linkages to

**Roger Feldman**, *Ph.D., Director of the Minnesota Health Care Financing Association Research Center, is a Professor in the Division of Health Services Research and Policy and the Department of Economics, University of Minnesota.*

**John Kralewski**, *Ph.D., Director of the Division of Health Services Research and Policy, holds the William Wallace Chair in Health Services Management at the University of Minnesota.*

**Janet Shapiro**, *B.A., is a Research Associate in the Division of Health Services Research and Policy at the University of Minnesota.*

**Hung-Ching Chan** *is a Ph.D. candidate in the program in Health Services Research, Policy and Administration at the University of Minnesota.*

This research was supported by contract no. 240-85-0053 from the Department of Health and Human Services, Health Resources and Services Administration.

the HMO after its inception. Not surprisingly, contracts between these hospitals and HMOs were designed to improve predictability of hospital costs and admissions rather than to achieve price concessions for the HMOs.[5]

These findings were supported by a national study conducted by the authors in 1981 with the Group Health Association of America (GHAA).[5] In a survey of GHAA members, we found that most HMOs paid full billed charges for hospital services, even though they had a formal agreement with their primary hospital. This study also found that HMOs seldom negotiated with more than one hospital when attempting to obtain a contract. Finally, it seems that price was not a major factor causing HMOs to develop alliances with their principal hospitals. Hospital location and the range of services offered were the major factors cited by HMOs as determining hospital selection, and price was a secondary consideration.

Other observers suggested that staff model and group practice HMOs typically engage in "one-time shopping" only.[6] Once a group or staff HMO has negotiated a contract with a hospital, the two organizations increasingly act as partners. Disrupting this relationship for any reason apparently involves too many transactions costs. This is especially true for HMOs organized around existing fee-for-service (FFS) group practices, which usually rely on the hospitals where FFS physicians have admitting privileges; these HMOs may not shop at all.

One problem with the existing studies of HMO-hospital contracts is that they were conducted largely in the late 1970s and early 1980s. As health insurance markets become more competitive and as prepaid plans compete to gain or retain market share, they may increasingly attempt to reduce the costs of hospital services. In addition, most of the literature we reviewed

pertains to a single market area, often the Minneapolis-St. Paul metropolitan area. Although this area is often cited as an example of a competitive health care market, it would be instructive to compare data and results from several cities, each in a different stage of development in its HMO market.

Consequently, our goal was to provide information on HMO–hospital contracts that was up-to-date and that represented HMOs in different market areas. This article will present the results of our descriptive analysis of hospital contracts. We focus on many of the same issues that have been addressed by previous studies (e.g., who initiates the contract, how many hospitals are involved in negotiations with each HMO, what factors are important in developing a contractual relationship with a hospital, and if the HMO obtains a discount from the hospital's full billed charge). In a companion article,[7] we examined the relationship between concentration of HMO services at a particular hospital and the hospital's price, and in general we found that hospitals have become much more willing to give discounts to HMOs than was shown in our analyses from the early 1980s.

## SELECTION OF HMOs AND DATA COLLECTION

In choosing optimum environments to assess the degree to which HMOs create competitive markets for hospital services, a number of factors were considered. Some of these relate to the environmental conditions that may affect the ability of an HMO to create price competition among hospitals. These include hospital occupancy rates, the number of beds per 1,000 people in the community, the size of the community, and the community's experience with HMOs.

TABLE 1

ATTRIBUTES OF CASE STUDY SITES, 1985

| Case study site | No. of HMOs | No. of hospitals | Beds/ 1,000 people | Average length of stay | Patient days/ 1,000 people | Average occupancy rate | HMO membership/ 1984 population (%) |
|---|---|---|---|---|---|---|---|
| 1 | 10 | 73 | 3.2 | 8.6 | 954.6 | 81.7 | 10.8 |
| 2 | 2 | 35 | 4.5 | 8.0 | 1,224.0 | 75.8 | 3.7 |
| 3 | 6 | 36 | 4.6 | 8.1 | 1,174.5 | 67.8 | 40.4 |
| 4 | 5 | 45 | 4.1 | 6.4 | 1,056.0 | 71.1 | 7.4 |

Four communities were chosen for inclusion in this study. Table 1 shows some of the environmental factors that went into consideration of site selection. It should be noted that all the attributes, such as patient days per 1,000 people in the community, refer to the community standard, not the HMO being studied. Although the four sites were all large metropolitan areas, they represented substantial differences in hospital market conditions. Site 1 had the study's lowest number of beds per 1,000, the highest average length of stay and, not surprisingly, the highest hospital occupancy rate. Site 2 was selected for its newness to the HMO market and its slight market penetration. It had the study's second highest number of beds per 1,000. The third study site was a mature HMO market that had the greatest HMO membership in the study and the lowest occupancy rate, conditions that should promote price concessions and other favorable contractual relations with HMOs. The fourth site was a rapidly expanding but immature HMO market with five HMOs (up from two in 1980), but only 7% of the area population enrolled in HMOs in 1985.

The following propositions were considered when selecting HMOs for inclusion in the study:

- HMOs that are able to concentrate the majority of their patients in fewer hospitals obtain lower prices for hospital services than those that must use many hospitals for inpatient services.
- Group, staff, and network HMOs are able to concentrate inpatients in fewer hospitals; therefore, they obtain lower prices for hospital services than individual practice association (IPA) HMOs.
- HMOs that are older are able to concentrate inpatients in fewer hospitals, thereby obtaining lower prices for hospital services than newer plans can.
- HMOs that are able to concentrate a majority of their patients in fewer hospitals will shift their patient workload from one hospital to another to obtain lower prices.

These propositions suggest that HMOs should be chosen on the basis of age (young versus old) and type of organization (more tightly organized versus more loosely organized). Ideally, enough HMOs would be included in the study so that variation in HMO characteristics would be observed within each type of market area. This would permit generalizations that are specific to a particular set of HMO and market characteristics; for example, IPA-model HMOs may obtain significantly different hospital contracts when the hospitals they negotiate with have lower occupancy rates than when the hospitals are fully occupied by non-HMO

*HMOs that are able to concentrate the majority of their patients in fewer hospitals obtain lower prices for hospital services than those that must use many hospitals for inpatient services.*

patients. However, the number of HMOs selected for the present study was limited by our contract with the funding agency to no more than 10 plans. Therefore, HMOs had to be selected carefully to represent as many different configurations as possible within the limits of the study.

When HMOs were selected for this study, no group practice HMOs were identified as suitable study HMOs in the communities that best matched the desired study environment. The plans selected for this study therefore included two staff-model plans, two networks, and three IPAs. The definitions of types of HMOs used for this study follow those used in a 1985 study by InterStudy.[8] They are as follows:

- *Staff*: A service is delivered through a physician group practice that is controlled by an HMO unit.
- *Group*: An HMO unit contracts with an independent group practice to provide service.
- *Network*: An HMO contracts with two or more independent group practices to provide contract services. It is primarily organized around groups, but may include a few solo practices.
- *IPA*: An HMO has one or more of the following characteristics: contracts directly with independent physicians; contracts with one or more associations of physicians; or contracts with one or more multispecialty groups, but is predominantly organized around single-specialty practices.

Table 2 lists the configuration of HMOs selected for this study. Each HMO's enrollment has been rounded to the next highest thousand, using 1985 enrollment figures. The new HMOs were under 5 years old; the old HMOs had been in existence for 6 to over 25 years. Four of the HMOs were not-for-profit, three were for-profit. There were two staff-model HMOs, two networks, and three IPAs. Two of the HMOs were nationally owned, one was acquired by a national organization after the study commenced, and one was managed by a national firm, although it was categorized as a local plan.

For this analysis, we needed information about both the contracting process and the discounts obtained

**TABLE 2**

HMO CHARACTERISTICS BY CASE STUDY SITE, 1985

| Case study site | HMO | Enrollment | New–old[*] | Profit status[†] | Model | Ownership[‡] |
|---|---|---|---|---|---|---|
| 1 | A | 198,000 | Old | NP | Staff | L |
|   | B | 115,000 | Old | NP | IPA | L |
| 2 | C | 42,000 | Old | P | Staff | N |
|   | D | 25,000 | New | P | IPA | L |
| 3 | E | 216,000 | Old | NP | Network | L |
|   | F | 201,000 | Old | NP | Network | L |
| 4 | G | 60,000 | New | P | IPA | N |

[*] New = Less than five years old; Old = More than five years old.
[†] P = For-profit; NP = Not-for-profit.
[‡] N = National; L = Local.

through the contracts. Although this information was available (at least in principle) from the hospitals, we chose to obtain it from the HMOs. It was deemed easier to obtain the data from HMOs than from hospitals, since some hospitals might have refused to cooperate with a study of this extremely sensitive nature.

Some HMOs in the study used almost every hospital in their market area. It was agreed that these HMOs would provide data for the hospitals where 95% of their admissions occurred. This probably resulted in less than complete information on tertiary care hospitals, but it did supply the needed data for the descriptive analysis.

Each participating HMO completed a form for every hospital where HMO patients were admitted (subject to the exclusion just noted). Forms were completed for 102 hospitals, 100 of which had contracts with the HMOs and two of which did not have contracts, but nevertheless admitted HMO patients. Sixty of the contracts were held by two of the study IPAs, and 42 were in the four staff and network plans. One IPA in case study site 4 was unable to complete the hospital contract forms because ownership and management changed midstudy. This IPA was dropped from the study, and no contract data from that plan is included in the study.

One of the two remaining IPAs was organized before 1980, whereas the other was less than five years old in 1985. In contrast, all of the staff and network plans included in the study were organized before 1980. Consequently, the dimensions of plan type and plan age are correlated in our study, with staff and network plans being somewhat more mature. This makes it difficult to decide whether observed differences in

hospital contracts (e.g., discounts) are due to the age of the HMO or its organizational form. However, most of the IPA contracts were provided by the more mature IPA.

Table 3 shows the number of completed hospital contract forms by case-study site and HMO. Case study site 1 included an IPA where hospitals throughout the entire market area were used, accounting for the large number of hospital contracts and the increase in 1984 and 1985, when the IPA added many new physicians. Case study site 2 was represented by only one HMO, accounting for the few hospital contracts. In case study site 3, neither HMO completed forms for all the hospi-

**TABLE 3**

COMPLETED HOSPITAL CONTRACT FORMS BY CASE STUDY SITE AND HMO

| Case study site | Health plan | Plan type[*] | No. of complete Contract forms |
|---|---|---|---|
| 1 | A | SN | 7 |
|   | B | IPA | 46 |
| 2 | C | SN | 8 |
|   | D | IPA | 0[†] |
| 3 | E | SN | 15 |
|   | F | SN | 8 |
| 4 | G | IPA | 18 |
| Total |  |  | 102 |

[*] SN = Staff or network.
[†] This HMO was unable to complete the hospital contract forms.

**TABLE 4**

NUMBER OF CONTRACTS INITIATED, BY HMO TYPE, IN YEAR OF CONTRACT INITIATION

| HMO type | 1969 | 1972 | 1973 | 1976 | 1977 | 1978 | 1979 | 1980 | 1981 | 1982 | 1983 | 1984 | 1985 | 1986* | Total |
|---|---|---|---|---|---|---|---|---|---|---|---|---|---|---|---|
| IPA | 0 | 0 | 0 | 0 | 0 | 1 | 3 | 4 | 5 | 3 | 3 | 25 | 18 | 1 | 63 |
| Staff or network | 2 | 1 | 1 | 2 | 1 | 1 | 0 | 2 | 4 | 2 | 6 | 2 | 7 | 4 | 35 |
| Total | 2 | 1 | 1 | 2 | 1 | 2 | 3 | 6 | 9 | 5 | 9 | 27 | 25 | 5 | 98 |
| Percentage | 2 | 1 | 1 | 2 | 1 | 2 | 3 | 6 | 9 | 5 | 9 | 28 | 26 | 5 | 100† |

* Incomplete.

† Percentages are based on the number of cases where complete data is available for each question; therefore, the sum of percentages always equals 100 (subject to rounding off).

tals under contract, selecting only the hospitals that accounted for 95% of its hospitalizations. Case study site 4 was represented by one HMO that covered an extensive geographic area.

## RESULTS OF THE STUDY

### Contract initiation

In 51.5% of the cases, the HMO initiated the contract; in 48.5%, both the hospital and the HMO were responsible for initiating the agreement. There were no cases where a hospital initiated the contract.

The numbers of the hospital–HMO contracts initiated each year from 1969 to 1986, disaggregated by HMO type, are exhibited in Table 4. Because the data were gathered in 1986, the numbers for 1986 are incomplete.

Over 81% of all contracts were initiated from 1981 to 1986, with 58% of the contracts commencing in the last three years. By type of HMO, 87% of the IPA hospital contracts were initiated from 1981 to 1986, compared with 71% of the staff and network contracts. This is consistent with the fact that the two IPAs in the study were new entrants to the prepaid health plan market; therefore, their major contract negotiations had been recently completed. The number of contracts initiated by the staff and network models also appears to have been increasing. In part, this reflects the expansion of these HMOs into new market areas. It also reflects their efforts to increase access to services in order to compete with the more decentralized IPAs.

### Contract termination and negotiation

Ninety percent of the contracts had specific provisions for the termination of the agreement or contract

before its normal ending date. Table 5 shows the terms of notification with and without cause, by number of days. It is interesting to note that cause does not seem to be an issue in termination. In the majority of cases, contracts could be ended at similar times without or without cause. In 13 cases, termination without cause required 60 days notice, whereas termination with cause needed only 30 days notice. Apparently neither the HMOs nor the hospitals wished to hold the other party to a contract if that party wanted to be released from it.

There is a considerable difference in the frequency of contract negotiation by HMO type (see Table 6). In the IPAs, 70% of the hospital contracts were renegotiated automatically or had an open-ended arrangement. This means that these contracts tended to be restructured or at least reconsidered each year. The nature of IPAs apparently calls for a more flexible business arrangement between HMOs and hospitals. Staff and network HMOs appear to have established more stable relation-

**TABLE 5**

CONTRACT TERMINATION WITH CAUSE AND WITHOUT CAUSE BY TERMS OF NOTIFICATION IN DAYS

| No. of contracts (%) | No. of days with cause | No. of days without cause |
|---|---|---|
| 13.0 (18.3) | 30 | 60 |
| 8.0 (11.3) | 60 | 60 |
| 44.0 (62.0) | 90 | 90 |
| 1.0 (1.4) | 120 | 120 |
| 4.0 (5.6) | 180 | 180 |
| 1.0 (1.4) | 365 | 365 |
| 31.0 | Not specified | Not specified |

**TABLE 6**

FREQUENCY OF HMO–HOSPITAL CONTRACT NEGOTIATION, BY HMO TYPE

| HMO type | Open-ended automatic renewal | Number of years | | | | | | Total |
|---|---|---|---|---|---|---|---|---|
| | | 1 | 2 | 3 | 4 | 5 | 6 | |
| IPA | 44 (69.8%) | 19 (30.2%) | 0 | 0 | 0 | 0 | 0 | 63 (100%) |
| Staff or network | 0 | 19 (54.3%) | 5 (14.3%) | 6 (17.1%) | 3 (8.6%) | 1 (2.9%) | 1 (2.9%) | 35 (100%) |

ships, and in some instances keep the same contract for an extended period of time. Thirty-one percent of their hospital contracts were negotiated for a three-to-seven year period.

**Reasons for contractual agreements**

Table 7 shows the factors that were important in developing a contractual relationship with a hospital. A list of possible factors was presented to the respondent with instructions to rank the three most important factors in order of importance (1 being the most important).

Affiliation of HMO physicians was ranked as the most important factor in hospital selection in 73% of the cases. This reflects the dominant number of IPA contracts in our sample: IPAs normally contracted with hospitals where their physicians are affiliated, and 63% of the hospital contracts were in the IPA category. Convenience to plan enrollees ranked as the second most important reason for the selection of a hospital, and the reputation of the hospital was ranked third. The fact that price was not shown to be a major factor factor in selecting a hospital validates interview findings that stated repeatedly that price becomes an issue only after a hospital has been selected for other reasons.

**TABLE 7**

FACTORS BY RANKED IMPORTANCE FOR CONTRACTUAL RELATIONS WITH A HOSPITAL

| Factor | | Importance | | | |
|---|---|---|---|---|---|
| | | Not ranked | 1 | 2 | 3 |
| Affiliation with HMO physicians: | No. | 22 | 74 | 4 | 1 |
| | % | 21.8 | 73.3 | 4.0 | 1.0 |
| Convenience to plan enrollees: | No. | 16 | 2 | 61 | 22 |
| | % | 15.8 | 2.0 | 60.4 | 21.8 |
| Reputation of hospital: | No. | 42 | 5 | 6 | 48 |
| | % | 41.6 | 5.0 | 5.9 | 47.5 |
| Range of services: | No. | 82 | 5 | 6 | 8 |
| | % | 81.2 | 5.0 | 5.9 | 7.9 |
| Price of services: | No. | 63 | 1 | 21 | 16 |
| | % | 62.4 | 1.0 | 20.8 | 15.8 |
| Have a needed service: | No. | 99 | | 1 | 1 |
| | % | 98.0 | | 1.0 | 1.0 |
| Organizational linkages: | No. | 101 | | | |
| | % | 100 | | | |
| Other:* | No. | 87 | 14 | | |
| | % | 86.1 | 13.9 | | |

* Quality of service, proximity to HMO clinics, nature of services provided, physicians' desire to use the hospitals, organizational compatibility, and ability to work together.

**TABLE 8**

RANKINGS OF FACTORS BY IMPORTANCE FOR DEVELOPMENT OF CONTRACTUAL RELATIONSHIPS WITH SPECIFIC HOSPITALS, BY HMO TYPE

| HMO type | | Ranks of importance | | | | Total |
|---|---|---|---|---|---|---|
| | | Not ranked | 1 | 2 | 3 | |
| *Affiliation with HMO physicians* | | | | | | |
| IPA: | No. | 0 | 64 | 0 | 0 | 64 |
| | % | 0 | 100 | 0 | 0 | 100 |
| Staff or network: | No. | 22 | 10 | 1 | 1 | 34 |
| | % | 65 | 29 | 3 | 3 | 100 |
| Total: | No. | 22 | 74 | 1 | 1 | 98 |
| | % | 22 | 76 | 1 | 1 | 100 |
| *Convenience to plan enrollees* | | | | | | |
| IPA: | No. | 0 | 0 | 47 | 17 | 64 |
| | % | 0 | 0 | 73 | 27 | 100 |
| Staff or network: | No. | 16 | 2 | 14 | 5 | 37 |
| | % | 43 | 5 | 38 | 14 | 100 |
| Total: | No. | 16 | 2 | 61 | 22 | 101 |
| | % | 16 | 2 | 60 | 22 | 100 |
| *Reputation of hospital* | | | | | | |
| IPA: | No. | 18 | 0 | 0 | 46 | 64 |
| | % | 28 | 0 | 0 | 72 | 100 |
| Staff or network: | No. | 24 | 5 | 6 | 2 | 37 |
| | % | 65 | 14 | 16 | 5 | 100 |
| Total: | No. | 42 | 5 | 6 | 48 | 101 |
| | % | 42 | 5 | 6 | 48 | 101 |

Interestingly, having a needed service was not considered important by any of the respondents, and under 20% ranked range of services as important. Table 8 shows the three top factors influencing hospital selection by HMO type (1 being the most important). These data indicate that selection of hospitals by IPA HMOs is largely based on the existing affiliations of their physicians and convenience to plan enrollees. Conversely, staff and network HMOs appear to weigh the reputation of the hospital more heavily, with convenience to plan enrollees a close but second-level consideration.

The split among the staff and network HMOs regarding the importance of convenience to plan enrollees probably reflects the difference between HMOs with new contracts and those with old contracts. For HMOs with old contracts, enrollee convenience was not an issue, and thus 43% of those respondents did not include this factor in their top three rankings. An equal number, however, listed enrollee convenience as their first or second most influential factor. These answers probably show the influence of newer contracts resulting from expansion into new market areas as well as initiatives designed to improve staff and network competitiveness with IPA plans.

It is clear from these data that enrollee convenience is playing an increasingly important role in HMO decision making. Interview data indicate that this is especially true in mature markets, where HMOs must compete on the basis of access to care as well as price. Since IPA models rely heavily on access to care as a major competitive edge over staff and network HMOs, it is not surprising that they ranked enrollee convenience as highly important in all market areas.

## Organizational relationships

We were interested in the organizational relationships between HMOs and the hospitals with which they had contractual relationships. A list of 20 organizational arrangements derived from previous studies was presented to the HMOs, and they were asked to check those that were included in their contracts. The unit of analysis was the individual contract. Table 9 lists these items and the number of contracts that included each provision.

Contrary to expectations, few interorganizational arrangements were found, even in mature markets. The lack of organizational relationships may be attributed to the circumstances under which the survey forms were completed. The questions were framed and answered in the context of formal written contracts. Therefore, many of the relationships listed might exist informally between the HMO and the hospital or the

### TABLE 9

HMO/HOSPITAL ORGANIZATIONAL RELATIONSHIPS

| Arrangement | No. of instances |
|---|---|
| Joint ventures | 0 |
| HMO physicians represented on hospital board | 1 |
| HMO administrators represented on hospital board | 1 |
| Hospital represented on HMO board | 0 |
| Interlocking boards | 0 |
| Joint strategic planning | 1 |
| Shared management | 0 |
| Hospital-owned HMO | 0 |
| HMO-owned hospital | 0 |
| Leasing or operating agreements | 1 |
| Joint teaching programs | 2 |
| Joint utilization review | 10 |
| Major stockholders | 0 |
| Frequent meetings between management | 3 |
| HMO medical staff hold key hospital positions | 1 |
| Joint medical staff conferences (continuing education) | 1 |
| Arrangements for shared use of equipment, facilities, etc. | 2 |
| Exclusive arrangement so that hospital cannot contract with other HMOs | 0 |
| Exclusive arrangement so that HMO cannot contract with other hospitals | 3 |
| Exclusive arrangements for some services | 4 |

HMO and the physicians. For instance, HMO physicians represented on hospital boards and HMO physicians holding key hospital positions are prime examples of situations that may be more prevalent than they look from the single reported case. In the category, "exclusive arrangement so that the HMO cannot contract with other hospitals," the three cases were instances where a single specialty service was utilized at the hospital. All three cases were reported by one HMO. It appears from these data that HMOs prefer to maintain an arm's-length relationship with hospitals.

### Contract negotiation environment

For each hospital contract, respondents were asked, "Did you negotiate with other hospitals in competition with the hospital under discussion before entering into the current agreement?" We were surprised to find that 88% answered affirmatively, which initially suggested much more rigorous negotiations than were implied in the structured in-person interviews with those who negotiated the contracts. However, given the dispersion of hospital contracts (see Table 3) and the frequency with which affiliation of HMO physicians was ranked as the most important reason for a contractual relationship with a particular hospital (see Table 7), it is apparent that negotiations were conducted primarily with other hospitals in the neighborhood of the chosen hospital. Furthermore, these hospitals were often selected because of affiliations with HMO physicians. Thus the extent of marketplace competition may be overstated by the response to this question. Even so, this finding represents a major shift from our previous studies.[3,4] It appears that HMOs are becoming more aggressive in placing hospitals in competition with each other for HMO patients.

### Contract adjustments

Financial arrangements in 87% of the contracts were changed during the past five years, and organizational arrangements were changed in 75% of the contracts. Most of the financial changes involved the amount paid, although some also altered the method of payment by shifting from a discount on charges to a per diem rate. Most of the organizational changes were minor adjustments in admitting procedures and utilization-review mechanisms.

Our past HMO studies have found that HMO needs and expectations of hospitals change as the HMOs become more established in a community and increase their market share.[3,4] Therefore, we were interested in

TABLE 10

MAJOR AREAS FOR CONTRACT CHANGES BETWEEN
HMOS AND HOSPITALS

| Area of change | Frequency | Percent |
|---|---|---|
| Type of service | 46 | 63.0 |
| Price | 12 | 16.4 |
| Payment arrangement | 8 | 11.0 |
| Simplify administrative procedures | 3 | 4.1 |
| On site utilization review | 2 | 2.7 |
| Organizational relationship | 1 | 1.4 |
| Other | 1 | 1.4 |
| Missing | 29 | |
| Total | 102 | 100.0 |

whether there were parts of the arrangements with the hospitals that the HMOs would like to change. Consequently, we asked what areas they were changing or would like to change and how they were proceeding to make those changes.

The HMOs reported that for 73% of their contracts, they were either in the midst of change or desired some kind of change. Table 10 shows the major areas for contract changes between HMOs and hospitals. The most frequent change to occur was in type of service. This resulted largely from IPAs trying to concentrate mental health and clinical lab work in fewer hospitals, to control costs. The next two most important areas where change was desired were price and payment arrangements. This finding parallels the interview finding that price is not the primary reason for selecting a hospital, but is attended to and frequently revised after a relationship is established.

The chief executive officers (CEOs) in the newer HMOs in the study described similar phases in their pursuit of hospital contracts. Initially, most hospitals in their area were not interested in even meeting with the CEOs. Consequently, they concentrated on developing single admission agreements. Then hospital occupancy rates began to drop and, at the same time, the HMOs' enrollment increased. Hospitals then became interested in talking. Yet the HMOs' primary interest was still in gaining access to key hospitals, regardless of price. Once a relationship was established, the HMO would begin to examine its admissions and gather data on utilization and costs. Then the HMO began serious negotiations with the hospitals for price concessions.

## Utilization and concentration of hospital services

Services were divided into inpatient and outpatient services (see Table 11) so that hospital utilization could be examined by specific service. Two thirds of the hospitals were used for pediatrics and obstetrics. Almost every hospital was used for medical–surgical admissions and over 50% were used for mental health, but only one third were used for chemical dependency. The small percentage of hospitals used for tertiary services reflects the fact that it is easier for HMOs to concentrate those patients in fewer institutions. This is also the case for chemical dependency, although in this case it also results from hospital specialization. Most hospitals were used for ambulatory surgery, nearly all for emergency department care, and 70% for other outpatient services such as physical therapy.

Table 12 shows the concentration of services by case study site using Herfindahl indices. The Herfindahl index (H-index) is the sum of squared market shares of admissions for each HMO.[9] Commonly used in studies of industrial concentration, the Herfindahl index attains a maximum value of 1.0 when the HMO admits patients to only one hospital. The H-index declines as more hospitals are used and increases with rising inequality of admissions among a given number of hospitals.

Table 12 illustrates that concentration of services varies considerably within geographic areas (case study sites), within services (such as pediatrics or obstetrics), and by type of HMO (IPA versus staff or network), but less so among similar HMO types. Clearly, staff and network HMOs can concentrate patients more effectively than IPAs. The lowest overall

TABLE 11

NUMBER OF HOSPITALS USED BY SERVICE (N = 102)

| Service | No. | Percent |
|---|---|---|
| Inpatient | | |
| Pediatric | 69 | 67.6 |
| Obstetrics | 65 | 63.7 |
| Medical–surgical | 97 | 95.1 |
| Mental health | 59 | 57.8 |
| Chemical dependency | 35 | 34.3 |
| Tertiary care | 38 | 37.3 |
| Outpatient | | |
| Ambulatory surgery | 86 | 84.3 |
| Emergency department | 95 | 93.1 |
| Other | 74 | 72.5 |

**TABLE 12**

CONCENTRATION OF ADMISSIONS BY SERVICE FOR CASE STUDY SITE AND HMO*

| Case study site | Health plan† | No. of contracts | Total admissions | Pediatrics | Obstetrics | Medical–surgical | Mental health | Chemical dependency‡ | Tertiary‡ | Emergency department | Pediatrics–medical–surgical§ |
|---|---|---|---|---|---|---|---|---|---|---|---|
| 1 | A(SN) | 7 | 8066 [.3125] | 1095 [.3393] | 4005 [.4966] | 2964 [.2687] | 1 [1.000] | 1 | 0 | (7) | 4059 [.2041] |
|   | B(IPA) | 46 | 8739 [.0377] | 0§ | 2285 [.0685] | 6140 [.0348] | 314 [.0739] | 0 | 0 | 61249 [.0375] | 6140 [.348] |
| 2 | C(SN) | 8 | (1)1769 [.2094] | (2)66 [1.000] | (1)549 [.6045] | (3)720 [.3497] | 0 | 0 | 0 | (4)1495 [1.000] | (3)786 [.3005] |
| 3 | E(SN) | 15 | 13191 [.3598] | 1237 [.2515] | 4085 [.6270] | 6492 [.3680] | 570 [.8025] | 281 | 526 | 9953 [.2309] | 7729 [.3021] |
|   | F(SN) | 8 | 15438 [.3459] | 3225 [.3100] | 3824 [.3315] | (1)8068 [.3951] | (2)274 [1.000] | 47 | 0 | [.2807] | (1)11293 [.3673] |
| 4 | G(IPA) | 18 | 2748 [.1143] | (10)61 [1.000] | (1)710 [.2077] | 1905 [.1129] | (1)72 [.2481] | 0 | 0 | (7) | (10)1966 [.1449] |

* ( ) = No. of missing contracts by service.
† SN = Staff or network.
‡ Herfindahl indices were not calculated for chemical dependency and tertiary care due to the small number of cases.
§ Health Plan B combined pediatrics and medical–surgical in its reports.

H-index calculated for a staff or network HMO plan, .2094, exceeded the highest index reported by an IPA in our case study. The highest overall H-indices, .3459 and .3598, were achieved by the two network plans in case study site 3, the market with a surplus of hospital beds and the lowest hospital occupancy rate. These HMOs appeared to be able to exploit both their strong organizational structure and the weaknesses of hospitals in this market in order to obtain a high concentration of patients. The H-index of .3598, for example, is about three times as large as the value that would occur if plan E spread its admissions evenly over the eight hospitals used.

In case study site 1, there was great variance in concentration of services between the HMO plans. This can probably be attributed to the fact that the two plans were organizationally at opposite ends of the HMO structure. One was a centralized, well-established plan and the other was a decentralized, relatively new plan. In case study site 3, the concentration index was similar for all services except obstetrics and mental health.

From these comparisons of case study sites, one can infer that HMO type is very influential in determining an HMO's ability to concentrate cases. Yet health plan C in case study site 2 was a staff HMO, and its concentration of services varied greatly depending on the service. This is a direct result of this plan's expansion into new geographic market areas.

## Discounts

For each hospital contract, the HMO supplied information on the number of admissions and the number of patient days for the last full year, price paid to the hospital per admission prior to any coordination of benefit adjustments, and full billed hospital charge per admission for the following inpatient services: pediatrics, obstetrics, medical–surgical, mental health, chemical dependency, and tertiary services. Medical–surgical and pediatrics were subsequently combined to accommodate one HMO that could not disaggregate pediatrics from medical–surgical.

For outpatient services (specifically the emergency department), the number of emergency department visits or authorizations for the last full year, price paid to the hospital per emergency department visit or authorization, and full billed hospital charge per emergency department visit or authorization were reported.

Table 13 shows the percentage discount from full billed charge by service and HMO type. Staff and network HMOs got larger discounts for inpatient services than did IPAs, as shown in Table 13, and some of the differences were dramatic. For example, in medical–surgical contracts (where the data are most complete) staff and network HMOs got a 26% discount, on average, compared to a discount of 4% in the IPA contracts. When looking at the inpatient cases reported, differences are statistically significant in every instance where there were data for both HMO types. Staff and network HMOs also received larger discounts than IPAs for emergency department services. However, the average difference is not as large as originally hypothesized and is not statistically significant.

### Reimbursement methods

Table 14 shows the reimbursement method by service for IPAs and staff and network HMOs. Inpatient reimbursement methods seem to be related to type of plan. IPAs' predominant method of paying for general acute inpatient care was a specified percentage discount from charges. This accounted for 69% of medical–surgical contracts, 63% of pediatrics contracts, and 59% of obstetrics contracts. On the other hand, staff and network HMOs tended to use flat per diem payments regardless of length of stay. Seventy-four percent of their medical–surgical contracts, 55% of their pediatrics contracts, and 47% of their obstetrics contracts used this method. A flat per diem rate was seldom used by IPAs.

*Staff and network HMOs got larger discounts for inpatient services than did IPAs, and some of the differences were dramatic.*

This notable difference in reimbursement arrangements may be explained by differences between the IPA and staff and network model plans. The staff and network HMOs in the study were all more mature plans and probably had more accurate historical knowledge of their hospital utilization, as well as firmer control over their physicians. Therefore, the flat per diem rate was a comfortable means of reimbursement.

A substantial number of IPA contracts paid full billed charges for hospital inpatient care. These contracts were generally new ones where the HMO had little leverage to obtain discounts. If an IPA wants to use a specific hospital, it is sometimes willing to accept full billed charges and renegotiate at a later time. This is substantiated by the findings that price was a major

TABLE 13

DISCOUNT FROM FULL BILLED CHARGE BY SERVICE AND HMO TYPE

| Service* | Type of HMO | | | | |
| | IPA | | Staff or network | | |
| | $N^†$ | % | $N^†$ | % | $p^‡$ |
|---|---|---|---|---|---|
| Pediatrics (67) | 1 | 0 | 18 | 18.5 | |
| Obstetrics (65) | 41 | 1.5 | 13 | 29.0 | .000 |
| Medical–surgical (97) | 62 | 3.8 | 20 | 25.7 | .000 |
| Mental health (59) | 43 | 2.5 | 11 | 28.0 | .000 |
| Chemical dependency (35) | 0 | | 8 | 39.0 | |
| Tertiary (33) | 0 | | 8 | 17.5 | |
| Emergency department (95) | 43 | 4.6 | 22 | 9.1 | .124 |
| Total inpatient (356) | 64 | 3.5 | 22 | 24.0 | .000 |

* The number following each service is the number of hospitals where this service was used.
† $N$ = The number of cases where an HMO reported the price paid to the hospital per admission and the full billed charge per admission.
‡ $p$ = Probability value.

**TABLE 14**

REIMBURSEMENT METHOD BY SERVICE AND HMO TYPE (%)*

| Reimbursement method | Medical–surgical IPA | Medical–surgical S/N | Pediatrics IPA | Pediatrics S/N | Obstetrics IPA | Obstetrics S/N | Chemical dependency IPA | Chemical dependency S/N | Mental health IPA | Mental health S/N | Tertiary IPA | Tertiary S/N | Ambulatory surgery IPA | Ambulatory surgery S/N | Emergency department IPA | Emergency department S/N | Other outpatient IPA | Other outpatient S/N |
|---|---|---|---|---|---|---|---|---|---|---|---|---|---|---|---|---|---|---|
| Full billed charge | 11 (16) | 0 | 8 (20) | 1 (5) | 6 (18) | 1 (5) | 2 (10) | 0 | 2 (7) | 0 | 7 (29.2) | 0 | 19 (32) | 1 (5) | 20 (35) | 0 | 14 (25) | 0 |
| Specified percentage discount from charge | 43 (69) | 6 (22) | 26 (63) | 8 (40) | 20 (59) | 5 (26) | 15 (75) | 1 (10) | 26 (84) | 2 (29) | 13 (54.2) | 4 (36.4) | 40 (68) | 17 (77) | 37 (65) | 20 (83) | 42 (74) | 22 (88) |
| Flat per diem charge regardless of length of stay | 7 (11) | 20 (74) | 6 (15) | 11 (55) | 7 (21) | 9 (47) | 3 (15) | 5 (50) | 3 (10) | 5 (71) | 4 (16.7) | 7 (63.6) | 0 | 2 (9) | 0 | 1 (4) | 1 (2) | 3 (12) |
| Staged per diem charge depend on length of stay | 1 (2) | 0 | 1 (2) | 2 (10) | 1 (3) | 2 (11) | 0 | 1 (10) | 0 | 0 | 0 | 1 (9.1) | 0 | 0 | 0 | 0 | 0 | 0 |
| Per admission rate | 2 (3) | 0 | 0 | 0 | 0 | 0 | 1 (5) | 2 (20) | 2 (7) | 0 | 1 (4.2) | 3 (27.3) | 1 (2) | 0 | 0 | 0 | 0 | 0 |
| Per visit–procedure rate | 0 | 2 (7) | 0 | 0 | 0 | 0 | 0 | 1 (10) | 0 | 0 | 0 | 2 (18.2) | 1 (2) | 6 (27) | 1 (2) | 5 (21) | 1 (2) | 9 (36) |
| Capitation | 0 | 1 (4) | 0 | 0 | 0 | 2 (11) | 0 | 0 | 0 | 0 | 0 | 0 | 0 | 0 | 0 | 0 | 0 | 0 |
| Negotiated method | 0 | 0 | 0 | 0 | 0 | 0 | 0 | 0 | 0 | 0 | 0 | 0 | 0 | 0 | 0 | 0 | 0 | 0 |
| Other | 0 | 1 (4) | 0 | 0 | 0 | 1 (5) | 0 | 2 (20) | 0 | 1 (14) | 0 | 0 | 0 | 0 | 0 | 0 | 0 | 0 |
| Applicable | 62 | 27 | 41 | 20 | 34 | 19 | 20 | 10 | 31 | 7 | 24 | 11 | 59 | 22 | 57 | 24 | 57 | 25 |
| Missing | 1 | 7 | 0 | 8 | 8 | 4 | 2 | 3 | 14 | 7 | 1 | 2 | 1 | 3 | 4 | 10 | 2 | 0 |
| Not applicable | 1 | 4 | 23 | 10 | 22 | 15 | 42 | 25 | 19 | 24 | 39 | 25 | 4 | 13 | 3 | 4 | 5 | 13 |
| Total | 64 | 38 | 64 | 38 | 64 | 38 | 64 | 38 | 64 | 38 | 64 | 38 | 64 | 38 | 64 | 38 | 64 | 38 |

* S/N = Staff and network.

reason for wishing to change an arrangement with a hospital (see Table 10). Also, one administrator pointed out that it is not unusual for full billed charges at one hospital to be less than discounted charges at another hospital. Full billed charges are never used by staff or network HMOs.

Reimbursement methods used by IPAs and staff–network plans were more closely aligned for hospital outpatient services (e.g., emergency department or ambulatory surgery) than for inpatient services. Table 14 shows that more than 70% of all contracts used a specified percentage discount to pay for outpatient services. In the remaining 30% of the contracts, IPAs almost always paid full billed charges, whereas staff and network plans generally used per-visit or per-procedure rates.

We also looked at reimbursement method by case study in the two sites represented in our study, each of which had two HMOs. In case study site 1, the home of an IPA and a staff HMO, a specified percentage discount from charges was used over 86% of the time, except for obstetrics, where it was still the predominant reimbursement method. The use of the specified discount by two disparate plans suggests reimbursement mechanisms are at least partially market driven, relating to the atmosphere of the environment as well as the type of HMO plan.

In case study 3, the site of two mature network models, reimbursement for about two thirds of the contracts was a flat per diem rate regardless of length of stay; the other one third of the contracts specified a percentage discount from charges. Chemical dependency was reimbursed in a number of ways, apparently depending more on the hospitals involved than on the HMOs. This was also the case with tertiary care, suggesting that availability of unique services rather than HMO model type dictates reimbursement modes in this market.

## CONCLUSION

Several important trends are evident from these data. The HMOs have taken a very proactive role in initiating and negotiating contracts. About one half of the 102 contracts were initiated by the HMOs, and the rest were jointly initiated. Provisions in the contracts made them easy to terminate, with or without cause. The contracts were also easy to change; most were reviewed annually, renegotiated on a yearly basis, or maintained as an open-ended arrangement.

Seventy-three of the contracts were in the midst of change, according to the HMOs. The most frequent change to occur was for the IPAs to concentrate services; the next two most important areas where changes were desired were price and payment arrangements. This substantiates our finding that price is not a matter of initial concern, but that after a relationship with a hospital is established, price and payment methods are attended to and frequently changed.

Almost all of the 102 hospitals with contracts were used for medical–surgical admissions, but fewer were used for mental health, and only one-third were used for chemical dependency. In terms of patient concentration, we found that staff and network plans concentrated patients more effectively than IPAs, even though they were increasingly being pressured to expand access.

Ability to concentrate patients appears to be related to size of discounts received. For example, in medical–surgical contracts (where the data are most complete), staff and network HMOs got a 26% discount, on average, compared to a discount of 4% in IPA contracts. Differences in discounts are statistically significant in every case where inpatient data were reported by staff and network plans and IPAs.

Inpatient reimbursement methods also appear to be contingent on the type of plan, with IPAs using a specified percentage discount from charges, and staff and network HMOs using a flat per diem payment. A substantial number of the IPA contracts, but none of the contracts negotiated by staff or network plans, still pay full billed charges.

●    ●    ●

Our study was limited because only a few HMOs could be asked to participate. Therefore, the results may not be fully generalizable. Nevertheless, by selecting HMOs of different model types in different market environments, we were able to observe that patient concentration and discounts are largely determined by HMO model type, whereas reimbursement methods appear to be at least partially market driven.

In general, we conclude that HMOs are becoming more aggressive in placing hospitals in competition with each other for HMO patients. The degrees of patient concentration and discounts received by some HMOs in our study are impressive. These results, which differ from those of studies done 5 or 10 years ago, provide new evidence of competition in the market for hospital services.

## REFERENCES

1. Manning, W.G., et al. "A Controlled Clinical Trial of the Effect of Prepaid Group Practice on Use of Resources." *New England Journal of Medicine* 310, (1984): 1505–10.

2. Dowd, B., et al "Use of Health Care Services in Twin Cities Health Plans: A Tobit Model With Selectivity." Paper presented at the 115th Annual Meeting of the American Public Health Association, New Orleans, La., October 18–22, 1987.

3. Kralewski, J.E., Countryman, D., and Shatin, D. "Patterns of Interorganizational Relationships Between Hospitals and HMOs." *Inquiry* 19 (1982): 357–62.

4. Kralewski, J.E., Countryman, D. and Pitt, L. "Hospital and Health Maintenance Organization Financial Agreements for Inpatient Services: A Case Study of the Minneapolis/St. Paul Area." *Health Care Financing Review* 4, no. 4 (1983): 79–84.

5. Kralewski, J.E., Doth, D.S., Rosenberg, R.G., and Burnes, D.G. "HMO–Hospital Relationships: An Exploratory Study." *Health Care Management Review* 8, no. 2 (1983): 27–35.

6. Aquilina, D., and Appel, G.L. "HMOs' Real Competitive Role." *Hospitals* 57, no. 17 (1983): 80–92.

7. Feldman, R., et al. "Effects of HMOs on the Creation of Competitive Markets for Hospital Services." Paper presented at the Fifth Annual Meeting of the Association for Health Services Research, San Francisco, Calif., June 26–28, 1988.

8. *HMO Summary: June 1985.* Excelsior, Minn.: InterStudy, 1985.

9. Scherer, F.M. *Industrial Market Structure and Economic Performance.* Chicago: Rand McNally, 1971.

# Product lines in a complex marketplace: Matching organizational strategy to buyer behavior

William N. Zelman
and
Curtis P. McLaughlin

*Product-line strategy should be developed in relation to markets. This article focuses on designing product-line strategy in relation to four purchaser types: (1) traditional purchasers, (2) motivated purchasers, (3) HMO-type purchasers, and (4) PPO-type purchasers. In many cases, product-line strategy may have to adopt various combinations of the above.*

*Health Care Manage Rev*, 1990, 15(2), 9–14
© 1990 Aspen Publishers, Inc.

**Product-line management** has two very important concerns: the product and the market.[1] In developing product lines, hospitals can be product-driven or market-driven or can accommodate both perspectives.[2,3] By tradition, hospitals have tended to be product-oriented and have tended to focus on producing services as opposed to servicing markets. However, introduction of the prospective payment system (PPS), increased competition, alternate delivery systems, and growing acceptance of strategic planning and marketing have all contributed to an increased focus on marketing.

A fundamental attribute of the health care field is that health care organizations must serve many markets, including patients and potential patients, payers, caregivers, regulators, and the community. Each of these markets can serve as the basis for organizing product lines. This article discusses organizing product lines around purchasers.

## BUYER BEHAVIOR

Figure 1 illustrates two important characteristics of health care buyer behavior: the segmentation of the services purchased and the contractual arrangement thereof. The first dimension, segmentation, is shown on the vertical axis of Figure 1 and refers to whether services are purchased in a bundle or as discrete services: that is, whether the purchaser (patient or third party) chooses to purchase a comprehensive set of services from one source or to shop among providers for specific services on the basis of price and quality.

The second dimension, contractual arrangement, shown on the horizontal axis of Figure 1, refers to the nature of the relationship between the payer and provider of services, whether or not there is a specific, prearranged contract between the provider and the insurer covering the care of the patient.

### The traditional purchaser

The historical pattern for the purchase of health care is represented in the upper left-hand quadrant of Figure 1. In this pattern, a purchaser of care pays on a noncon-

**William N. Zelman**, *Ph.D., C.P.A., is an Associate Professor in the Department of Health Policy and Administration, School of Public Health, University of North Carolina at Chapel Hill.*

**Curtis P. McLaughlin**, *D.B.A., is a Professor in the School of Business Administration and the Department of Health Policy and Administration, School of Public Health, University of North Carolina at Chapel Hill.*

---

FIGURE 1

---

TYPES OF BUYERS OF HEALTH CARE SERVICES

---

|  | Segmentation decision | |
|  | **Bundled** | **Discrete** |
| **Noncontractual (indemnity insurance)** | Traditional purchaser | Motivated purchaser |
| **Contractual (managed care)** | HMO-type purchaser | PPO-type purchaser |

*Contractual arrangement* (row axis label)

---

tractual basis for a bundle of services that has already been provided. In such instances, the amount paid will be all or a portion of the amount billed by the provider, who has been chosen by the patient and who determines what services are necessary. The situation represented in this quadrant is thought of with nostalgia by many providers.

The traditional purchaser frequently "pays the first dollar" of physician and hospital fees and leaves all of the health-related decision making to the provider. This quadrant is characterized by few controls: no provider contracts, no peer review, no preadmission screening, and low deductibles and copayments. It is similar to the original indemnity policy, which was popular in the 1940s.

**The motivated purchaser**

The upper right-hand quadrant of Figure 1 represents a cost- and quality-motivated buyer who seeks care through a number of providers and whose payment relationship with the provider is noncontractual. These motivated buyers may, however, provide any number

---

*The traditional purchaser frequently "pays the first dollar" of physician and hospital fees and leaves all of the health-related decision making to the provider.*

---

of incentives, disincentives, and constraints to motivate patients or potential patients to be more judicious in their health care choices. For instance, employers and insurance companies have added a number of inducements to indemnity policies to increase buyer awareness of costs and to reward rational purchase behavior. To capture patients' attention, insurers have increasingly relied on copayments and deductibles and have increasingly put constraints on specific provider behaviors, such as stipulating that certain procedures must be done on an outpatient basis unless prior approval is received and requiring second opinions.

The federal government also is directly involved in such activities. For example, large-scale buyers like the Health Care Financing Administration (HCFA) have emphasized that hospital costs and death rates should be published (the latter is presumably a measure of quality). This information may be aimed at individuals, corporate buyers, and referring physicians, but in all cases, the motivation of the purchaser is similar: to influence provider behavior or the decision maker's choice of providers.

**The health maintenance organization (HMO)–type purchaser**

While the services in the top row of Figure 1 are purchased without a previously negotiated financial arrangement, contractual purchasing of services before they are needed can be appealing to the sophisticated corporate purchaser. Such options, frequently referred to as *managed care,* are depicted in the bottom row of Figure 1.

The lower left-hand quadrant of Figure 1 represents services purchased in a bundle under contract. The best example of this is the employer who contracts with an HMO, which agrees to completely manage and provide the health care of its enrollees. In such instances, the employer usually does not have to manage use or take on the risks of cost overruns, because the HMO does. This option shifts many decisions and risks to the provider and is a major contractual option for smaller employers and insurers.

### The preferred provider organization (PPO)–type purchaser

The lower right-hand quadrant of Figure 1 represents services purchased discretely with a separate contractual agreement covering each group of services. For example, many PPOs arrange physicals at previously negotiated rates through one provider and other services through other providers. The PPO-type purchaser should ideally be quite sophisticated in his or her ability to evaluate providers' past performance and capabilities in order to select among them and should have considerable clout in the marketplace to negotiate rates.

## BUYER BEHAVIOR AND PRODUCT-LINE STRATEGY

Focusing on product segmentation helps orient the provider toward product management strategy. Focusing on the contractual arrangement orients the purchaser toward market management (see Figure 2).

### Product concerns

Consider segmentation first. If the buyer is purchasing services as a bundle, then the product-line strategy must emphasize breadth or range of services, perhaps at the expense of depth. This focus requires considerable internal coordination among services and an emphasis on managing patients as well as services.

On the other hand, if the purchaser is purchasing services on a one-by-one basis, then product-line strategy must focus on strong product identification, management, and marketing. Primacy must be given to specialization, perhaps at the expense of being a full-service organization. In such instances, product lines should be conceptualized vertically, with emphasis on single services, their substitutes, and their complements. The numerous medical and surgical alternatives in the cardiovascular area offer a useful example.

---

**FIGURE 2**

---

PRODUCT-LINE STRATEGY IN RESPONSE TO BUYER BEHAVIOR

| | Segmentation decision | |
| | Bundled | Discrete |
|---|---|---|
| **Noncontractual** | Offer range of services. Focus marketing efforts on patients, potential patients, and referral sources. | Specialize. Focus marketing efforts on patients, potential patients, and referral sources. |
| **Contractual arrangement** **Contractual** | Emphasize continuity of care. Focus marketing efforts on patients, potential patients, employers, third parties, and enrollees. | Decentralize authority. Focus marketing efforts on patients, potential patients, employers, third parties, and enrollees. |

**FIGURE 3**

POSSIBLE PROVIDER RESPONSES TO MARKET STRUCTURES

| Contractual arrangement | Segmentation decision: Bundled dominant | Segmentation decision: Discrete dominant |
| --- | --- | --- |
| Noncontractual dominant | *1. Traditional purchaser* Develop broad service and general marketing capabilities. | *2. Motivated purchaser* Offer a narrow range of specialty services. Target marketing efforts. Strongly coordinate marketing and production functions. |
| Contractual dominant | *3. HMO-type purchaser* Develop broad service capability. Target marketing efforts primarily to employers, third parties, and enrollees. | *4. PPO-type purchaser* Offer a narrow range of specialty services. Target marketing efforts primarily to patients and potential patients, employers, and third parties. Set up strategic business units. |

### Market concerns

The contractual dimension emphasizes the marketing function as opposed to the product function of product-line management. Marketing in this case should include a broad range of marketing tasks including market identification, assessment, planning, development, and management.

As noted in Figure 2, the two types of contractual arrangements are noncontractual and contractual. If the purchase is to be noncontractual, then product-line strategy should direct marketing efforts to patients and potential patients and to referral sources. On the other hand, if the purchase is to be made on a contractual basis, then marketing efforts must be directed to patients, potential patients, employers, or other third parties influencing the contracting decision.

### Considering product and market concerns together

Both of these dimensions, product and market, come together in Figure 3, which shows appropriate strategies for each of the four logical combinations of product and market strategies. If the product-line strategy is to operate in quadrant 1, characterized by traditional purchasers, then the appropriate product-line strategy should be to provide a wide variety of services with marketing efforts directed to a wide variety of patients and referral sources.

*Many urban communities consist of many types of purchasers, no one of which dominates.*

If the product-line strategy is to operate in quadrant 2 with a preponderance of motivated purchasers, then the appropriate strategy is to identify, manage, and market specific services to specific potential patient markets and referral sources. The difference between these first two product-line strategies is one of degree: In the case of the motivated shopper, services will be

---

## FIGURE 4

---

### POSSIBLE PROVIDER RESPONSES TO MARKET STRUCTURES, INCLUDING MIXED BUYER BEHAVIOR

| | | Market structure | |
|---|---|---|---|
| | **Bundled dominant** | **Mixed** | **Discrete dominant** |
| **Noncontractual dominant** | Develop broad service and general marketing capabilities. | Offer a midrange of services, but focus on certain specialties. Target marketing efforts to general population and specific target groups. | Offer a narrow range of specialty services. Target marketing efforts. Strongly coordinate marketing and production functions. |
| **Contractual arrangement    Mixed** | Develop broad service capability. Target marketing efforts to general population, employers, third parties, and enrollees. | Offer a midrange of services, but focus on certain specialties. Target marketing efforts to general population, target groups, employers, third parties, employees, patients, potential patients, and enrollees. | Offer a narrow range of specialty services. Target marketing efforts to patients and potential patients, employers, and third parties. Strongly coordinate marketing and production functions. |
| **Contractual dominant** | Develop broad service capability. Target marketing efforts primarily to employers, third parties, and enrollees. | Offer a midrange of services, but focus on certain specialties. Target market efforts primarily to employers, third parties, patients, potential patients, and enrollees. | Offer a narrow range of specialty services. Target marketing efforts primarily to patients, potential patients, and third parties. Set up strategic business units. |

---

fewer and narrower and the number of targeted markets will probably be greater.

A product strategy that focuses on quadrant 3, characterized by HMO-type purchasers, should emphasize a broad range of services and managed care. Marketing strategy may be broad or focused as the market dictates but should target enrollees *and* employers. Finally, in quadrant 4, which is characterized by PPO-type buyers, product strategy should be specialized while market strategy should focus on patients, employers, and insurers.

### Serving several market segments at once

Note that each of the above four alternatives assumes a market largely dominated by one type of payer. However, many urban communities consist of many types of purchasers, no one of which dominates. If this is the case, a provider may want to appeal to various types of purchasers and thus operate in several market segments at once, adopting a hybrid product-line approach, with the added intermediate possibilities of a mixed position (see Figure 4).

As the market moves toward the bottom of Figure 4, more marketing energies have to focus on employers and third parties as well as patients. As the market moves to the right in Figure 4, more segmenting of product development and delivery is necessary. Finally, as one proceeds from the upper left toward the lower right of the matrix, one progresses from the status quo toward new marketing and organizational arrangements. The further the market moves toward the bottom right, the more marketing and product efforts should resemble those of strategic business units, characterized by high specialization, autonomy, and accountability.

## ORGANIZATIONAL IMPLICATIONS

Product-line strategy should vary with the characteristics of the buyer market. Five points should be considered as the organization maps out its product-line strategy.

First, "Business as usual," providing a wide range of services to a broad population together with generalized marketing efforts, is likely to be an inappropriate strategy in many markets. Second, to the extent that purchasers begin to buy care through negotiated contracts, development of the market management function of organizations will be crucial to organizational success.

Third, to the extent that purchasers purchase discrete services, the characteristics of key services rather than the breadth of the product line become important. This may mean that certain services may have to be expanded or modified, while others may have to be eliminated.

Fourth, the organization should realize that trying to serve a complex market may mean adopting many of the characteristics of a loosely coupled organization as suggested by Weick[4] and putting even more time, resources, and energy into coordinating its product-line efforts. Furthermore, earlier and more careful attention must be given to the use of coordinators, joint training, communication mechanisms, and effective committees to plan and implement product-line market and service components. Top committees must deal with broader issues affecting multiple product lines, while many operating decisions will be pushed down to a lower level. More people must participate in the governance process, not fewer.

Fifth and last, difficulties can be expected as the organization attempts to (1) move from a matrix organization to strong product-line control, (2) combine market and product manager functions in some product lines and keep them separate in others, (3) develop interdisciplinary product lines, and (4) make some services product lines and keep the organization functioning in a more traditional manner in others. Thus, there are likely to be problems no matter what changes are made in attempting to strategically position the organization in a complex marketplace.

The important first step is not to commit prematurely to one form of product-line organization but to prepare the organization for real product-line management, regardless of which form proves best. This preparation will include the following actions:

- get people to think about possible roles and organizational structures and unfreeze their thinking about how services could and should be organized and managed under various market structures.
- familiarize the staff and administration with the true role of the product-line manager, regardless of the organizational structure.
- select and train potential product-line managers, who must be individuals with professional knowledge, management skills, social standing, and interpersonal skills adequate to carry out the role of a true product-line manager.
- experiment with new product-line organizations within subunits of the hospital (such as the outpatient department and fitness programs) to give potential leaders a chance to grow and to acclimate people to new reporting systems, power structures, and working relationships.

Then, as the market picture becomes clearer, the organization can move decisively.

## REFERENCES

1. Zelman, W.N., and Parham, D.L. "Strategic, Operational, and Marketing Concerns of Product-Line Management in Health Care." *Health Care Management Review* 15, no. 1 (1990): 29–35.
2. Ames, B.C. "Dilemma of Product/Market Management." *Harvard Business Review* 49, no. 2 (1971): 66–74.
3. MacStravic, S. "Market Administration in Health Care Delivery." *Health Care Management Review* 14, no. 1 (1989): 41–48.
4. Weick, K. "Educational Organizations as Loosely Coupled Organizations." *Administrative Science Quarterly* 21, no. 1 (1976): 1–19.

# A hospital administrator's guide to successful HMO negotiations

Michael B. Matthews

*Many issues must be considered when hospitals negotiate with HMOs. Hospital administrators can improve negotiations with HMOs by understanding the philosophy and terminology of alternative delivery programs, as well as their hospital's own operating requirements.*

*Health Care Manage Rev*, 1987, 12(4), 77–79
© 1987 Aspen Publishers, Inc.

**Hospitals will become** increasingly dependent on health maintenance organizations (HMOs) for revenue streams as these programs continue their proliferation in the marketplace. Yet most hospital administrators have not committed resources sufficient to deal with these powerful new forces. The result of these two factors is that hospitals may engage in relationships not in their long-term best interest, or worse still, may make the critical mistake of being too passive and not get the opportunity to affiliate with these new payers in any manner whatsoever.

Nine steps can be used to assist a hospital in becoming a beneficiary—rather than a victim—of the transition to an alternative delivery systems environment.

## STEP 1. ANALYZE THE MARKETPLACE

In the near future, HMOs are not going to go away; nor are they going to represent 100 percent of a hospital's revenues. However, understanding what happens to the bottom line at various points between these extremes is critical in determining a hospital's range of options. Financial models should be developed to explore alternative market scenarios, addressed in the following questions.

- What if HMO market penetration grows from 5 percent to 25 percent or 50 percent? What factors influence such growth?
- What if the hospital's share of HMO business remains constant or shifts significantly?
- What if overall community admission rates fall as HMOs grow to influence the health care delivery system?
- What if the hospital must expand its outpatient activity to accommodate the HMO philosophies and procedures?

## STEP 2. ESTABLISH DECISION CRITERIA

HMOs are uniform neither in the way their programs are designed nor in the objectives they establish for hospital affiliation. Establishing criteria for deciding with whom and on what terms the provider wishes to affiliate can facilitate common understand-

**Michael B. Matthews,** *M.S.P.H., is Vice President of Corporate Planning and Marketing for Akron City Hospital, Akron, Ohio. He has been active in health systems analysis for ten years.*

ing among the board, medical staff, and management staff. Such criteria could include the following:

- impact on medical staff relations;
- financial impact on the hospital;
- marketability of the product;
- financial solvency of the program;
- model design, including presence of risks and incentives; and
- potential for increasing new business.

## STEP 3. UNDERSTAND THE FINANCIAL REQUIREMENTS

HMOs know what they can afford to pay for hospital services and still remain price competitive with their premiums. Hospitals must analyze their own data to know what flexibility they may have in establishing prices sufficient to attract the interest of HMOs. Linking financial requirements to incentives the HMO offers its members to use a particular facility is a good approach.

## STEP 4. EDUCATE THE BOARD

Board reaction to HMO developments can range from apathy to too much concern. To plan properly, board members should understand the value of appropriately designed relationships with alternative delivery programs. Seminars, outside consultation, and retreats have been used successfully for this purpose.

## STEP 5. INVOLVE THE MEDICAL STAFF

An HMO cannot succeed without physician participation, and most physicians cannot act without proper information. Establishing good channels of communication with the medical staff can facilitate physician decision making. Physicians have established advisory committees regarding alternative delivery systems at a number of hospitals to provide analyses and recommendations to their colleagues. Executing hospital–HMO contracts without having acceptable physician–HMO contracts can only lead to conflict with the medical staff.

## STEP 6. SPEAK THE HMO's LANGUAGE

Preferred provider organizations are usually easy to deal with because they typically want a simple discount of billed charges. HMOs, on the other hand, seek alternative financial arrangements, such as per diem, per case, or capitation contracts. The hospital's charges should be analyzed from these perspectives to satisfy the HMO's need for rate predictability and the hospital's need for appropriately priced services.

## STEP 7. RECOGNIZE THE RISKS AND REWARDS OF EACH PROPOSAL

Per diems, diagnosis related group schedules, and fixed-price outpatient surgery schedules each place the hospital at some risk. The assumptions that went into setting the rates may not hold in reality, and costs could actually be higher than expected. This is a problem since revenue is locked into the contracted rate structure for a negotiated time period. However, incentives can usually be worked into HMO contracts to reward the hospital for performance. The trade-off between incentives and risks within each individual contract must be judged from each hospital's philosophical constructs.

## STEP 8. INVOLVE THE OPERATIONS STAFF

What may seem like simple language in a contract could create nightmares for the operations staff. The medical records, admissions, billing, and utilization review staffs should review proposed contracts to determine operational problems. Also, following through with these departments after HMO contracts have been executed can significantly increase the chance of success for any program.

## STEP 9. MONITOR THE IMPACT OF THE HMO CONTRACTS

Most hospital information systems are ill prepared to handle the demands of multiple financial reimbursement arrangements. This compounds the problem of appropriately monitoring performance under HMO contracts. It is much better to develop this capability now than when the HMOs become 30 percent of the business.

● ● ●

These steps are by no means simple. But by developing a strategic plan that incorporates these steps, the hospital can move into a position of negotiating positively and not reacting to HMO negotiations out of fear or weakness. HMOs are beginning to recognize, to some extent, that for them to maintain long-term viability and success in the marketplace, they must establish positive negotiations with providers, resulting in win–win relationships in the long run. By the same token, hospitals must accept the notion that HMOs are here to stay. To engage in negotiations from a stance of hostility is to end any hope of establishing a long-term, fruitful relationship.

# Critical factors for successful hospital-based case management

Frank G. Williams,
Louise H. Warrick,
Jon B. Christianson,
and
F. Ellen Netting

*Six hospitals were funded to develop programs for long-term case management. Factors that should be considered when developing hospital-based case management are discussed within three areas: organizational placement, program management, and financial viability.*

A **major purpose** of case management is to maximize the effective use of resources by ensuring that individuals receive health and social services appropriate to their needs. It is a process that involves assessing the needs of individuals, agreeing on a plan of care, making referrals to appropriate services, monitoring, and evaluating outcomes.

Hospital-based case management can include both short- and long-term components. Short-term case management is used to facilitate transition of patients from hospitalization. The care of patients is managed by nursing and social service staff following discharge, typically for one to three months. Under prospective payment, short-term case management can be a cost-effective means to facilitate patient recovery.

In long-term case management, case managers continue to assist the disabled and frail elderly for extended periods, often two years or more. Some hospitals see it as a needed service in their communities that may have the potential to maintain ties with patients and generate revenues after hospitalization. Medicare's reported intent to hold hospitals financially responsible for services received following hospitalization will, of course, intensify hospital interest in case management.

From an administrative perspective, case management involves two elements: patient advocacy and resource control. Patient advocacy is the primary function of case managers in traditional community-based settings. Their task has been to find scarce resources for the frail elderly and physically and mentally disabled clients

*Frank G. Williams, Ph.D., Associate Professor in the School of Health Administration and Policy, College of Business, Arizona State University. His research interests are in the areas of rural health, long-term care, and reimbursement policy.*

*Louise H. Warrick, Dr.P.H., is Research Assistant Professor, Department of Family and Community Medicine, University of Arizona. Her areas of interest are maternal and child health and long-term care.*

*Jon B. Christianson, Ph.D., is Professor in the Division of Health Services Research at the School of Public Health, University of Minnesota. His research interests are in capitated financing and rural health care.*

*F. Ellen Netting, Ph.D., A.C.S.W., is Associate Professor of Social Work at Arizona State University. Her major areas of research focus on nonprofit organizations and the regulations and oversight of housing and health care for the elderly.*

Funding for this project was provided by the Flinn Foundation of Phoenix, Arizona. The authors express their appreciation to the hospitals who participated in this demonstration.

with chronic needs. In hospital and managed care environments more emphasis is placed on resource control.

Hospital-based case management usually begins at the time of discharge or at the completion of home health or rehabilitative care. However, prospective payment has focused attention on controlling the use of resources during the course of treatment as well. Administrators are beginning to use the term "case management" to refer to a type of utilization review process that is more prospective and broader in scope. The goal is to plan and monitor a cost-effective course of treatment rather than wait to certify major services and additional days of hospital stay as requested.

In this article the authors identify factors that should be considered by hospitals in developing case management programs. The authors' observations are based on an evaluation of a demonstration program in which six hospitals in Arizona and New Mexico established long-term case management programs with foundation support. The Flinn Foundation's Hospital-Based Coordinated Care (HBCC) program was designed to assess the feasibility of acute care hospitals providing continuous intensive case management and coordination of community-based resources. The overall objective was for the hospital-based case management programs to become sufficiently cost effective and integrated into their parent organizations so as to be continued after grant funding ended.

Four hospitals in Arizona were selected to participate in the demonstration program in October 1985. In January 1987, two New Mexico hospitals were awarded similar grants. Table 1 provides a summary of the characteristics of the six programs.

Unlike most previous publicly supported case management demonstration programs,[1] the Flinn HBCC sites were expected to attract clients who could pay for at least some of their services. HBCC case managers did not have funds to purchase services. Consequently, their activities were focused primarily on service coordination and care planning. Evaluation of the HBCC program yielded evidence that the hospitals were able to provide case management of acceptable quality and enhance the continuum of services in their communities. However, the demonstration programs confronted a variety of problems that made it difficult for them to be integrated into their hospitals and to become financially viable.[2] These problems, and the way in which they arose, suggest some important considerations for hospitals considering the implementation of case management programs.

## METHODS

Several data sources were used in this analysis. Two sets of structured interviews were conducted at each site. These interviews occurred during the first and last six

## TABLE 1

### CASE MANAGEMENT PROGRAM SITE CHARACTERISTICS

| | Hospital* | | | | | |
|---|---|---|---|---|---|---|
| | A | B | C | D | E | F |
| Licensed beds | 282 | 203 | 380 | 129 | 477 | 265 |
| Program located in or out of hospital | | | | | | |
| Beginning of grant | In | In | Out | Out | Out | In |
| End of grant | Out | In | Out | In | Out | In |
| Staffing† | Mix | RN | RN | Mix | SW | SW |
| Utilized volunteers | No | No | Yes | Yes | Yes | Yes |
| ALOS in case management program (days) | 351 | 280 | 384 | 363 | 293 | 262 |

*Hospital D was rural, the others urban.
† Case manager staffing:
RN=Program used registered nurses as case managers.
SW=Program used social workers as case managers, with a nurse consultant.
Mix=Program used both RNs and SWs as case managers.

months of program operations. Common interview protocols were developed for comparable positions across sites, with 12 to 15 interviews conducted at each site during each visit. Program directors, case managers, social service directors, discharge planners, home care directors, volunteer coordinators, and administrators were interviewed at all hospital sites. In addition, community-based individuals were interviewed, including referral sources, service providers, and Area Agency on Aging staff. After each site visit, interview notes were summarized and returned to respondents so they could correct inaccuracies and expand on previous answers. In addition, the authors conferred with program staff on an ongoing basis during the demonstration and visited each site at least once every six months.

## RESULTS

The overall objective of the case management programs becoming permanently integrated into their parent organizations was only partially met at best. When the grant ended, two of the programs were terminated by their host hospitals, two were downsized and inte-

---

*The overall objective of the case management programs becoming permanently integrated into their parent organizations was only partially met at best.*

---

grated into hospital utilization management, one was merged into an alternative case management program, and one evolved into a shorter-term model of case management. What factors explain these different outcomes with respect to integration of the programs into their sponsoring hospitals? From evaluation, factors were grouped into three categories: organizational placement, program management, and financial viability.

### Organizational placement

The organizational placement of programs reflected whether case management was viewed as integral to the total management of a hospitalized patient. The majority of the programs were located organizationally as a separate department. Only one program was placed as part of a continuum of care for hospital patients in its coordinated care department. At the end of the demonstration when hospital administrators looked for evidence of cost savings to the hospital, many were surprised to learn that

their programs had not targeted exclusively hospital patients at discharge. In fact, several programs drew the majority of their patients from referrals by community agencies. In an effort to refocus program efforts on ways in which hospitals might financially benefit from case management, three of the programs were organizationally relocated back into the hospital within their respective utilization review departments.

Physical location and relocations of the programs also reflected whether case management became viewed as a part of the hospital. Initially, only two programs were located within their parent hospitals. While this separation did not directly interfere with case management activities, it lessened the opportunity for case managers to work with hospital discharge planners and may have been symbolic of lack of hospital commitment to the program or understanding of its goals. Both of these hospitals terminated their programs at the end of the demonstration.

Physical and organizational proximity to hospital functions facilitated program integration by promoting a focus on hospitalized patients, enhancing program visibility, and encouraging relationships with hospital providers. Table 2 provides a summary of the design characteristics deemed successful by hospital administrators.

### Program management

At the end of the demonstration there were two programs without directors, two with full-time directors, and two with part-time directors. The amount of time program directors devoted to the program varied, and half of the programs experienced turnover of program directors. The programs that did not have a program director at the end of the demonstration were also those programs that experienced director turnover, and that operated in an environment of severe fiscal restraint and several upper-level administrative restructurings. At the end of the demonstration, one of these programs was closed and one was under consideration for closure.

The type of person selected to be program director was important to program development. Some program directors were selected because of their clinical skills, with the expectation that they would play an important role in ensuring the quality of client care. While this was true to some extent, the more effective directors appeared to be those who were able to relate closely to the hospital's primary mission, irrespective of their professional backgrounds. These directors also developed ready access to hospital or corporate administrators with whom there was a mutual understanding of program objectives and strategies to achieve self-sufficiency. For the hospital ad-

## TABLE 2

CHARACTERISTICS OF CASE MANAGEMENT PROGRAMS JUDGED TO BE SUCCESSFUL BY HOSPITAL
ADMINISTRATORS

|  | Successful | Unsuccessful |
|---|---|---|
| Program location | In-hospital<br>Within utilization management | Out-of-hospital<br>Separate department |
| Program focus | Hospital mission | Undefined or on community development |
| Case management focus | Short-term, nurse intensive | Long-term, community-based support services |
| Client recruitment | Hospital clients | Community clients* |
| Outreach | To hospital staff, discharge planners, and medical staff | To community |
| Program director | Program as the primary responsibility | Part-time or absent |
| Hospital financial environment | Fiscally stable | Fiscally unstable |
| Hospital administration | Involved in defining program objectives and strategies to document program effectiveness | Uninvolved, late emphasis on documenting program effectiveness |

*Unless these clients were a source of revenue sufficient to sustain program.

ministrator, case management could be seen as a program that was very time consuming with little personal payoff. With limited administrative attention, the capability of the program director as a manager appeared to be more important to program success than the director's clinical skills.

In all cases the introduction of the new case management program disrupted established professional relationships. Continuous efforts were needed on the part of program directors and case managers to convince discharge planners, social workers, and physicians of the value of case management and to educate them concerning the role of the case manager. Where lack of clarity over professional responsibility for patient care persisted, program integration was hindered. In two programs strained relationships between case management staff and discharge planners were never resolved. In one there was a difficult relationship with the home health program that persisted throughout the demonstration. At the end of the funding period, hospital administrators at two sites noted the problem and its negative impact on the lack of referrals of high-risk hospital patients to the case management program. They addressed the issue by reorganizing these programs into their utilization review

units. Failure to successfully negotiate interdepartmental relationships was a major factor that impeded successful program development.

Complex interdepartmental relationships also led to complex and time-consuming processes for recruiting case management clients. Case managers at the sites used several creative methods to obtain hospital-based referrals. They reviewed admission records, attended discharge planning conferences, and met with home health nurses and hospital social workers to identify appropriate clients. At one site a case management nurse walked the floors looking for potential clients.

Community-based referrals were obtained by professional networking with senior advocacy groups and agencies. One site targeted outreach efforts to physicians through periodic columns in newsletters, personal visits from the program's nurse consultant, presentations at clinical meetings, and a yearly marketing survey.

Upper-level management understanding of, and commitment to, the program clearly, and not surprisingly, were important factors related to program survival. Except for one site, hospital-based case management was a new concept for the hospital's administrators. All the sponsoring organizations over the demonstration period experienced fiscal problems resulting in organization-wide staff reductions, program closures, and administrative restructuring. In order for the demonstration programs to survive the fiscal and administrative turmoil in their host hospitals, they required visibility and support from upper-level administrators.

The potential benefits of case management in discharge planning and managed care programs attracted the interest of most hospital administrators, and they looked for documentation of cost savings in these areas. Program attempts to measure productivity and cost effectiveness occurred when upper-level management was involved in the demonstration on an early and continuing basis. Without ongoing top-level administrative input, programs tended to lose their focus on hospital needs, shifting to a broader community focus over time. When administrators were committed to senior services as part of the hospital mission and were able to define how case management could contribute to cost savings, programs developed in a quite different way. In this case, the program would focus on recruiting at-risk hospital discharged patients; staff felt they were part of the larger organization and their purpose was explicitly defined; staff was supportive of the need to document the effects of case management, and there was less uncertainty about the future of the program, thereby raising staff morale.

In three programs, case managers were concerned that their hospital administrators lacked an understanding of how case management functioned and how it could benefit patients. This lack of understanding, in their opinion, was reflected in a lack of institutional support for the case management program as evidenced by isolation from hospital departments and frequent changes in program leadership.

### Financial viability

Case management is not generally covered by third party reimbursement. It was hoped that the case management programs could achieve financial viability by directly charging patients for their services and by generating increased hospital admissions and outpatient services. The programs could also benefit hospitals through avoided medical costs if the programs facilitated earlier discharge of Medicare patients or avoided non-reimbursable readmissions.

The decisions made to discontinue or merge the programs at the end of the grant, however, were based on data relating only to direct revenues from patient charges, which were very small. Little or no data were collected by the hospitals concerning indirect revenues

*Even with optimistic assumptions about indirect revenues and avoided costs, none of the programs appeared capable of reaching break-even levels when the grant ended.*

generated by the programs or costs avoided. Nevertheless, even with optimistic assumptions about indirect revenues and avoided costs, none of the programs appeared capable of reaching break-even levels when the grant ended. The average annual cost of operating a coordinated care program in the six demonstration hospitals was approximately $200,000, with a range from $157,000 to $284,000. Approximately 95 percent of these costs were borne directly or indirectly by the hospitals, with the remaining 5 percent reflecting the estimated value of donated volunteer time. Of the hospital costs, 87.5 percent were direct costs associated with program operations. These expenditures ranged from $115,000 to $214,000, and consisted largely of salaries and fringe benefits. The remaining 13.5 percent of costs were support services provided by the hospitals to the allocated programs, including rent or physical plant depreciation, the value of accounting and administrative time, and equipment. Hospital direct costs were offset by grant funding of up to $100,000 per year.

The costs for each of the case management programs and the average costs are displayed in Table 3. The costs are reported in two categories. Direct costs include all expenditures that would normally appear in a departmental expense report, such as salaries, fringe benefits, equipment, and supplies. The indirect costs include expenditures that would not necessarily appear on an expense report but nevertheless represent resources utilized to operate the programs.

The first category of indirect costs, called hospital resources, includes items that are part of overall hospital expenses but may not be allocated to program level budgets. They include the implicit (or explicit) rental value of the space occupied by the case management program, shared equipment, and the time of upper-level administrators and of accounting staff devoted to program operations. The second category of indirect costs consists of the value of volunteer time utilized by the program. This value was estimated by multiplying estimated volunteer hours for each program by $7.50 per hour, the assumed market value of this time. Volunteers trained as friendly visitors or companions are included in program (as opposed to service) costs as they performed monitoring

## TABLE 3

ANNUAL COSTS OF HOSPITAL-BASED CASE MANAGEMENT PROGRAMS*

| | Hospital | | | | | | |
|---|---|---|---|---|---|---|---|
| | A | B | C | D | E | F | Average |
| Dates covered | 1/88–12/88 | 7/88–6/89 | 9/88–8/89 | 3/88–2/89 | 7/89–6/90 | 4/89–3/90 | |
| Direct costs | | | | | | | |
| Salaries and fringe benefits | $114,942 | $123,405 | $145,596 | $100,030 | $203,167 | $185,914 | $148,912 |
| Other expenses | 8,214 | 14,224 | 25,074 | 15,015 | 10,926 | 27,005 | 16,743 |
| Subtotal | 123,156 | 137,629 | 170,670 | 115,045 | 214,093 | 212,919 | 165,655 |
| Indirect costs | 13,453 | 18,999 | 25,601 | 25,220 | 32,114 | 27,000 | 23,580 |
| Volunteer time | | | 15,756 | 740 | 37,500 | 3,000 | 9,499 |
| Subtotal | 13,453 | 18,999 | 41,357 | 25,960 | 69,614 | 30,000 | 33,079 |
| Total costs | $136,609 | $156,628 | $212,027 | $141,005 | $283,707 | $242,919 | $198,734 |

*To facilitate comparison among time periods, all cost figures were updated to 1990 using a 5 percent inflation rate.

and surveillance functions that otherwise would have required additional case manager time. Except at one program, volunteers were not trained to provide direct services (e.g., housekeeping, personal care) and, in fact, were cautioned against doing so.

Costs per demonstration client varied greatly from $150 to $531 per month. However, these per-client costs are overstated because the programs also provided services to many nondemonstration clients. Nondemonstration clients were those who received some case management services but who were not sufficiently frail to need long-term case management. When nondemonstration clients are considered, the cost of Flinn HBCC programs are comparable with the upper range of similar programs, at about $200 per client per month.

## RECOMMENDATIONS

At the end of the demonstration most hospital administrators appeared willing to support short-term, skilled, nursing-intensive case management as an extension of the discharge planning function. Many were supportive of a case management program with a broader focus as long as it was financially self-sufficient and could be viewed as part of a continuum of services for seniors consistent with the mission of the parent organization.

The most important lesson that hospital administrators can learn from the difficulties faced by the HBCC

sites is the need for a clear understanding of program objectives. While the HBCC programs, subsidized with grant funding, were modifying and expanding to meet client needs, hospital administrators operating under increasing fiscal pressure expected the programs to narrow their focus to utilization control. This contradiction is not simply an artifact of the demonstration setting. Because of the uncertain financial payback of hospital-based case management, it will be important for hospital administrators in any setting to specify and quantify direct and indirect financial and mission-related objectives.

Clarification of objectives will encourage more careful identification of information needs, particularly concerning financial viability. If an objective of case management is to facilitate earlier discharge to less expensive levels of care or to reduce unreimbursed Medicare readmissions, a focus on methods to track and compare utilization and cost data is required. It may also be desirable to track the number of additional client referrals to other in-house revenue-producing programs. This requires a system to monitor and evaluate referrals and associated revenues.

If case management is to be an integral part of a comprehensive seniors program, the information system must capture demographic, marketing, and outside referral data as well. Fee-for-service billing to support case management requires detailed activity and productivity data for cost analysis. Outcome measurement requires data collection to evaluate the effect of case management services on clients. This typically means more frequent assessments that are expanded to include a broad scope of psychosocial and environmental variables.

If a valued objective of the hospital-based case management program is to contribute to a continuum of care, then that program needs to be a fully integrated part of the hospital system. Supporting this objective is the assumption that case management can perform an important "bridging" function between the acute care received in an institutional setting and chronic health and social services received in a community setting. For this bridging to be effective, it must begin while the patient is still in the hospital so that needed services are in place on the day of the patient's discharge. In this case, specific policies and procedures are required to screen patients for case management.

In most situations it is expected that hospital-based case management would be short term (e.g., three months postdischarge) and intensive with an emphasis on utilization control. The logical administrative placement of the service is within the utilization review and quality assurance functions of the hospital in coordination with discharge planning. There are two primary reasons for this recommendation. First, a case management program needs to have a strong identity. It needs to be able to define and measure its benefit to the system. In order to demonstrate cost savings to the hospital, the referral base should be the high-risk or high-cost clients who may exceed the diagnosis related group (DRG) length of stay or may require readmission within 15 days. Documentation of program effectiveness, a major obstacle to the continuation of some programs after the demonstration, seems most likely to be accomplished in this administrative structure.

Second, and most important with respect to establishing a continuum of care, is that a partnership with discharge planning is critical to identify the patients who could potentially benefit most from case management; those individuals at risk of posthospital discharge breakdowns who might avoid rehospitalization through health monitoring, health education, and agency supports. With the typical short hospital stays under DRGs, discharge planners do not have adequate time to complete comprehensive posthospital plans and find community services that can start immediately. Under these circumstances, the case management process would begin prior to hospitalization in order to develop comprehensive treatment, discharge, and follow-up care plans. It would then continue in the community to ensure that patient care needs are met during the crucial postdischarge period.

It appears that case management does not need to be a 24-hour, on-call system, but can be a regular weekday program. Case management is not designed to be an emergency response system. It functions to create the support systems necessary to provide full coverage for clients. When these services are in place the appropriate providers should respond to the sudden changes in client needs. The three HBCC programs supporting an on-call system reported that it was infrequently utilized by clients. On-call case management might be considered if case managers were to staff emergency rooms. This becomes important as hospitals participate in managed care programs and need to decrease hospitalizations with the emergency room as the entry point.

The assessment of clients should be initiated in the hospital and be carried out to complement the discharge planning functions. Completion of the assessment in the client's home is critical to understanding client support systems and functional status out of the acute care setting. The assessment instrument needs to contain a strong medical component without losing the data on financial, demographic, environmental, psychosocial, activities of daily living, and informal caregiver functions. Care plan development needs to include physician input when medical and rehabilitative needs predominate at hospital discharge.

In addition to coordination of patient care there are administrative advantages to placing case management within the utilization review/quality assurance department. In this structure, case management can be coordinated with and have easy access to the hospital's information system, medical records, inpatient units, and policies and procedures of the parent organization. Conversely, case management records can be integrated into the hospital record system. Accomplishing these tasks was identified by case managers and program directors as problematic when the demonstration programs were not closely integrated with the hospital.

With respect to the staffing of case management units, both social workers and nurses are needed. Nurse case managers are required to assess the immediate and long-term medical, nursing, and health information needs of clients. While nurse case managers should take the lead in assessment and participate in care planning, case managers with a social work background need to be available to further assess the social service needs and to broker and coordinate community-based services. The HBCC case managers who had experience managing posthospitalized clients on a short-term and intensive basis recommended a caseload size of 25 as appropriate in this setting. Based on the experience of the HBCC programs, the authors suggest that the director of the program be hired primarily based on managerial capability. In order to appreciate implementation and operational problems, program directors should also carry a limited caseload at least until the program is well established.

•  •  •

The results of this demonstration program suggest that the most viable model of hospital-based case management depends on reimbursement incentives. In the past cost-based reimbursement encouraged hospitals and physicians to keep frail elderly patients in the hospital until they were completely recovered and ready to go home or be discharged to a nursing care facility. Hospital-based case management was not seen as necessary, especially with the growth of home care.

Case management became of interest to hospitals with the implementation of prospective payment, which caused patients to be discharged much sooner. Something more than discharge planning was needed to extend the recovery process and help frail patients adapt to their changing health status. The HBCC grant program implemented a long-term case management program so that frail patients would receive continuous monitoring and support. However, the hospitals were reimbursed only for inpatient care. During periods of economic difficulty it did not prove financially viable for the grantee hospitals to maintain long-term care case management programs that extended significantly beyond the treatment for which they were reimbursed. In retrospect, given the reimbursement incentives in place at the time of the grant, a shorter-term case management model focusing on transitioning the patient from hospitalization would have proved more viable. Indeed, that is the approach adopted by the HBCC program that was most viable when the grant funding ended.

The longer-term case management models implemented in this grant were likely premature rather than inappropriate. As hospitals become more at risk as a result of capitation and managed care, they will likely become more interested in continuous case management as a means to ensure appropriate and cost-effective delivery of inpatient care and positioning the hospital as a "full-service" provider for the elderly. Nevertheless, the implementation and management of these programs will require careful attention by hospital administrators to the clear definition of program objectives, close management supervision with respect to staffing relations with other hospital units, and the evaluation of performance. Without this input, these programs can easily

develop in ways that are not congruent with the hospital's overall goals and, as a result, have a brief and unsatisfactory life.

## REFERENCES

1. Applebaum, R.A. "The Evaluation of the National Long-Term Care Demonstration: Recruitment and Characteristics of Channeling Clients." *Health Services Research* 23, no. 1 (1988): 51–66.
2. Christianson, J.B., et al. "Hospital Case Management: Bridging Acute and Long-Term Care." *Health Affairs* 10, no. 2 (1991): 173–84.

Part IV

# PHYSICIANS and MANAGED CARE

# Factors for success: Capitated primary physicians in Medicare HMOs

J. Kevin McCurren

*Since their introduction in 1985, Medicare health maintenance organizations (HMOs) have had mixed results, and little research has been completed on what factors lead to a successful experience for capitated physicians in Medicare HMOs. The pilot study discussed in this article was conducted in early 1989 in an attempt to identify those factors. The study involved structured individual diagnostic interviews with successful capitated Medicare HMO primary physicians, revealing that they share common characteristics in practice philosophy, attitudes, and administrative control.*

*Health Care Manage Rev*, 1991, 16(2), 49–53
© 1991 Aspen Publishers, Inc.

## INTRODUCTION

In the spring of 1985, TEFRA-authorized HMOs began providing full, capitated health services to enrolled Medicare beneficiaries. By December of 1986, there were 121 risk contracts with a total of 945,135 enrollees. Though many of the HMOs had existing membership from earlier Medicare demonstration projects, the dramatic growth in these plans indicated a new trend in HMO development and growth.[1] However, as of January of 1989, the number of Medicare HMOs stood at only 136 plans representing 1,560,510 enrollees, a 1.3 percent decrease from the June 1988 high enrollment of 1,581,054. The number of participating HMOs was 22 percent less than the June 1987 high of 179 participating plans.[2]

Contrary to early expectations, Medicare risk contracting has been a rocky road for many HMOs. There have been numerous nonrenewals of participating plans. Despite the difficulties experienced by many, some HMOs have had very favorable experiences. FHP International, a Fountain Valley, California-based HMO, aggressively continues to pursue HMO participation, having derived more than half of its revenue in fiscal 1988 from Medicare. FHP experienced a fiscal 1988 net income of $16.4 million, a $9.5 million increase over 1987's net income of $6.9 million. Other notable successful Medicare risk contractors include Pacificare Health Systems in California, and Humana, Inc. in Florida.[3]

From its origin, the Medicare HMO market has provided a base of research on the trends, techniques, and experiences of Medicare HMOs. However, given the uncertain nature of Medicare HMOs and the high risk associated with participation, little research has developed conclusive work on the success factors of Medicare HMO contracting. Likewise, little research has been published on how Medicare risk contracting affects contracting physicians and the factors that contribute to a successful contracting physician experience.

Harrington and associates explored factors that HMO risk contractors considered to be associated with successful Medicare enrollment. Important factors for enrollment success included age and size of plan, broad geographic coverage, aggressive and sophisticated marketing, and competitive pricing. Their study, like several others, focused on enrollment success from the plan's perspective.

More recent articles have focused on the Medicare HMOs' effect on the contracting physician and medical practice. These articles indicate that similar to the HMOs' experiences, Medicare HMO contracting has provided mixed results for physicians, and specifically for group practices. A January/February, 1988 article in Group Practice Journal, the journal of the American Group Practice Association, suggested that the high nonrenewal rate for group practice HMOs was attributable to the uncertainty of legislative changes and inadequacy of the reimbursement rates.[4] However, a subsequent article in the same journal suggests that Medicare HMO contracting can be a successful proposition for group practices, generating enormous revenues in a short time.[5]

---

*There is clearly a need to identify factors that will predict and determine the success of contracting physicians under Medicare risk.*

---

Given the importance of the primary physician in the overall success of the Medicare HMO, there is clearly a need to identify factors that will predict and determine the success of contracting physicians under Medicare risk. This study explores the relationship of a primary physician's HMO Medicare success with two factors: (1) attitude toward Medicare HMOs and managed care, and (2) operational changes within the practice setting.

The pilot study used qualitative analysis, employing individual diagnostic interviews and supported with statistical data, to develop an overview of factors related to a physician's success as a Medicare risk provider. Preliminary discussions were conducted with Medicare HMO medical directors and experienced providers as a formative process for refining the interview format. These interviews revealed a general belief that the most important factors for a primary physician's success under Medicare risk contracting were attitudinal and operational. With this direction, interview guidelines were designed in two parts. The first segment involved questions to elicit the physician's attitude toward capitated managed care, Medicare HMOs, and impacts of these on the physician's practice, the patient, and relationships with other physicians. The second segment was a series of fact-gathering questions designed to elicit information about the physician's history, practice statistics, operational facts, and practice methodologies.

The consolidated findings of the interviews were tested through focus groups composed of Medicare risk physicians.

## METHODOLOGY

The interviews were conducted in two major markets. Two health plans were represented. A total of 17 interviews were conducted at the offices of the physicians. Physicians chosen for the study were all successful, capitated primary care providers under at least one Medicare risk contract. Names of physicians were submitted by the provider relations department of the participating HMOs. Successful physicians were defined as having the following characteristics:

- Medicare HMO enrollment of 50 members or more,
- positive financial performance under the Medicare risk contract, and
- favorable quality assessment as indicated by the plan's quality assurance programs and member relation services.

The interviews generally lasted from one to three hours and often included discussions with the physician's office manager.

Following conclusion and analysis of the interview, the findings were retested in each market through focus groups with primary care Medicare HMO physicians. The focus groups did not include any of the interviewed physicians but were designed to act as a sounding board to test the conclusions of the original interviews.

## FINDINGS

### Physician Profiles

The interviewed physicians were responsible for a designated Medicare enrollment. Though several types of practice structures were represented including solo, small group, and large single specialty structures, the responses were elicited as the opinion or attitude of the individual physician.

The average Medicare enrollee practice was 618 enrollees. This average represented a Medicare enrollment from as small as 50 members to an enrollment as large as 2,300 members for a physician representing a group practice. The enrollment percentage of the physician's practice dedicated to Medicare HMO patients ranged from approximately 98 percent to approximately 20 percent.

Most of the physicians participated in multiple HMOs. However, the participating Medicare HMO generally represented the largest HMO plan within the physician's practice. Almost all of the practices could be classified as private practices, though two of the practices had teaching affiliations with local hospitals.

The relationship between the physician and the Medicare HMOs was as a contracted, capitated primary physician. Though the capitation arrangements varied by plan, in both plans the primary physician was at risk in the primary care pool, the specialty pool, and a portion of the hospital pool. While it is believed that the level of physician risk–gain may affect the physician's attitude and practice methodologies, it was not the intent of this study to assess this impact.

All physicians, except one, had been involved in the Medicare HMO for at least a year. Many of the physicians had been involved in the HMO business for several years, often having been originators of managed care in their market.

Fifteen of the physicians were trained in either internal medicine or family practice, with one physician trained in a medical subspecialty but practicing in primary care and another trained as a surgeon and also practicing as a primary physician. Of the primary care–trained physicians, 10 were internists and 5 were family practitioners. The family practitioners generally had practices oriented toward the older population. In fact, the family practices were more reflective of the typical internal medicine practice, which generally has 50 percent of average weekly visits with Medicare patients. These statistics indicate that Medicare HMO enrollees naturally tend to enroll with the physician population that typically provides the Medicare primary care, the internists and older adult family practitioners.[6]

Operationally, the practices of the physicians have not changed dramatically because of Medicare capitation. The level of services and equipment are characteristic of a typical Medicare-oriented, fee-for-service practice.

Because of the capitation revenue, however, the total revenue of the practices commonly exceeded industry norms for family practice and internal medicine. In practices with a higher concentration of Medicare capitation, office staff, who would be dedicated to billing functions in a fee-for-service practice, are reassigned to assist the physician in monitoring the medical care system and improving the coordination of the components of the medical system.

## ATTITUDE ASSESSMENT

### Founders and Followers

In response to questions about why the physicians decided to participate in Medicare HMOs, and how they felt about managed care, the physicians tended to fall into two classifications of responses. These classifications are labeled founders and followers.

The founders' responses to these questions showed motivations beyond monetary gain or practice growth. They reflected strong intrinsic values. Their responses also indicated little regard for the status quo and a bent toward risk taking. In response to questions about why they decided to participate in the Medicare HMO, their answers were characterized by such statements as

- "I saw it as a challenge,"
- "It was a better way to serve my patients," or
- "I liked the concept."

Following physicians' responses to this question were characterized by extrinsic values. The reasons given by following physicians indicate that the decision to participate was economically driven. Examples of their reasons include

- "a new source of patients or income,"
- "protecting my practice," or
- "participate or lose the business."

Though some of the following physicians were early participants in HMOs, more often the founding physicians had been involved in HMOs for a longer time. Likewise, in an analysis of financial performance, the stronger performers tended to be founding-type phy-

*Perhaps their natural tendency to explore new methods led them also to find more cost-effective techniques for managing the care.*

sicians. Perhaps their natural tendency to explore new methods led them also to find more cost-effective techniques for managing the care.

### Forest versus Trees

The interviews included questions about whether the Medicare risk contract was profitable, whether it offered value to their practice, and how they made this assessment.

Though 13 physicians indicated that their Medicare risk contract was profitable, the more successful physicians displayed a more cognitive understanding of their practice as a business unit. The successful Medicare HMO provider discusses profitability as return on invested time, incremental revenue, and total profitability. Instead of focusing on their practices as piecemeal service, they see the HMO contract as offering a pool of funds to be expended in the most cost-effective allocation that will meet their members' health needs.

The physicians consistently agreed that Medicare HMO patient management was more demanding and time consuming than fee-for-service. When asked to quantify how much more demanding, their responses ranged from 3 to 10 times more demanding. At the same time, the physicians were comfortable with the increased demands, as they improved the quality of care.

When asked how they felt about Medicare capitation versus traditional fee-for-service—did they view Medicare capitation as a necessary evil or embrace it as a cost-savings device—their responses focused on the positive aspects of the program. They did not dwell on Medicare HMOs as a loss of the fee-for-service system, but emphasized the positive aspects: a steady source of revenue, revenue without hands-on services, and another source of patient financing. Several physicians expressed an opinion that Medicare capitation is not positive or negative, but simply another source of health care financing. Again, this attitude reflects a broader understanding of their practice as a larger economic unit.

### Likes and Dislikes

When asked what aspects of Medicare capitation they liked the most, the respondents strongly stated that one of the most favorable characteristics of the program is the comprehensive, continuous care they are able to deliver, especially to patients who would be unable to afford the care under the fee-for-service system. The physicians believe that the gatekeeper, capitated payment system provides a continuity and comprehensiveness of services that improves the quality of care. Also, the financing mechanism of capitation allows them to focus their attention and resources on the aspects of patient care where there is the greatest need. Several physicians stated that the Medicare capitation with its financing flexibility provided a more rewarding professional and personal experience. The physicians also indicated that they like the financial remuneration and growth potential that Medicare capitation provided.

In responding to the least-liked aspects of Medicare capitation, the physicians consistently mentioned excessive utilization of services by some members and their inability to control or disenroll abusive, noncompliant, and overdemanding patients. Excessive paperwork was also commonly mentioned.

It is interesting to note that in responding to least-liked aspects, only one physician mentioned increased financial risk associated with the capitation. It appears that once a physician becomes successfully comfortable with capitation, the risk aspect is not a major factor in attitude.

### Relationship Management

To identify how Medicare capitation has changed their practice patterns and methodology, the physicians were asked a series of questions about how their participation in Medicare HMOs changed the services or procedures provided to patients. The respondents stated that managed care has not significantly changed the way they practice medicine or the services provided within their offices. Besides limited lab and ancillary medical services, most practices have not added services. However, the physicians did state that the level of responsibility for the patients' medical needs has changed. This additional responsibility requires more physician attention to the patients' needs, more responsive after-hours care, and greater use of the physicians' clinical and diagnostic skills.

The physicians were asked if and how Medicare capitation has changed their specialist network and referrals. Almost all physicians stated that Medicare capitation did not significantly change their referral patterns. Except in isolated cases, they continue to refer to the same specialists used in fee-for-service practice. However, many physicians indicated that while their specialist network did not change, their relationship with their specialists did change dramatically. Because of the increased need for precise, quality communication between the primary physician and the specialist, the physicians stated that Medicare capitation has enhanced their understanding of the specialists' capabilities and charges and has improved communication between physicians. The physicians emphasized the importance of a limited specialist network, not for negotiated fees, but for better communication. As one physician stated, "It took me two years to train the specialists before they understood the requirements of treating *my* HMO patients."

Several of the more successful physicians stated that the key to a successful managed-care practice is the specialist relationship. They talked of changing the traditional primary specialist relationship in which the specialist has the dominant role. In the Medicare HMO, the primary physician must play a stronger role in the decision making. They emphasized that the management of the medical care must never leave the control of the primary physician.

**Administrative Management**

To identify how the physicians have adapted administratively or changed practice management techniques, the physicians were asked what administrative changes, if any, were required for Medicare capitation.

Many physicians mentioned the additional staff required for managing HMO paperwork and the need for more attention to practice financials. Three patterns surfaced as the size of the physicians' Medicare HMO enrollment increased. In larger multiphysician practices, a designated physician is consistently responsible for managing and monitoring utilization of outside medical services. This physician, for example, will review all admissions or specialty referrals before or immediately after the referral. Second, as the number of HMO patients increases, the physicians tend to appoint an HMO coordinator. This is a staff person responsible for tracking referrals, monitoring membership information, tracking communications between physicians, and serving as an information resource for members. Third, the physicians involved with larger memberships also emphasized the impor-

---

*The physicians stated that strong practice management allows them to focus their attention on the medical management of the patient.*

---

tance of a strong practice manager. This individual is responsible for all administrative issues of the practice. The physicians stated that strong practice management allows them to focus their attention on the medical management of the patient.

**CONCLUSION**

The physicians interviewed for this study represented many different practice scenarios, including

- diverse geographic, cultural, and practice structures;
- varying contractual arrangements with the Medicare HMOs; and
- varied professional background and training.

Even with their considerable differences, the successful Medicare HMO primary physicians display similar characteristics in philosophy, attitude, and administrative controls. Likewise, as the successful Medicare HMO practices increase their concentration of Medicare capitated patients, they exhibit common evolutionary characteristics in clinical and administrative management. To duplicate the successful Medicare HMO practice, a solid foundation must be established. That foundation will involve selection of the physician with the right attitude and education to reinforce the successful attitude and communicate techniques for developing a successful practice.

**REFERENCES**

1. Harrington, C., Newcomer, R.J., and Moore, T.G. "Factors That Contribute to Medicare HMO Risk Contract Success." *Inquiry* 25 (1988): 251–62.
2. Interstudy. 1989 *January Update of Medicare Enrollment in HMOs* Excelsior, Minn.: Interstudy, 1989.
3. "For Some HMOs, The Risk of Medicare Is Paying Off." *Modern Healthcare* (January 13, 1989); 47–49.
4. Rasmussen, B. "Reagan Looks Toward MECA To Solve Medicare Capitation Dilemma." *Group Practice Journal* 37, no. 1 (1988): 16–22.
5. Barnett, B. "Medical HMO Management." *Group Practice Journal* 38, no. 5 (1989): 29–36.
6. American Medical Association. "Total Visits with Medicare Patients per Week, 1987." In *Physician Marketplace Statistics*. Chicago, Ill.: American Medical Association, 1988.

# Lessons learned hiring HMO medical directors

David J. Ottensmeyer,
and
M. K. Key

*A medical director has enormous influence on medical cost and quality in managed care organizations. Little empirical work has been done on the attributes of an effective HMO medical director. The survey discussed in this article sought to examine those desirable traits from the perspective of medical directors who have risen in the ranks to become employers of medical directors. Mailed questionnaires asked 30 experts to rate skills and personality qualities based on what they would look for in a prospective hire. The factors that emerged as significant were communication and interpersonal skills, clinical credibility, ego strength, concern about quality, motivation, data orientation, and leadership qualities, along with organizational/systemic variables. Implications for hiring and physician education are drawn.*

*Health Care Manage Rev*, 1991, 16(2), 21–30
© 1991 Aspen Publishers, Inc.

**Hiring and maintaining** competent, effective medical directors for health maintenance organizations (HMOs) is a challenge. Based on our experience and that of colleagues, we see certain HMO medical directors rapidly cycling from job to job, without successful experiences. Why? Is it that they lack the proper background, training, attitude, or motivation? This curiosity led to the present study, in which we sought an answer to the question, "What qualities make a good hire for an HMO medical director?"

The field of managed care is growing, creating more opportunities for medical directors. Trends are toward 76 percent of the insured populace being covered by managed care in 1995, with only 11 percent in straight fee-for-service plans.[1] At the end of 1988, there were 32.6 million persons enrolled in 614 HMOs nationwide.[2] HMOs' market share for large- and medium-sized employer–provided health insurance grew to 19 percent in 1988 from 13 percent in 1986 and 7 percent in 1985.[3] Short of going to national health insurance, America would appear to be banking on managed care as the solution to the rising cost of health care. Managed care is basically an approach that superimposes organizational structure, control, measurement, and accountability upon the health care system to effect a balance in the utilization of health care resources, cost containment, and quality enhancement. It does so by employing three strategies: (1) the alteration of financial incentives for providers, (2) the introduction of management control, and (3) the use of information systems to facilitate operational decisions.[4] To accomplish those strategies, the HMO medical director is expected to understand health care and to have a management orientation in a managed care system.

**David J. Ottensmeyer,** *M.D., is the President of the Travelers Health Company and Chief Medical Officer of the Managed Care and Employee Benefits Division of The Travelers Companies in Hartford, Connecticut. At the time of this work, he was Executive Vice President and Chief Medical Officer of EQUICOR, Inc. in Nashville, Tennessee.*

**M. K. Key,** *Ph.D., is a consultant for the Center for Continous Improvement, QUORUM Health Resources, Inc. in Nashville, Tennessee. While this research was conducted, Dr. Key was Director of Administration, Research and Development of EQUICOR, Inc., also in Nashville.*

The authors wish to thank Dr. Howard M. Sandler for his consultation on study design and analysis and Ms. Denise Fenchel for her administrative assistance.

The medical director in an HMO plays the lead role in the management of medical costs. Functions of the HMO medical director were examined in a 1985 survey by Witt Associates.[5] Even though the newly established independent practice associations (IPAs) were underrepresented and larger staff model HMOs were overrepresented in their study, the functions all types held in common were utilization review, quality assurance, and medical staff affairs. Most were active in physician recruitment as well. The HMO medical director has responsibility for the control of medical management costs, which can approximate 85 percent of a plan's budget. The director, in order to be successful, must manage utilization, assure quality standards of care, and influence providers to change the way they practice medicine.

Medical management has become a formalized specialty, owing to the efforts of the American Academy of Medical Directors and the American College of Physician Executives (ACPE). The medical director is one evolving and expanding role of the physician executive.[6] The medical director of the future will have an increasingly important role in speaking the languages of medicine and business and interfacing between the two disciplines.

Permut is one of many authors to note the difference in skills required of managers and clinicians, many of which are contradictory. Others to note manager–clinician role conflict are Doyne,[7] Forkosh,[8] Hartfield,[9] Kurtz,[10] Ottensmeyer and Key,[11] Porter and Royer,[12] and Stearns and Roberts.[13] Many maintain that the crossover from clinician to manager is made more difficult by medical school training. Others point to basic clinician–manager differences in personality and workstyle (autonomous versus teamwork; crisis-oriented versus long-range planner; conflict avoiders versus conflict managers). Others argue that physicians are inadequately prepared to be managers[9] and prescribe programs of managerial training to remedy that deficiency.[12,14,15]

There are many thoughtful pieces about what makes a good physician manager, though not many devoted to the HMO medical director,[6,16] and not many empirical studies about either. One study by Jacobs and Mott[17] surveyed HMO executives with responsibility for physician selection. Two major questions were posed: (1) what emphasis should be given to 21 predefined areas at some time during the medical education process, and (2) what rating should be given to 17 criteria for recruiting or employing physicians. Although the study did not focus on physician manag-

ers, it did find that personal attributes and interpersonal skills were nearly equal in weight to items like board certification.

The present study was designed to explore the desirable traits of a prospective HMO medical director. The perspective sought was that of the seasoned medical director, experienced in both managed care and the hiring of HMO medical directors.

## METHOD

### Instrument

The survey tool was inductively developed through structured interviews with persons who have been medical directors and who are not in management roles, supervising medical directors. These consultants were asked in interviews to define the qualities of the ideal or most effective HMO medical director they could imagine. They produced a list of traits, some of which resembled "Qualifications" for the job (i.e., those items looked for before the hire), while others described an effective medical director by performance on the job—these we entitled "Characteristics." Finally, some traits were more generic personality "Attributes."

Likert-type scales[18] were constructed for the items described as Qualifications and Characteristics. The six-point scales asked for the amount of agreement–disagreement with statements about the hypothetical medical director. A semantic differential scale was created for the Attributes, pairing bipolar opposites. Open-ended questions asked experts to list important traits that had been missed in the questionnaire.

The instructions asked participants to assume that they were hiring a medical director for a 50,000-member metropolitan-area IPA or group model plan that is beyond the initial start-up phase. They were requested to consider the combination of skills and personality characteristics they would look for in a prospective hire. They were asked to keep in mind medical directors they had known who were effective in their roles, as evidenced by such criteria as quality standards and utilization statistics.

*The experts were selected because of experience in the field as medical directors, familiarity with the strengths required to perform the job, and their roles in selecting and supervising medical directors.*

Questionnaires were delivered by mail or facsimile with a cover letter asking for participation from a group of experts. There were no incentives offered other than feedback on the results of the study. Thirty out of 34 in the sample responded with complete questionnaires.

## Panel of Experts

The experts were selected because of experience in the field as medical directors, familiarity with the strengths required to perform the job, and their roles in selecting and supervising medical directors. As portrayed in Table 1, there were 30 people surveyed (29 males, 1 female) with an average age of about 54 years. The ages ranged from 38 to 68. The major positions held by the experts were medical director (13) and vice-president (8), with 2 additional people describing themselves as VP–medical director. These physicians had held their current positions from 2 months to 21 years with a mean of 3.83 years. The mean number of medical directors hired was slightly over 7 (with a range from 0 to 28). Those surveyed had over 13 years of experience in managed health care on the average (M = 13.276, with a range from 5 to 38). Ten had Fellow of the ACPE certification, one had an M.B.A., and another, an M.S. in health care administration. In short, the group was older and experienced both in managed health care and in the hiring of medical directors.

In 1985, Kindig and Lastiri[19] found the average age of physician administrators was 54 years, their tenure in administration was 18 or more years, and HMO administrators spent the highest percentage of time in administration. Nash[20] in 1987 added 3 other studies' data to the Kindig work and found the HMO physician executive to be younger (average age 45) and more likely to possess a management degree (10 percent). Our sample was more like that of Kindig and Lastiri.

Table 2 shows the medical specialty of the respondents. The proportions in each specialty are similar to those of all HMO medical directors, as reported in the Witt survey.[5]

## RESULTS

Means and standard deviations were calculated for the Likert scale items. Table 3 presents a rank ordering by means of the Qualifications. A score of five or above reflects moderate or strong agreement with the statement that "It is important that a medical director (have this qualification)." Topmost in the estimation of our experts were *communication skills, a clear philosophy of managed care, a minimum of five years' clinical experience,* and the *willingness to see oneself as different.* Least important were *maintaining a private practice* and *planning to retire in the position.*

Table 4 ranks the means of characteristics of an effective medical director, as described by the experts. Many more Characteristics than Qualifications were strongly rated (meaning more than moderate agreement). These included *concern about quality of care, easy to communicate with,* being *willing to take a stand, able to influence providers to change practice,* having a *medical license,* having the *respect of other providers, using data effectively,* being *skilled at committee work,* having *regular contact with network physicians, working with nurses as peers,* being *flexible in dealing with others, improving utilization statistics,* being *intellectually curious, good at documentation,* and *comfortable in a bureaucracy.*

It is of interest to observe the conformity in opinion; there is very little variance in most of the items. By contrast, a few items earned wide disagreement.

## TABLE 1

### DESCRIPTION OF THE GROUP*

| Attribute | Mean | Range |
|---|---|---|
| Age | 53.6 yrs. | 38–68 |
| Years in current position | 3.8 yrs. | 2 months–21 yrs. |
| Number of medical directors hired | 7.1 | 0–28 |
| Total years' experience | 12.9 yrs. | 4–38 |

*Gender: 29 males and 1 female.

## TABLE 2

### MEDICAL SPECIALTY*

| | | Witt Survey[5] |
|---|---|---|
| Internal medicine | 11 (36%) | 33% |
| Pediatrics | 8 (26%) | 19% |
| Family practice | 6 (20%) | 18% |
| Other | 5 (16%) | 30% |

*N = 30.

## TABLE 3

### QUALIFICATIONS

|      |                                   | Mean |
| ---- | --------------------------------- | ---- |
| Q8   | Communication skills              | 5.93 |
| Q9   | Clear philosophy                  | 5.73 |
| Q4   | Min. 5 yrs. clinical experience   | 5.46 |
| Q10  | Willing to see self as different  | 5.00 |
| Q2   | UM experience                     | 4.96 |
| Q13  | Financial skills                  | 4.93 |
| Q1   | QA experience                     | 4.63 |
| Q12  | Salesmanship                      | 4.56 |
| Q11  | IPA/group model experience        | 4.53 |
| Q7   | Sees self as career administrator | 4.53 |
| Q5   | Formal management training        | 3.66 |
| Q3   | Is in primary medical specialty   | 3.23 |
| Q6   | Maintains private practice        | 2.26 |
| Q14  | Retire in position                | 2.26 |

Those traits with scores ranging from 1 to 6, with a standard deviation of 1.25 or more, included being in a *primary medical specialty*, having *management training*, *planning to retire in the position*, *seeing self as career administrator*, being *intellectually curious, computer literate*, and *maintaining hospital privileges* (the most disagreed-upon item). Our experts disagree with the necessity of these traits. From discussions with the respondents, it seems that *planning to retire* and *career administrator* were misunderstood. Some read these as tongue-in-cheek indices of poor motivation and lack of clinical expertise; other participants probably took them as indicative of commitment to the profession of medical administration, thus the wide disagreement.

Table 5 displays the mean scores on Attributes. It argues that the effective medical director must be *persuasive, people-oriented* (contrasted to *solitary*), *confident, proactive, a team player* and *quality-oriented* (as opposed to *hard dollar-oriented*). There were certain items for which the experts would not commit either way: *patient or physician advocate, intrusive versus retiring, autocrat versus democrat, listener versus talker, peacemaker versus confrontative, product-oriented versus process-oriented, people-oriented versus data-oriented*. This suggests that the effective medical director should possess a combination of these personality dimensions.

The responses were analyzed by the expert's primary HMO experience—staff–group versus IPA (18 versus 10). Staff–group types would be expected to

## TABLE 4

### CHARACTERISTICS OF AN EFFECTIVE MEDICAL DIRECTOR

|      |                                          | Mean        |
| ---- | ---------------------------------------- | ----------- |
| C14  | Is concerned about quality of care       | 5.96        |
| C1   | Is easy to communicate with              | 5.80        |
| C16  | Is willing to take a stand               | 5.76        |
| C20  | Influences providers to change practice  | 5.70        |
| C21  | Licensed physician                       | 5.70        |
| C2   | Respected by providers                   | 5.63        |
| C9   | Uses data effectively                    | 5.63        |
| C4   | Skilled at committee work                | 5.60        |
| C3   | Challenges physicians                    | 1.50 (5.55)* |
| C13  | Has regular contact with network physicians | 5.53     |
| C18  | Works with nurses as peers               | 5.50        |
| C10  | Flexible in dealing with others          | 5.50        |
| C17  | Can improve utilization statistics       | 5.43        |
| C6   | Intellectually curious                   | 1.66 (5.33)* |
| C2   | Good at documentation                    | 5.13        |
| C11  | Comfortable in a bureaucracy             | 5.06        |
| C22  | Regularly phones network physicians      | 4.96        |
| C12  | Entrepreneurial                          | 4.60        |
| C15  | Detail-oriented                          | 4.40        |
| C8   | Computer literate                        | 3.26 (3.73)* |
| C19  | Needs hospital privileges                | 2.90        |
| C5   | Paperwork is a priority                  | 2.20        |

*Reflected value (i.e., 7–original value).

behave more like managers, with more bureaucratic and organizational interests, whereas IPA types would value more political and persuasive aptitudes. After identifying respondents whose backgrounds could be labeled primarily staff–group model or IPA-type, *t*-tests were conducted on differences in each item and overall scores. No differences were found; they did not look at the qualities in materially different ways. Jacobs and Mott[17] also found no difference in a majority of areas across staff, group, IPA, and network HMOs when they were asked about physician training needed.

### DISCUSSION

#### Communication and Interpersonal Skills

Communication skill was rated the most important qualification, not unlike the findings of Cummings,[21]

## TABLE 5

### ATTRIBUTES OF AN EFFECTIVE MEDICAL DIRECTOR

|  |  | Mean |
|----|----|----|
| A15 | Persuasive (vs. unconvincing) | 5.73* |
| A10 | People-oriented (vs. solitary) | 5.40* |
| A1 | Confident (vs. hesitant) | 5.33* |
| A2 | Proactive (vs. reactive) | 5.26 |
| A9 | Team-player (vs. autonomous) | 5.15* |
| A11 | Quality-oriented (vs. oriented to hard dollars) | 5.12* |
| A4 | Flexible (vs. rigid) | 4.93 |
| A8 | Planner (vs. crisis manager) | 4.90* |
| A12 | Generalist (vs. specialist) | 4.85 |
| A7 | Listener (vs. talker) | 4.33 |
| A5 | Intrusive (vs. retiring) | 4.24* |
| A3 | Patient advocate (vs. physician advocate) | 4.02* |
| A13 | Peacemaker (vs. confrontative) | 3.96 |
| A16 | People-oriented (vs. data-oriented) | 3.95 |
| A14 | Product-oriented (vs. process-oriented) | 3.86 |
| A6 | Democratic (vs. autocratic) | 3.72* |

*Reflected value (i.e., 7—original value).

Fine,[22] Hartfield,[9] and Staley and Staley.[23] Hartfield surveyed nonphysician supervisors of physician executives and found that, next to time and task management, physician executives suffer most from communication problems. An ACPE survey of 185 physician executives asked what they thought about their own communication effectiveness.[23] They agreed that managerial communication skills across the board are vital to the success of the health care organization; of the complex communication skills, managing conflict was rated most important both on the job and in achieving a managerial position; listening and speaking were consistently rated most important and most in need of enhancement; and speaking skills were rated higher than were writing skills. In our own study, writing and oral skills, both one-to-one and with groups, were mentioned in the open-ended questions. On the Attributes, respondents indicated that the medical director must be both a *listener* and a *talker*.

Several of the other highly rated traits cluster with communication skills. *Easy to communicate with, regular contact with physicians, persuasive,* and comments about being a *tough negotiator* all pertain to effective communication for influencing providers. Being a good com-

municator makes this easier. Even being *skilled at committee work*—a talent physicians lack and an activity few of them relish[8]—is an essential and highly rated communication form.

Interpersonal skills, discussed also by Cummings[21] and Ferguson,[24] describes another cluster of items: *flexible in dealing with others, people-oriented, works with nurses as peers,* and is a *team player.* Flexibility is the key to successful management, according to Doyne.[7] Brown and McCool found that orientation to employees, patients, and visitors is essential to managers in care-giving settings. In dealing with others, networking rather than using formal authority characterizes

> *The ideas, resources, and power to get something done in complex situations must come from a wide variety of sources, and interpersonal skills are a real advantage.*

the successful health care leader of today.[16] The ideas, resources, and power to get something done in complex situations must come from a wide variety of sources, and interpersonal skills are a real advantage.

*Working with nurses as peers* links to the *team player* concept. Open-ended comments made were: "able to have people work with him, not for him", being "group-oriented" and "creating harmonious working relationships", being "nonelitist toward non-physicians," "must be willing to give up the autonomy they had in private practice in order to be an effective team player," and "able to work in a team environment rather than being in control as they were as practitioners." These physicians must not be characterized by the "MDeity syndrome." Doctors have been found to be notoriously poor team players.[7,12] Jacobs and Mott also found that the ability to relate to nonphysician staff members and to work in a team rated high in importance in hiring.[17]

### Clear Philosophy

A *clear philosophy of managed care* was the second highest–rated Qualification. As one respondent put it:

[this is] a belief that health care can be delivered and practiced in a different way—one that is more cost effective; a way that is equitable and acceptable to patients; a way that retains the quality of the present health care system without its excesses and extravagances.

[It is] a belief that most physicians want to do the right thing for their patients and for society; a belief that physicians can change their style and practice patterns if shown other effective ways to do it; a belief that physicians will change if given credible information on which to base decisions.

[The philosophy] incorporates an understanding of the role and limitations of the managed care organization as it attempts to organize, staff, and control delivery systems. That results in a belief in the job of the medical manager as a change agent, a coach to the profession and a leader ready to confront the hard issues.

### Clinical Credibility

A minimum of five years in clinical practice was the third highest–rated Qualification. Clinical experience is needed for technical competence, to render good clinical decisions for an HMO patient, and for the credibility it carries with other clinicians. Managers need a good knowledge of medicine in order to deal with physician providers effectively (Ailes, R.J.; pers. com.; 1989) as well as a strong understanding and sensitivity to physician problems.[22] For this reason, many of our panel did not want a *career administrator* in this position. Our experts did feel that the HMO medical director should be licensed, but need not be from a *primary medical specialty*, although there was disagreement about this. This is an interesting finding, as three fields still predominate among physician executives: internal medicine, pediatrics, and family practice.[25] There is an old debate about whether physician administrators should keep up their clinical skills,[26] but our sample did not value *maintaining a small private practice*, nor did many see the utility of having *hospital privileges*.

Tied in with the idea of clinical credibility was a set of comments by respondents that pertained to respect and regard. For example, "The medical director must be recognized by others as a highly qualified physician"; and "They should have attained some status as a clinician (board certification, advanced training, reputation)." Furthermore, "if managing in a community where he/she has practiced, their clinical skills should be known to be good." Respected by providers was the sixth highest Characteristic—there is clear value to reputation here. Jacobs and Mott[17] found also that the reputation of a physician's place of residency and his or her training in a U.S. medical school were important hiring criteria.

### Ego Strength

Another group of items appears to relate to a phenomenon variously characterized as backbone, security, resilience—a factor we have called ego strength. In other management literature, this has been described as hardiness. In our respondents' words, "being able to take an unpopular position and stand alone," "to take extreme criticism and profit from it," "willing to take flak [sic] and not worry about being popular or loved," "can handle daily crisis, hostility, and anger without...burnout," "can laugh at self and handle constructive criticism." This idea received the most comment in the open-ended inquiry.

Ego strength appears to relate also to the fourth highest Qualification, *willing to see self as different*, and the third highest Characteristic, *willing to take a stand*. As Ailes puts it, "Too many medical doctors have been unable to cut the umbilical cord to clinical practice. Until they make this separation, they generally are not effective in representing the views of their employer in the position of medical director" (Ailes, R.J.; pers. com., 1989). Medical directors must be secure enough to separate their identities from those of the clinical community, to be able to confront others, to take criticism, and to hold differing views.

Many indicated that an effective medical director *challenges physicians* (ninth from highest Characteristic). Physicians as opposed to managers are typically described as conflict avoiders.[9] High-performing managers, on the other hand, respect the rights and integrity of others, while knowing how to stimulate people in conflict situations.[16] The HMO medical director cannot shy away from confrontation and conflict, but our sample rated both *peacemaker* and *confrontative* as required. Confidence was the third highest Attribute, "even to the point of being a risk-taker," said one expert. In the Hartfield[9] study, the author also found that whatever physician executives do, they do with conviction and confidence.

### Concern About Quality

The number one Characteristic was *concern about the quality of care*. In the Attributes, the experts valued *quality-orientation* over *hard dollar–orientation*. One of our respondents commented that the medical director needed training, knowledge, and judgment to make proper decisions about appropriateness (of care) without interfering with quality. In a typical HMO, medical review services include those managers qualified to guard quality. As administrators, physicians are unique because they understand the requirements of quality care—they speak the language of patient care, and embody both corporate and clinical cultures.[27]

## Motivation

Another group of items pertained to the motivation or ambition to choose the career of medical director and not use it to escape medical practice; to make a "positive move toward management and not away from clinical practice." There were many comments about having a career orientation and desiring to succeed as a medical director and have others do the same. Another commented that the medical director must passionately *want* to change provider behavior and convince others to do the same. Motivation is probably why *planning to retire in this position* was rated so low in this survey and why there was confusion about the value of having a *career administrator* in the position.

This finding agrees with the literature. Cummings[21] mentions desire to become a manager; Doyne[7(p.13)] warns a potential physician executive to not flee to management, but to enter it "…because you want to be there." Ferguson[24(p.1117)] says that "…unless you have a thorough and convincing reason for wanting to become an administrator, don't become one." When Kindig and Lastiri[19] surveyed physician administrators, they found that the reasons for choosing administration had changed over time. The majority these days seek administration for positive reasons—impact on health care delivery, new opportunities and challenges, and managerial enjoyment and talent.

Motivation or drive may link to qualities described by our experts as high energy (4 respondents), optimistic (2), hard-working (2), enthusiastic (1), and having perseverance (1). Brown and McCool[16(p.70)] interviewed health care leaders and found being "…healthy, energy-giving, hard-working" to be an essential trait.

## Data Orientation

The proficiency in *using data effectively* rated seventh, and the ability to *improve utilization statistics* ranked number 13 in Characteristics of an effective medical director. Others have cited the value of abilities to interpret data and offer recommendations based on characteristics unique to an organization.[22] Brown and McCool,[16] interviewing primarily high-performing hospital administrators, found that leaders seem to enjoy sampling and testing ideas, using conceptual and analytic constructs, organizing data points and concepts. Our sample reminded us that the medical director must be people-oriented as well as data-oriented.

## Formal Management Training

*Formal management training* was rated very low by the panel, although there was disagreement over this item. In Kindig and Lastiri,[19] 83.6 percent of 2,393 physician administrators said formal graduate coursework in management was required or advisable. Our results are at variance with this. In our evaluation of the study group, it appears that many of this group have grown up in the field and have learned on the job—an apprenticeship system. There were comments about on-the-job training's being superior to formal education; another mentioned that a high-quality clinical background has quality assurance (QA) and utilization review (UR) in it. There were, however, remarks that a medical director "must have a good business sense" and "must be able to understand and work with financial and marketing people." Some felt that management, computers, financial skills, and marketing could all be learned and need not be prerequisites for the job, but acquired through continuing education and on-the-job training.

## Leadership Qualities

A constellation of qualities seemed to describe leadership. Cummings'[21(p.7)] "failure to lead" describes one of the reasons managers fail. The panel commented on the importance of being a futurist, having vision and purpose; leadership and management ability; observing the big picture; being mature in judgment, and not capricious. Brown and McCool[16] also describe being mission-oriented, visionary, and entrepreneurial as leadership attributes for the 1990s.

There were two comments about adaptability to change. Brown and McCool[16] wrote that high-performing managers at work are open to change. Our panel rated the effective medical director as proactive, agreeing with Fine.[22] The physician is taught to react and is poor at proactive planning and thinking, whereas a manager must be proactive.[7,12]

The effective medical director *influences providers* (the fourth highest–rated Characteristic). The influence of clinical leadership has been clearly demonstrated in setting practice patterns and determining group norms of practice style. This is particularly prominent in the acceptance of innovations.[28]

## The sine qua non's

The survey did not ask about intelligence and integrity, but the panel was quick to point out that these were prerequisites we had not asked about. Comments about intelligence included the need to be smart, able to form concepts as well as put them in operation, analytic, detail and product oriented. The *intellectually curious* Characteristic was rated fairly high by the panel.

---

*Health care professionals are strongly identified with their professional norms and codes of ethics . . . .*

---

Comments about honesty (3); being ethical (2); having the "ability to persist for what is professionally correct regardless of consequences to company" formed a cluster of items having to do with integrity. Health care professionals are strongly identified with their professional norms and codes of ethics; it is not unusual that this would be valued in the present study.

### Organizational–Systemic Variables

Most HMOs exist in an organizational environment quite different from the autonomy the clinical practitioner enjoys. Many in fact are owned by large organizations that could be characterized as bureaucracies. Our sample agreed with the supposition that effective medical directors need to be *comfortable in a bureaucracy*. This factor describes a special set of skills—for meetings, paperwork documentation, adherence to policy and procedure, multitiered management, and political influence tactics—that are typical of a bureaucracy. The *good at documentation* Characteristic ranked one place above the *bureaucracy* item. This form of communication is critical for continuity of care, audit trails, and legal liability. In our experience, medical directors take a keen interest in the documentation of medical practice; yet our panel seemed to feel that paperwork is a low priority. Paperwork may have a negative connotation not borne by documentation (e.g., insignificant memos as opposed to patient records).

Comments were made that the medical director must have an organizational sense of purpose; must strongly identify with and understand the provider community; and, at the same time, have strong organizational skills that facilitate the use of the managed health care system.

We were reminded that the *organization* is also responsible in some part for the success of its medical directors. Managers often fail because of poorly defined institutional goals, poorly defined criteria by which the results of their efforts will be measured, and inadequate resources, according to Cummings.[21] Ailes[25] asserted that maintaining competent, effective medical directors is a function of the employer (Ailes, R.J.; pers. com.; 1989). It is the organization's responsibility to define what it wants the medical director to accomplish (be specific about job descriptions, too often written like "walk on water") and provide on-the-job training.

## COMPARISON WITH NON-M.D. EXECUTIVES

In a survey subsequent to the one described above, the authors presented the same questions to non-M.D. HMO executives with experience hiring medical directors. The instructions asked the respondents to make the same assumptions about a prospective hire as posed in the physician survey, and to keep in mind effective medical directors they had known. Of the 20 people surveyed (19 men, 1 woman), the average age was 41.9 years—considerably younger than the physicians surveyed earlier. They had hired about 8 medical directors each (M=8.1) and, as a group possessed almost 12 years experience in managed health care (M=11.7). Most described themselves as vice presidents (N=11); some cited the job title of president/ CEO (N=6). Eight held master's degrees, three held J.D. degrees, with the rest described as holding B.A. or B.S. degrees or none. Although their years of managed care experience were comparable to the physicians', the extent of their formal education was less—thus their ability to start their careers earlier.

When compared to the physician responses, the non-M.D. results were essentially similar. For the most part, they agreed with the M.D.s on which Qualifications, Characteristics, and Attributes were important in the person they hire. On the Qualifications scale, for example, they gave *communication* and *clear philosophy* (in that order) their highest ratings. On the Characteristics scale, the non-M.D.s rated *quality of patient care* (M=5.95) second only to *licensed physician* (M=6.0), while the M.D. group rated *quality of care* the highest (M=5.976). Both groups included *confident, persuasive, people-oriented, a team player,* and *proactive* in their top five most-desired Attributes.

There were a few minor, but interesting, differences between the two groups on the Characteristics scale. The M.D.s rated both *easy to communicate with* (5.8 vs. 5.45, $t(48)=2.117$, $p<.05$) and *skilled with committees* (5.6

vs. 4.9, $t(48=3.36, p<.005)$ higher than the non-M.D.s, perhaps indicating that these were areas of difficulty for the M.D.s. This is somewhat supported by the larger difference on *feeling comfortable in a bureaucracy* (5.067 vs. 3.100, $t=6.837, p<.001$), with the M.D.s' apparent discomfort being reflected in the importance they placed on this item. The only other difference was found on *low priority for paperwork*, where the M.D.s rated this slightly lower than did the non-M.D.s (2.2 vs. 2.9, $t(48)=-2.158, p<.05$).

On the whole, both groups were in substantial agreement about which Qualifications, Characteristics, and Attributes were important in choosing a medical director. The small differences may be reflective of uneasiness with some aspects of the management role, as expressed by the physicians. If this is the case, hiring processes might best be directed to an exploration of factors like comfort with bureaucracy, paperwork, and committees as well as ease of communication.

For a more complete summary of the non-physician survey findings, write to Dr. M.K. Key, 1857 Laurel Ridge, Nashville, TN 37215.

## CONCLUSIONS

Most of these areas of managerial competence can be classified as Edgar Schein[29] described them: analytical, interpersonal, and emotional. They are personal traits rather than formal credentials. Communication, interpersonal skills, ethics, intelligence, clear philosophy, data orientation, motivation, and ego strength all surfaced in this exploration. Technical competence was also identified in the form of clinical and managerial skill, but not as achieved through formal management training. This reflects how the panel acquired their training, for the most part. The panel seemed to feel that most of the requisite management skills could be learned on the job and that the employer should be, in large part, responsible for that training. The majority of this group developed the field of medical management over many (13) years, with on-the-job training and experience plus continuing education. To meet the high demand for medical directors today, there now may be a need to standardize, formalize, and abbreviate the length of time spent acquiring the prerequisite skills.

Most of these factors cannot be determined by resume-type qualifications, but must be teased out and verified during interviews and by checking references. One obvious predictor of future success is past behav-

ior, as one respondent reminded us. An understanding of local market or local community experience is useful for an IPA medical director, another panelist maintained. But for the longer haul, the experience needed comes from being on the job, and that outweighs local knowledge of the community or medical politics.

Based on the results of this study, licensed physicians with more than five years of clinical practice, sound clinical skills, and good reputations should be sought to fill HMO medical director positions. They need not be in a primary medical specialty, have a degree in management, maintain hospital privileges, or plan to keep up a private practice. They need data skills as well as people skills, and should have demonstrated ability to control utilization and influence providers. Their motivation is important: they must have chosen management and not fled medicine, and have status among physicians but be secure enough to separate their identities from those of physicians. They must demonstrate concern for quality of care over hard dollars. Their communication skills are of utmost importance, from being a team player to being persuasive to being willing to confront. They must understand and believe in managed care, have leadership skills, be able to work within organizations, and possess a certain hardiness to perform in this role.

This is just an exploratory study, much akin to anthropological inquiry, so the next steps could include tightening and refining of criteria into factors and validation of these traits in the hiring process. Future efforts might also include prospective research on their relationship to medical director success criteria. Studies could then examine the relative predictive power of each factor to performance on the job, and this information be used to modify hiring criteria.

Medical directors could have enormous influence on the future success of managed care organizations. In their management of utilization, they are concerned with approximately 85 percent of the expenditures of the organization, that is, medical benefits. Because they blend clinical knowledge with managerial acumen, they are uniquely positioned to influence providers to change their patterns of practicing medicine, as one peer to another. One panelist remarked that medical directors must passionately *want* to change provider behavior and convince others to do the same; as another said, they must have the ability to move and change other physicians.

No single trait or characteristic identifies an outstanding medical director, yet the composite painted here is imposing. There will clearly be trade-offs for any one candidate. But look keenly for communicators with clinical credibility, leadership ability, the proper personality, character, and motivation, and all the rest will follow—provided they are adept at working within large organizations, and those organizations support the medical director with clear direction and training.

## REFERENCES

1. Ward, B. "Medical Meetings: Wilkerson Group Symposium." *In Vivo: The Business and Medicine Report* 25, no. 12 (1987): 11–13.
2. Group Health Association of America. *National Directory of HMOs 1989.* Washington, D.C.: GHAA, 1989.
3. Bureau of Labor Statistics. *Employee Benefits in Medium and Large Firms.* Bulletin 2236, 36. Washington, D.C.: U.S. Department of Labor, 1989.
4. Key, M.K., and Ottensmeyer, D.J. "Managed Health Care: The Benefits Approach to Cost and Quality." *Personnel* (1990): 67(9): 29–30, 32.
5. Belton, D.G., and Baron, C.R. "Profile of the HMO Medical Director." *Medical Group Management* 34, no. 2 (1987): 17–22.
6. Permut, R. "Medical Director, and Evolving and Expanding Role of the Physician Executive." *Group Practice Journal* 38 (1989): 52, 54, 59–60.
7. Doyne, M. "Physicians as Managers." *Healthcare Forum Journal* 30, no. 5 (1987): 11–13.
8. Forkosh, D.S. "Good Doctors Aren't Always Good Managers." *The Hospital Medical Staff* 11, no. 5 (1982): 2–5.
9. Hartfield, J.E. "Physicians in Management: The Costs, Challenges, and Rewards." In *The Physician Executive.* Tampa, Fla.: American Academy of Medical Directors, 1988.
10. Kurtz, M.E. "The Dual Role Dilemma." In *The Physician Executive.* Tampa, Fla.: American Academy of Medical Directors, 1988.
11. Ottensmeyer, D.J., and Key, M.K. 'The Unique Contribution of the Physician Executive to Health Care Management." In *The Physician Executive.* Tampa, Fla.: American Academy of Medical Directors, 1988.
12. Porter, R.D., and Royer, T. "Physician Managers—A Challenge for Training and Teamwork." *Medical Group Management Association Journal* 35 (1987): 42–47.
13. Stearns, N.S., and Roberts, E.B. "Why Do Occupational Physicians Need to be Better Managers?" *Journal of Occupational Medicine* 24 (1982): 219–24.
14. Fink, D.J., and Goldhar, J.D. "Management for Physicians: An Annotated Bibliography of Recent Literature." *Annals of Internal Medicine* 92 (1980): 269–75.
15. Hillman, A.L., et al. "Managing the Medical Industrial Complex." *The New England Journal of Medicine* 315 (1986): 511–13.
16. Brown, M. and McCool, B.P. "High-Performing Managers: Leadership Attributes for the 1990s." *Health Care Management Review* 12, no. 2 (1987): 69–75.
17. Jacobs, M.O., and Mott, P.D. "Physician Characteristics and Training Emphasis Considered Desirable by Leaders of HMOs." *Journal of Medical Education* 62 (1987): 725–31.
18. Nunnally, J.C. *Psychometric Theory.* New York, N.Y.: McGraw Hill, 1967.
19. Kindig, D.A., and Lastiri, S. "Administrative Medicine: A New Medical Specialty?" *Health Affairs* 5 (1986): 146–56.
20. Nash, D.B. "Growing Demand for an Emerging Subspecialty." *Consultant* 27, no. 11 (1987): 97–108.
21. Cummings, K.C. "Why Some Managers Fail." *Physician Executive* 14, no. 4 (1989): 6–8.
22. Fine, A. "New Challenges for Medical Directors." *Physician Executive* 16, no. 2 (1990): 36–7.
23. Staley, S.S., and Staley, C.S. "Physician Executives and Communication." *Physician Executive* 15, no. 2 (1989): 15–17.
24. Ferguson, G. "Advice for Physicians Considering Careers as Administrators." *Canadian Medical Association Journal* 134 (1986): 1177–8.
25 Ailes, R.J. Qualities of an Effective Medical Director. Written communication. October 9, 1989.
26. Nelson, S. "The Rising Incomes—and Numbers—of MD Execs." *Hospitals* 61, no. 18 (1987): 63.
27. Friedman, E. "Physician-Administrators Making a Comeback." *Medical World News* 1 (1986): 34–43.
28. Nash, D.B., and Hillman, A.L. "Physician-Executives Can Be Mediators." *Modern Healthcare* 16, no. 24 (1986): 49.
29. Eisenberg, J.M. *Doctor's Decisions and the Cost of Medical Care.* Ann Arbor, Mich.: Health Administration Press, 1986.
30. Schien, E. *Career dynamics: Matching Individual and Organizational Needs.* Reading, Mass.: Addison-Wesley, 1978.

# Critical factors in recruiting health maintenance organization physicians

Nancy B. Fisher,
Howard L. Smith,
and
Derick P. Pasternak

*What factors facilitate successful physician recruiting by health care organizations? Answers surfaced in a study of physician recruiting by a large HMO in the Southwest. Professional networking and word-of-mouth advertising appear to be the prominent means by which physicians learn of attractive staff positions. Successful recruiting also depends on a practice setting that fosters quality care, emphasis on patient care delivery, and collegial interaction.*

*Health Care Manage Rev*, 1993, 18(1), 51–61
© 1993 Aspen Publishers, Inc.

What are the critical factors that facilitate successful recruitment of medical staff members? This question is very important to many health care organizations. Over 80 percent of hospitals with up to 399 beds report recent physician recruitment activity, while over 76 percent of hospitals with 400 or more beds are actively recruiting staff members.[1] Health maintenance organizations (HMOs) are expanding rapidly and as a result are recruiting physicians at unprecedented rates.[2] The situation may be most challenging for rural areas, which continue to have problems in attracting physicians despite changes in the national physician supply.[3] In sum, most health care organizations are vitally interested in recruiting high-quality medical staff members. Nonetheless, there is limited information available on effective recruitment practices. Health care executives face a difficult problem for which few innovative strategies have been proposed.

Physician recruitment is an especially perplexing challenge confronting HMOs. Although recent medical school graduates are more likely to pursue practice opportunities with HMOs than before, a recruitment problem remains.[4] Family practitioners, internists, pediatricians, obstetrician-gynecologists, and general surgeons are in high demand due to HMO enrollment growth.[5] Primary care practitioners normally provide a case management function essential to utilization and cost controls.[6] In the past, these physicians were difficult to recruit because of negative attitudes associated with HMOs and their tendency to view HMO care delivery as inferior to that in other practice settings.[7,8] Additionally, physicians have perceived a significant loss of autonomy and independence in HMOs.[9] Possibly as a result of the above factors, there is a tendency for HMO physicians to be younger, concerned about practice location and off-hour coverage, and less interested in income issues.[10]

*Nancy B. Fisher, M.S.W., M.B.A., is a planning analyst with Presbyterian Healthcare Services in Albuquerque, New Mexico. Her interests include health care strategic planning and marketing.*

*Howard L. Smith, Ph.D., is Professor and Associate Dean at the Anderson Schools of Management, University of New Mexico. His primary research interests include health services administration and strategic management. He has published and consulted extensively in these areas.*

*Derick P. Pasternak, M.D., M.B.A., is President of Lovelace, Inc., a federally qualified HMO and group medical practice in Albuquerque, New Mexico. An internist by training, he previously served as medical director at Lovelace. He has published widely on health care and medical topics.*

The purpose of this article is to address the issue of physician recruitment in HMOs by clarifying critical factors involved in the recruitment process. A study of medical staff members associated with the Lovelace Health Plan, an HMO comprised of approximately 300 physicians in Albuquerque, New Mexico, is used to define salient concerns in recruitment. The study also examines medical practice attributes important to Lovelace physicians, and to physicians who declined medical staff positions with Lovelace. The implications of this investigation for physician recruitment in HMOs and other health delivery settings are discussed.

## BACKGROUND

Limited research is available on physician recruitment. Most of the literature is experientially based and reported in professional journals. Some authorities indicate that physicians make practice location decisions based on income potential, geographic factors, perceived quality of medical care at the prospective site, quality of potential colleagues, and institutional reputation.[11,12] These criteria are similar to those used by physicians in ranking hospital attributes.[13] While these decision criteria influence whether a physician joins a health care organization, the recruitment process itself also may become an obstacle. Health care organizations may fail to adequately plan for the physician visit and subsequently create a poor impression that undermines recruitment.[14] Normally overlooked are invitations for family members and a concluding session to market the distinctive qualities of the organization.[15]

Although more than a decade old, a study by Fink[16] of 69 HMOs in the United States suggests that many of the recruitment issues noted above apply to HMOs. Fink's findings indicate that almost 75 percent of all HMOs studied recruit physicians who have just completed their residencies. More than one-third of the HMOs studied expressed concern that physicians were biased against group practice arrangements, an attribute that inhibited the recruitment process. However, new data do not necessarily support this finding.[17] Additionally, the HMOs indicated that they were at a distinct advantage in meeting salary and compensation offered by fee-for-service practices. The HMOs target new physicians who may be more amenable to group settings and may have lower salary expectations.

Fink's investigation confirmed the efficacy of personal contacts as well as advertisements in periodicals when recruiting physicians. Physician recruiters were not specifically mentioned as a prevalent strategy. It was also observed that 27 percent of the HMOs reported unsolicited inquiries from physicians. Fink concluded that this reflected greater acceptance of HMOs by physicians in general.

Potential resistance to group and managed care plans is a salient recruiting issue that has changed significantly in recent years. Formerly, physicians anticipated limitations on earning potential, lower quality of care, and decreased autonomy relative to HMOs. However, a study of 850 HMO physicians in Wisconsin discovered that physicians' expectations for lower earnings and quality of care were not realized.[18] The HMO physicians reported that their autonomy had decreased, which could lead to dissatisfaction and hesitancy to embrace systems designed to achieve efficiencies.[19] The implication for recruitment is significant. HMOs must work to keep medical staff members satisfied in order to prevent them from conveying negative messages to medical staff candidates.

## AN INVESTIGATION INTO PHYSICIAN RECRUITING

The Lovelace Health Plan (LHP) is New Mexico's largest HMO with over 128,000 enrollees. The LHP is an integral element of a complex health delivery system. Health plan members receive primary care at a main medical center and 12 satellite clinics in Albuquerque, New Mexico. Two clinics serve Santa Fe. The clinics are staffed by the physicians employed by Lovelace, Inc., a 300-physician-member medical staff offering multispecialty care. Lovelace, Inc. includes LHP as well as a for-profit hospital, clinical facilities, equipment, and all necessary personnel supports. The hospital facility consists of 235 inpatient beds and generally maintains an occupancy rate greater than 85 percent.

The market for managed care in Albuquerque has approximately doubled in the last five years. Total enrollment in 1986 was over 107,000 and by 1990 exceeded 193,000. In 1990, LHP's market share was 56 percent of all HMO enrollees. LHP's strategy is to maintain quality of care as well as economic viability. It is not particularly concerned about being the largest HMO solely because it has enrolled the highest number of members.

With 300 physicians assigned directly to the LHP medical staff, it is inevitable that annual recruiting must be undertaken. Turnover is very low—in the range of 5 percent—when considering retirements and those who have left for other professional opportunities. Nonetheless, when turnover is added to growth, LHP inevitably seeks to fill several medical staff positions yearly. Having

*The study began with a review of the literature and telephone interviews with five other nationally visible multispecialty group practices to obtain information on their recruitment processes.*

historically maintained a strong reputation for high quality of care, LHP is interested in attracting the finest candidates. Consequently, LHP has recently reviewed its physician recruitment process. This article assesses the current recruitment process and suggests several recommendations for other providers to consider when developing recruitment strategies.

From a methodological perspective, the study began with a review of the literature and telephone interviews with five other nationally visible multispecialty group practices to obtain information on their recruitment processes. On the basis of this information, a physician recruitment survey questionnaire was designed with the input of key medical and administrative personnel at Lovelace. (Copies of the questionnaire are available from the authors.) The questionnaire was then mailed to all physicians who interviewed for positions at Lovelace during 1989 and 1990. The responses included 76 physicians who were subsequently hired at Lovelace and 29 physicians who were offered positions at Lovelace but declined them. The response rate for the survey was 84 percent among physicians subsequently hired and 51 percent for physicians not hired by Lovelace. All data were collected over a one-month period.

## FINDINGS

Physicians were asked to indicate their specialty, means of learning about Lovelace, the Lovelace representative who made the first recruiting contact, and length of time that passed until a final hiring decision was made. Respondents indicated their perceptions of eight critical factors in the recruitment process (Table 1). Additionally, the physicians were asked to rate the overall coordination of the recruitment process. Finally, a five-interval rating scale (1=not important; 5=extremely important) was used to assess various practice attributes (e.g., salary, location, quality of care). In rating practice attributes, physicians were requested to indicate how important each attribute is to them (as physicians). They also indicated on a five-interval scale (1=very poor; 5=ex-

cellent) their perceptions of how Lovelace rates on each attribute.

## Recruitment process perceptions by physicians employed at Lovelace

Table 1 presents perceptions of the recruitment process by the 76 physicians employed by Lovelace. The data indicate a wide variety of clinical specialties among the respondents; no single clinical orientation dominates. Given the rapid growth of the LHP, this finding is anticipated. Both primary and specialty care received attention in physician recruiting. The predominant method of learning about the opportunities at Lovelace was through a colleague. Forty percent of the physicians hired at Lovelace indicate the importance of word of mouth in identifying placement opportunities. It should also be noted that only 11 percent learned about Lovelace through a recruitment firm. Thus, a good reputation remains a key basis for effective physician recruitment.

Clinical department chairpersons, division chairpersons, or administrators were the representatives most likely to make initial contact with a prospective recruit in 66 percent of the cases. Again, a physician recruiter was less likely to be the representative making the initial contact. These data underscore the relative value of professional networking and socialization in the recruitment process. Table 1 also confirms the importance of decision making at the completion of the interview. Forty-five percent of the physicians indicate that Lovelace contacted them within 1 to 7 days with a final decision, 29 percent indicated the decision took 8 to 14 days after the interview, and 13 percent indicated that a decision was made on the spot. In only 13 percent of the cases did it take more than 2 weeks to make a decision. Ability to deliver a quick decision appears to have some importance in retaining candidates.

The physicians hired by Lovelace were asked to express their perceptions of the recruitment process. As Table 1 suggests, almost 90 percent of the respondents answered affirmatively relative to the following:
- adequate information being provided in the first recruiting contact,
- accessibility to the department chairperson within a reasonable amount of time,
- provision of adequate information about the practice opportunity during the on-site interview,
- adequate information being provided on salary and benefits during the on-site interview, and
- adequate information on when Lovelace would contact the candidate with a final decision.

**TABLE 1**

PERCEPTION OF ISSUES SURROUNDING THE RECRUITMENT PROCESS BY PHYSICIANS EMPLOYED AT LOVELACE*

| Specialty | % |
|---|---|
| Other | 21 |
| Family practice | 16 |
| Other surgical specialty | 14 |
| Internal medicine | 12 |
| Other medical specialty | 12 |
| Urgent care | 9 |
| Obstetrics-gynecology | 8 |
| Pediatrics | 8 |
| **Means of learning about the Lovelace Medical Center** | |
| Colleague | 40 |
| Other | 32 |
| Professional journal | 12 |
| Recruitment firm | 11 |
| Residency program | 5 |
| Professional meeting | 1 |
| **Lovelace representative who made first recruiting contact** | |
| Lovelace department chairperson | 35 |
| Lovelace division chairperson | 18 |
| Lovelace physician | 17 |
| Lovelace administrator | 13 |
| Other | 12 |
| Physician recruitment firm | 5 |
| **At completion of the interview, how many days did it take until Lovelace contacted you with the final decision?** | |
| 1–7 days | 45 |
| 8–14 days | 29 |
| Immediate | 13 |
| 2–4 weeks | 7 |
| More than 4 weeks | 6 |

| Perceptions of recruitment process | Yes % | No % | No response % |
|---|---|---|---|
| Was adequate information provided by the Lovelace representative who made the first recruiting contact? | 91 | 9 | 0 |
| Were you able to speak with the department chairperson within a reasonable amount of time? | 95 | 1 | 4 |
| Did you receive a recruitment packet prior to your on-site interview? | 54 | 45 | 1 |
| Were all decision makers (spouse, significant other, children) invited to accompany you on the interview? | 47 | 36 | 17 |
| During the on-site interview were you provided adequate information on the practice opportunities? | 94 | 5 | 1 |
| During the on-site interview were you provided adequate information on salary and benefits? | 93 | 7 | 0 |
| At the completion of your interview were you provided adequate information on when Lovelace would contact you about a final decision? | 89 | 7 | 4 |
| Was the contact on a final decision made by the department chairperson? | 75 | 20 | 5 |

| How do you rate the overall coordination of the physician recruitment process at Lovelace? | % |
|---|---|
| Good | 67 |
| Excellent | 21 |
| Fair | 9 |
| Very poor | 0 |
| Poor | 0 |
| No response | 3 |

*n=76

These data suggest that Lovelace has effectively managed physician recruiting by presenting important information to candidates at key points over the course of the process. In this manner, Lovelace is not only able to communicate its strengths, but it also establishes confidence that there is nothing to hide.

Lovelace's recruiting process did not produce similar results on two recruiting issues. Only 54 percent of the physicians agree that they received a recruitment packet prior to on-site interviews. This failure is of limited practical significance to this particular group of respondents because they eventually were hired. However, the same conclusion may not hold true for other candidates. A recruitment packet may be valuable to both physician candidates and to Lovelace. It can establish a basis for further discussion and identify an inappropriate match. Effective recruiting takes time and effort from existing staff. Therefore, the ability to identify a poor match early in the process (either by Lovelace or by the candidate) may prevent unnecessary expenditures.

Only 47 percent of physicians indicated that Lovelace invited decision makers such as a spouse, significant others, and children to accompany the candidate on first interviews. It must be remembered that an institution is often recruiting the entire ensemble. Obviously, transportation and housing costs associated with recruitment can escalate rapidly if a candidate is accompanied by a large entourage. Therefore, there must be prudent decisions on who should be invited, but such decisions should be relatively easy when recruiting for positions that are traditionally difficult to fill. If there is uncertainty about the suitability of the candidate or the prognosis for a good fit, then an invitation to others associated with the physician can also be extended after the initial recruiting visit.

Finally, the physicians rated the overall coordination of the physician recruitment process at Lovelace. Eighty-eight percent rated the process as good or excellent. None of the physicians rated the process as poor or very poor. However, it must be remembered that these respondents were eventually employed by Lovelace, which is the optimal measure of recruiting success.

### Recruitment process perceptions by physicians declining employment

Table 2 displays the perceptions of physicians who were recruited and made an offer but who did not accept the offer. Similar to the physicians who were hired (Table 1), there is no specific pattern by specialty. Primary care specialists appear to be more prevalent in this group than

physicians who actually were employed by Lovelace. Twenty-nine percent of the physicians who did not accept a job offer are family practitioners and 17 percent are internists. A wide variety of clinical specialties are represented among the respondents.

Similar to the comparison group of physicians hired at Lovelace (Table 1), those declining an offer also indicate that they primarily learned about Lovelace from colleagues. Forty-one percent became acquainted with Lovelace's opportunities from colleagues, and 17 percent learned about Lovelace through professional journals. Again, only a small percent (i.e., 10 percent) became familiar with Lovelace through professional recruiters. Another similarity between the comparative groups is found in Lovelace representatives who made the first recruiting contact. Fifty-two percent of the physicians who did not accept a job offer by Lovelace indicate that a department chairperson, division chairperson, or administrator made the first contact regarding the position. This is similar to the results for Lovelace medical staff in Table 1. However, there appears to be greater initial contact made by professional recruiters in the case of physicians who did not accept Lovelace's job offer. It may be that recruiters are less able to identify and forge a match to the same extent as Lovelace staff.

A final similarity is found in the length of time required before being contacted about a decision. Forty-eight percent of the physicians who did not accept the job offer indicate that Lovelace contacted them within 1 to 7 days with a decision, 28 percent indicated the decision took 8 to 14 days, and 14 percent report the decision was immediate. In conclusion, Lovelace is able to reach a quick decision on a potential affiliation.

The physicians who did not accept a job offer perceive that the recruitment process was effective in

- providing adequate information in the first recruiting contact,
- enabling candidates to speak with the department chairperson in a reasonable amount of time during the recruitment process,
- providing adequate information on practice opportunities, and
- having the department chairperson contact the candidate about a final decision.

Lovelace's physician recruitment process also appears to deliver in a timely manner a recruitment packet prior to an on-site visit, to provide adequate information on salary and benefits, and to provide an indication at the end of the interview as to when a final decision will be made. In sum, there are only minor differences between response levels in Tables 1 and 2. This suggests that varia-

**TABLE 2**

PERCEPTION OF ISSUES SURROUNDING THE RECRUITMENT PROCESS BY PHYSICIANS DECLINING EMPLOYMENT*

| Specialty | % |
| --- | --- |
| Family practice | 29 |
| Internal medicine | 17 |
| Other | 17 |
| Pediatrics | 10 |
| Other medical specialty | 10 |
| Other surgical specialty | 10 |
| Obstetrics-gynecology | 7 |
| Urgent care | 0 |

| Means of learning about the Lovelace Medical Center | % |
| --- | --- |
| Colleague | 41 |
| Other | 29 |
| Professional journal | 17 |
| Recruitment firm | 10 |
| Professional meeting | 3 |
| Residency program | 0 |

| Lovelace representative who made first recruiting contact | % |
| --- | --- |
| Lovelace physician | 35 |
| Lovelace department chairperson | 24 |
| Lovelace administrator | 14 |
| Lovelace division chairperson | 14 |
| Physician recruitment firm | 10 |
| Other | 3 |

| At completion of the interview, how many days did it take until Lovelace contacted you with the final decision? | % |
| --- | --- |
| 1–7 days | 48 |
| 8–14 days | 28 |
| Immediate | 14 |
| 2–4 weeks | 7 |
| More than 4 weeks | 3 |

| Perceptions of recruitment process | Yes % | No % | No response % |
| --- | --- | --- | --- |
| Was adequate information provided by the Lovelace representative who made the first recruiting contact? | 93 | 7 | 0 |
| Were you able to speak with the department chairperson within a reasonable amount of time? | 97 | 3 | 0 |
| Did you receive a recruitment packet prior to your on-site interview? | 72 | 24 | 3 |
| Were all decision makers (spouse, significant other, children) invited to accompany you on the interview? | 62 | 34 | 3 |
| During the on-site interview were you provided adequate information on the practice opportunities? | 100 | 0 | 0 |
| During the on-site interview were you provided adequate information on salary and benefits? | 83 | 14 | 3 |
| At the completion of your interview were you provided adequate information on when Lovelace would contact you about a final decision? | 79 | 17 | 3 |
| Was the contact on a final decision made by the department chairperson? | 93 | 4 | 3 |

| How do you rate the overall coordination of the physician recruitment process at Lovelace? | % |
| --- | --- |
| Good | 52 |
| Excellent | 31 |
| Fair | 10 |
| Very poor | 3 |
| Poor | 4 |
| No response | 0 |

*n=29

tions in Lovelace's recruitment process are not the primary determining factor relative to whether a physician is employed or not at Lovelace. This conclusion is further supported by the fact that 83 percent (compared with 88 percent in Table 1) of the physicians who did not accept the job offer by Lovelace rate the overall coordination of recruitment as good or excellent.

### Practice ratings by physicians employed at Lovelace

Table 3 reports ratings of the practice attributes at Lovelace. The physicians employed by Lovelace were asked to rate the attributes' importance to physicians (1=not important; 5=extremely important) and to rate the attributes as present at Lovelace (1=very poor; 5=excellent). The results indicate that (on average) all of the practice attributes were rated as at least fairly important (i.e., $\bar{X}$=3.00) to the physicians. Furthermore, 72.7 percent (i.e., 8 out of 11) of the practice attributes are rated as very important by the physicians. The most important practice attributes are quality of care ($\bar{X}$=4.66), amount of clinical time spent on patients per week ($\bar{X}$=4.19), number of hours worked per week ($\bar{X}$=4.18), and interaction with colleagues ($\bar{X}$=4.14). At least 80 percent of the physicians

## TABLE 3

### PRACTICE ATTRIBUTE RATINGS BY PHYSICIANS EMPLOYED AT LOVELACE*

| Practice attribute | $\bar{X}$† | S.D. | % Rating attribute as very or extremely important to them as physicians |
|---|---|---|---|
| Quality of care provided | 4.66 | 0.58 | 95 |
| Amount of clinical time spent on patients | 4.19 | 0.68 | 84 |
| Number of hours worked per week | 4.18 | 0.78 | 80 |
| Interaction with colleagues | 4.14 | 0.69 | 80 |
| Professional autonomy | 4.00 | 0.79 | 77 |
| Salary | 4.01 | 0.77 | 76 |
| Geographic location | 4.04 | 0.84 | 75 |
| Call schedule | 4.08 | 0.87 | 74 |
| Nonsalary fringe benefits | 3.87 | 0.75 | 71 |
| Input into managerial decisions | 3.70 | 0.87 | 55 |
| Amount of administrative time | 3.07 | 1.04 | 32 |

| Practice attribute | $\bar{X}$‡ | S.D. | % Rating practice conditions at Lovelace as good or excellent relative to attribute |
|---|---|---|---|
| Geographic location | 4.25 | 0.81 | 79 |
| Quality of care provided | 3.97 | 0.73 | 74 |
| Nonsalary fringe benefits | 3.92 | 0.86 | 74 |
| Number of hours worked per week | 3.93 | 0.78 | 71 |
| Call schedule | 3.86 | 0.92 | 70 |
| Interaction with colleagues | 3.83 | 0.81 | 66 |
| Amount of clinical time | 3.76 | 0.78 | 62 |
| Professional autonomy | 3.68 | 0.75 | 59 |
| Salary | 3.43 | 0.85 | 51 |
| Amount of administrative time | 2.97 | 0.90 | 28 |
| Input into managerial decisions | 2.65 | 0.88 | 18 |

*n=76
† Scaling: 1=not important; 5=extremely important
‡ Scaling: 1=very poor; 5=excellent

retained by Lovelace rate these attributes as very or extremely important.

Professional autonomy ($\bar{X}$=4.00), salary ($\bar{X}$=4.01), geographic location ($\bar{X}$=4.04), and call schedule ($\bar{X}$=4.08) are also important practice attributes listed by the physicians. At least 74 percent of the respondents indicate that these attributes are very or extremely important. Less important are nonsalary fringe benefits and input into managerial decisions. However, more than half of the physicians still view these attributes as fairly important on average. Only the amount of administrative time is rated relatively low by the physicians hired at Lovelace. Thirty-two percent view this as an important practice attribute.

The physicians hired by Lovelace were also asked to rate the practice attributes as they apply to Lovelace. Some differences in perspective emerge in this comparison. Only geographic location is rated as good ($\bar{X}$=4.25) relative to Lovelace's practice conditions. The other practice attributes are rated as fair. Quality of care ($\bar{X}$=3.97), nonsalary fringe benefits ($\bar{X}$=3.92), number of hours worked per week ($\bar{X}$=3.93), and call schedule ($\bar{X}$=3.86) are rated as good by at least 70 percent of the physicians. Interaction with colleagues ($\bar{X}$=3.83), amount of clinical time spent with patients ($\bar{X}$=3.76), professional autonomy ($\bar{X}$=3.68), and salary ($\bar{X}$=3.43) are also rated as good at Lovelace by at least half of the physicians. Again, amount of administrative time ($\bar{X}$=2.97) and input into managerial decisions ($\bar{X}$=2.65) are rated low by the physicians.

The overall impression from these findings is that many of the practice attribute factors that are rated as very or extremely important to physicians are, for the most part, present at Lovelace. Lovelace does offer good quality of care, geographic location, nonsalary fringe benefits, number of hours worked per week, call schedule, and interaction with colleagues. It appears that Lovelace could do a better job relative to clinical time spent with patients, professional autonomy, and salary.

### Practice ratings by physicians declining employment

Table 4 presents ratings of practice attributes by physicians who did not accept the job offer by Lovelace. There are many parallels with the results in Table 3. This set of physicians rate quality of care ($\bar{X}$=4.79), geographic location ($\bar{X}$=4.39), interaction with colleagues ($\bar{X}$=4.32), and amount of clinical time spent on patients ($\bar{X}$=4.08) as the most important practice attributes. Nonetheless, all of the other practice attributes are rated as at least fairly important. Salary, input into managerial decisions, profes-

*Quality of care, interaction with colleagues, and amount of clinical time spent with patients are the prominent common denominators between the two groups.*

sional autonomy, call schedule, nonsalary fringe benefits, and number of hours worked per week are rated as important by almost 60 percent of the respondents. Only the amount of administrative time required by a practice is not consistently rated as important by the physicians.

For the most part, there is substantial consistency between practice attributes rated as important by physicians hired at Lovelace and those who did not accept the job offer by Lovelace. Quality of care, interaction with colleagues, and amount of clinical time spent with patients are the prominent common denominators between the two groups. The physicians employed by Lovelace do indicate a greater number of very important or extremely important attributes; notably, number of hours worked per week, professional autonomy, salary, geographic location, and call schedule. However, high percentages of the physicians who did not accept the Lovelace job offer also rate these factors as important. The differences in mean scores are not statistically or practically different.

Furthermore, the physicians who did not accept Lovelace's job offer rate Lovelace quite positively on many of the practice attributes. Over 70 percent of these physicians view Lovelace's practice environment as good or excellent on geographic location, number of hours worked per week, quality of care provided, amount of clinical time, nonsalary fringe benefits, and interaction with colleagues. These findings suggest that Lovelace has done a very good job in cultivating an attractive practice setting. Again, there are many favorable comparisons with the evaluations of physicians employed by Lovelace (Table 3).

Call schedule, salary, professional autonomy, and input into managerial decisions are rated as good by 55 percent of the physicians who did not accept the job offer at Lovelace. Comparison of these results with Table 3 suggests that the physicians employed by Lovelace also believe that the practice attributes could be more fully developed. Input into managerial decisions is the only attribute not rated highly by the two groups of physicians. The overall view of Lovelace's practice setting by physicians who have visited Lovelace and those who ultimately were employed is quite comparable.

## TABLE 4

PRACTICE ATTRIBUTE RATINGS BY PHYSICIANS DECLINING EMPLOYMENT*

| Practice attribute | $\bar{X}$[†] | S.D. | % Rating attribute as very or extremely important to them as physicians |
|---|---|---|---|
| Quality of care provided | 4.79 | 0.50 | 93 |
| Geographic location | 4.39 | 0.57 | 93 |
| Interaction with colleagues | 4.32 | 0.67 | 86 |
| Amount of clinical time spent on patients | 4.08 | 0.63 | 76 |
| Salary | 3.89 | 0.63 | 72 |
| Input into managerial decisions | 3.86 | 0.93 | 72 |
| Professional autonomy | 3.89 | 0.59 | 69 |
| Call schedule | 3.74 | 0.94 | 62 |
| Nonsalary fringe benefits | 3.74 | 0.66 | 59 |
| Number of hours worked per week | 3.71 | 0.76 | 59 |
| Amount of administrative time | 3.07 | 0.83 | 24 |

| Practice attribute | $\bar{X}$[‡] | S.D. | % Rating practice conditions at Lovelace as good or excellent relative to attribute |
|---|---|---|---|
| Geographic location | 4.32 | 0.72 | 83 |
| Number of hours worked per week | 4.07 | 0.60 | 83 |
| Quality of care provided | 4.11 | 0.69 | 79 |
| Amount of clinical time | 3.96 | 0.69 | 79 |
| Nonsalary fringe benefits | 4.07 | 0.72 | 76 |
| Interaction with colleagues | 3.89 | 0.74 | 72 |
| Amount of administrative time | 3.67 | 0.68 | 59 |
| Call schedule | 4.00 | 0.65 | 55 |
| Salary | 3.39 | 0.92 | 48 |
| Professional autonomy | 3.41 | 0.84 | 45 |
| Input into managerial decisions | 3.33 | 0.87 | 34 |

*n=29
[†] Scaling: 1=not important; 5=extremely important
[‡] Scaling: 1=very poor; 5=excellent

In view of the similarities between the response sets, it is appropriate to ask why some physicians decided to join the staff at Lovelace and others did not. The physicians who did not accept Lovelace's job offer were asked to clarify their reasons for their decision. A variety of reasons surfaced (see box entitled "Primary Reasons for Not Accepting a Position at Lovelace"). Interestingly, many (20 percent) of the physicians discovered that after visiting Lovelace their desire to relocate had changed. This implies that they could not perceive sufficient comparative advantage to undertake a move. Eighteen percent cited inadequate or noncompetitive salary, while 14 per-

**Primary Reasons for Not Accepting a Position at Lovelace**

| | % |
|---|---|
| No response given by physician. | 28 |
| Discrepancy between Lovelace position and desired position. | 20 |
| Inadequate, noncompetitive salary. | 18 |
| Wish to remain in present position. | 14 |
| Personal (family, location). | 10 |
| Another opportunity was better. | 10 |

cent listed a desire to remain in their present position. These results suggest that on further examination, the physicians remained in their present practices. The "grass is greener" phenomenon may have been operating in these cases.

## IMPLICATIONS

What factors facilitate successful recruiting of medical staff members? Worthwhile answers to this question have surfaced in the course of examining the LHP's efforts to attract and retain physicians. In considering the implications of these findings for other HMOs and providers it should be remembered that Lovelace's experience may not be completely transferable to other settings. Clearly, Lovelace has carefully cultivated an HMO practice setting conducive to attracting physicians of the highest caliber. The practice opportunities themselves play an important role in recruitment. In short, simply following well-designed recruitment strategies will not always guarantee success. The nature of an organization, personal rewards, practice climate, linkages with teaching and research institutions, location, and other factors affect recruitment success. Lovelace has carefully attended to these practice attributes, which, in turn, has reinforced recruitment efforts.

Lovelace's experience suggests that when recruiting, health care organizations should consider several strategies. First, potential physician candidates are likely to learn about an opportunity from colleagues, professional journals, and other sources, but less often from professional recruiters (Tables 1 and 2). For difficult-to-recruit positions it may be essential to tap the professional network of the medical staff. For example, if an organization has trouble attracting a surgical specialty, it may be useful for all medical staff members to write several colleagues alerting them to the position. Word-of-mouth advertising seems to work in the case of Lovelace. It may work for other organizations if the professional network is exercised.

Second, Lovelace's experience suggests that candidates should be contacted with a final decision within 14 days (Tables 1 and 2). Exceptions to this strategy may arise where a clinical department is sensitive to a particular personality or where physician availability allows some slack in the hiring decision. Nonetheless, it appears that organizations should establish a recruitment process that can deliver a decision within two weeks. This approach capitalizes on the strengths of the visit and reinforces the clarity of thinking by the provider relative to

potential candidates and the requirements of the position.

Third, Lovelace has found that an effective recruitment process is highly capable of communicating critical information (Tables 1 and 2). Specific ingredients of this process include the following:

- providing adequate information during the first recruiting contact,
- communicating between the clinical department chairperson and candidate within a reasonable amount of time,
- providing a recruitment packet before the on-site interview,
- communicating adequate information on practice opportunities during the interview,
- clarifying specifics regarding salary and benefits, and
- indicating when a final decision will be made.

It is unlikely that these elements of effective recruiting are germane solely to Lovelace. Other organizations should consider incorporating these ingredients in their recruiting process if they wish to establish a basis from which successful recruiting can evolve.

Finally, Lovelace has discovered that some practice attributes are more important to physicians than others (Tables 3 and 4). Reputation for quality care, ability to spend time in delivering patient care, and collegial interaction appear to be the most important practice attributes to physicians. In order to achieve successful physician recruitment, it is necessary to cultivate those attributes. This may not be an easy task because quality care reputation and collegial interaction are professional issues that seldom are developed overnight. However, emphasis on visible organizational commitment to quality and team-building efforts may grow the sort of climate that supports recruitment.

In the case of Lovelace, it rates fairly well on these key practice attributes. Nonetheless, like most organizations, progress can still be made. Several strategies are already being implemented to improve the prospects of delivering a better practice environment relative to collegial interaction and patient care delivery. Meanwhile, Lovelace can capitalize on its other distinctive features such as geographic location, practice hours required per week, nonsalary fringe benefits, and call schedule. These attributes have provided Lovelace a strong measure of success in physician recruitment.

•    •    •

Health care organizations that face the challenge of recruiting physicians can reconfigure their strategies in view of the experiences described for Lovelace. At the heart of successful recruitment is laying a foundation of basics—a well-structured and informative process. Organizations should also contemplate means to tap the collegial and professional network of their physicians. Central in this effort is continual questioning of whether the existing medical staff members have contributed to the recruitment process by spreading the word in the professional and collegial grapevine. Furthermore, organizations should build on their distinctive qualities and assets in attracting candidates. Special attention can be focused on the collegial environment, quality of care, and emphasis on medical care delivery. With these ingredients in mind, the prognosis for successful recruiting improves.

## REFERENCES

1. Grayson, M.A. "Physician Recruitment Takes Center Stage." *Hospitals* 63, no. 7 (1989): 30–34.
2. Korcok, M. "U.S. Doctors Flocking to Salaried Employment." *CMAJ* 136, no. 1 (1987): 73–75.
3. Crandall, L.A., Dwyer, J.W., and Duncan, R.P. "Recruitment and Retention of Rural Physicians: Issues for the 1990s." *Journal of Rural Health* 6, no. 1 (1990): 19–37.
4. Jacobs, M.O., and Mott, P.D. "Physician Characteristics and Training Emphasis Considered Desirable by Leaders of HMOs." *Journal of Medical Education* 62, no. 9(1987):725–31.
5. Thomas, M.C. "Groups Are Still Bidding Top Dollar for the Doctors They Want." *Medical Economist* 67, no. 4 (1990): 52–60.
6. Steinwachs, D.M., et al. "A Comparison of the Requirements for Primary Care Physicians in HMOs with Projections Made by the GMENAC." *New England Journal of Medicine* 314, no. 4 (1986): 217–22.
7. Powills, S. "Physicians Join HMOs Reluctantly." *Hospitals* 61, no. 19 (1987): 100.
8. Taylor, H., and Kagay, M. "The HMO Report Card: A Closer Look." *Health Affairs* 5, no. 1 (1986): 81–89.
9. Zoler, M.L. "Salaried Physicians: Decent Money, Great Call Schedule, But. . . ." *Medical World News* 29, no. 2 (1988): 34–36, 39.
10. Shouldice, R.G., "Characteristics of Physicians in HMOs." *Medical Group Management* 36, no. 4 (1989): 6, 9.
11. Koska, M.T. "Physician Recruiting 101: Avoid the Classic Mistakes." *Hospitals* 64 (1990): 46–49.
12. Martinsons, J.N. "What's the Top MD Recruitment Incentive?" *Hospitals* 62, no. 3 (1988): 69.
13. Muller, A., and Bledsoe, P. "Physicians' Ranking of Hospital Attributes: A Comparison by Use Group." *Health Care Management Review* 14, no. 3 (1989): 77–84.
14. Ripley, R.A., and Nichols, R. "Hiring Winners." *Medical Group Management* 34, no. 1 (1987): 45–47.
15. Taylor, M.W. "The Interviewing Process." *Medical Group Management* 34, no. 2 (1987): 40–44.
16. Fink, R. "HMOs and Physician Recruiting: A Survey of Problems and Methods Among Group Practice Plans." *Public Health Reports* 96, no. 6 (1981): 568–73.
17. Hay Group Consulting. *Survey of Physician Attitudes.* Chicago, Ill.: Hay Group Consulting, 1991.
18. Schulz, R., et al. "Physician Adaptation to Health Maintenance Organizations and Implications for Management." *Health Services Research* 25, no. 1 (1990): 43–64.
19. McKinlay, J.B., and Stoeckle, J.D. "Corporatization and the Social Transformation of Doctoring." *International Journal of Health Services* 18, no. 2 (1988): 191–205.

# Career paths of physician executives

David A. Kindig,
Nancy Cross Dunham,
and
Li Man Chun

*Survey data from a sample of physicians whose primary professional activity is administration were used to examine their previous administrative positions and career paths. Forty percent reported administrative positions in more than one type of health care organization, and time spent in administration increased with age and years in administration. Most responders with senior titles had four or more positions in a single type of organization or two positions in different types of organizations. These findings should be useful for further investigation on the physician executive role, as well as in career planning.*

The emergence of physicians' roles in key administrative and executive positions within many U.S. health care organizations has represented a major change in the medical profession over the last two decades. As the health care system grows ever more complex and competitive, there is a growing need to balance the inherent tensions between health care as a social good and health care as an economic good. The recognition of this boundary-spanning role is reflected in the growth of physician involvement in decision-making processes in health care institutions.

These changing roles for medical professionals are reflected, nationally, in the number of physicians who identify themselves as physician administrators or physician executives. For example, data from the 1986 American Medical Association's (AMA) Physician Masterfile indicate that there were 14,075 physicians who reported that their primary professional activity involved administration.[1] These physician administrators represented approximately 3 percent of all active, practicing U.S. physicians in that year.

Kindig and Lastiri-Quiros have examined and reported on various aspects of the roles physicians now play in the administrative arena of many health care organizations. In one study, it was found that physician executives often have responsibilities for a wide scope of general management issues in health care institutions.[2] Study results highlighted the boundary-spanning roles of today's physician executives; their job functions do not necessarily focus primarily on physician and/or medical staff issues, as they may have in the past.

A second study found that the majority of physician executives surveyed reported that they had entered administrative medicine for positive reasons.[1] In that survey, 39 percent of respondents reported that their primary reason for choosing an administrative career was to have a broad impact on health care delivery and to ensure quality of care. Another 13 percent reported a general enjoyment of management as the primary reason for choosing an administrative career.

**David A. Kindig,** *M.D., Ph.D., is Professor and Director of Programs in Health Management, Department of Preventive Medicine, University of Wisconsin, School of Medicine, Madison, Wisconsin.*

**Nancy Cross Dunham,** *M.S., is the Project Director for the John A. Hartford Foundation, Programs in Health Management, Department of Preventive Medicine, University of Wisconsin, School of Medicine, Madison, Wisconsin.*

**Li Man Chun,** *M.D., is a Lecturer from Beijing Medical University, Health Management Training Center, Beijing, China.*

*Health Care Manage Rev,* 1991, 16(4), 11–20

In a third study, using national aggregate data, it was found that the number of physicians whose primary professional activity was reported as administration increased by 19.2 percent from 1977 to 1986.[3] While this analysis found a significant increase in the number of young physicians who report being actively involved in administrative activities on a part-time basis, the biggest increase in those who report their primary professional activity is administration was found for older physicians. It was speculated that such growth in the numbers of older physician administrators may indicate that a shift of professional activities from clinical duties to managerial roles is becoming an increasingly common career move for physicians as they near retirement age.

Beyond these studies, very little is known about the career paths that physicians who work in executive capacities in health care organizations have followed during their professional lives. Most previous studies of physicians working in administration are dated or limited to one type of organization or group.

Information on the career paths of physician executives would be important to develop for at least two reasons. First, it was speculated that "administrative medicine" or "medical management" was becoming a new medical specialty.[1] The educational implications of that development have also been discussed.[4-6] Secondly, for those physicians who are thinking about becoming more actively involved in administrative activities in the health care field, such information on the "typical" career path and professional mobility of today's physician executives could be helpful in making important career decisions.

For example, students in the M.S. degree program in Administrative Medicine at the University of Wisconsin–Madison School of Medicine often ask about employment opportunities and career mobility for physician executives.[7,8] These authors' professional opinion is that the opportunities for increased responsibility and promotion of physician executives may be more common within an existing organization than for non-physician health care executives, particularly in community hospitals and multispecialty medical groups. Having a firmer basis on which to give such advice and direction would be useful to students and faculty alike.

---

*This study presents information that relates to the career paths and mobility of today's physician executives.*

---

This article, therefore, presents information that relates to the career paths and mobility of today's physician executives. In particular, the following issues are examined: (1) patterns of career moves among health care organizations, (2) years of clinical and management experience of physician executives, (3) differences in clinical and management experience between "senior"-level and "junior"-level executives, (4) average amount of professional time spent in administrative and clinical activities, and (5) the relationship of seniority to professional mobility.

## DATA AND METHODS

The identification and selection of the sample of physicians surveyed for this analysis have been previously described.[1,2] The study consisted of a telephone survey of a randomly selected sample of 878 physicians from the total number of 13,828 who were reported in the 1985 AMA masterfile as having their primary professional activity in administration. The survey sample represented over 6 percent of physician administrators in the United States at the time the survey was conducted. Complete data on number and types of organizations worked for and on seniority level of present administrative positions were available for 867 of the survey respondents (98.7 percent of the sample). Tables A-1–A-6 in the Appendix present data on these 867 physician executives.

Survey respondents were asked a wide variety of questions relating to their professional careers, including

- the number of years in practice,
- the number of years spent working in administration,
- the type of organization they worked in,
- their past and present administrative titles,
- the relative proportion of their professional time spent in administrative and clinical activities, and
- the number of job changes they had made in their administrative careers.

One way to examine the career paths of these physician executives is to classify respondents' administrative positions with respect to their level of executive authority within the organizations they work for. To do this classification, data were obtained that related to the job title and/or job description of the specific positions held by each respondent (their current position and up to three previous positions). These job classifications were then categorized as being either senior- or junior-level positions, depending on the degree of overall authority that a physician executive was likely to wield within the organization. Senior-level positions were those that included presidents, vice presidents, or chief executive officers of health care corporations or other institutions; presidents, vice presidents, or deans of academic institutions; and ranking governmental or military officials. Titles designated as indicating more junior-level positions included chairman/chief of academic departments or clinics; medical directors of health care organizations; middle-level officers in the military, public health service, or the Veterans Administration; directors or supervisors of nonacademic units; and health care consultants and others.

Another way of analyzing the career paths of physician executives is to classify and examine the data on the "stage" of their career at the current time, that is, the number of years in practice (defined as years since completing graduate medical education) and the number of years the respondent has been working in some type of administrative position. Data on the number of years in practice were categorized as follows: less than 10 years, 10 to 19 years, 20 to 29 years, 30 to 39 years, and 40 or more years. Data on the number of years in administration were categorized as follows: less that 5 years, 5 to 9 years, 10 to 14 years, 15 to 19 years, and 20 years or more.

Respondents were asked to report the type of health care organization they worked for at the time of the survey, as well as the types of organizations worked for in as many as three previous positions (if applicable). Data on type of organization worked for were classified into hospitals, educational institutions, government agencies, and "other" organizations (which included health maintenance organizations, group practices or clinics, health care corporations, nursing homes, insurance companies, and home health care organizations). Changes in types of organizations worked for were then tracked by noting the type of organization worked for at the time of the survey, and comparing that data to type of organizations worked for in previous positions.

## RESULTS

### Type of organizations worked for and moves among organizations

The distribution of survey respondents was first examined according to the type of organization they were working for at the time. Table A-1 shows that, with respect to their current positions, the 867 physician executives in the sample were distributed as such: 33.7 percent (292) were working in hospitals, 21.8 percent (189) were working in academic institutions, 21.2 percent (184) were in government agencies, and 23.3 percent (202) were working in other types of organizations.

*Almost 60 percent of the survey respondents reported having worked for only one type of organization in an administrative capacity.*

Table A-2 presents distributions according to whether or not the respondents presently (within each of the four classifications of organizations) have held all of their administrative positions within the *same type* of organization or have held administrative positions within *more than one type* of organization, and whether they have worked in one specific organization throughout their administrative career or worked for two, three, and four or more separate organizations. These data indicate that the physician executives in the sample tend to have had a fair amount of job stability throughout their administrative careers. Almost 60 percent (516 of 867) of the survey respondents reported having worked for only one type of organization in an administrative capacity. Of those, 57 percent (294 of 516) have worked for only one organization, 24 percent (124) have worked in two organizations, 12 percent (62) have worked in three organizations, and 7 percent (36) have worked in four or more organizations in an administrative capacity. Respondents in all types of organizations were generally similar in this regard, although, of those physician executives working in academic institutions, a full 70 percent (71 of 101) reported having worked only for their present organization in an administrative capacity.

The data also indicate that those physician executives working in hospitals and governmental organizations were most likely to report having worked for only one type of organization throughout their administrative careers. A total of 65 percent (191 of 292) of the respondents working in hospitals reported having worked *only* in hospitals throughout their administrative careers, while 67 percent (124 of 184) of those working in government organizations reported having worked *only* for government organizations.

Regarding the 351 respondents in the sample who did move across types of organization in their administrative careers, 70 percent (246) had worked for only two separate organizations, 22 percent (77) had worked for three organizations, and 8 percent (28) had worked for four or more separate organizations in an administrative capacity. As with those who had worked for only one type of organization, those in academic institutions were found to have, generally, had more job stability; 77 percent of those in academic institutions who had changed the type of organization they worked for had made only one such change (i.e., had worked for only two separate organizations) throughout their administrative careers.

### Practice and administrative experience of physician executives

In addition to examining the types and numbers of organizations worked for, data were also analyzed on the distribution of survey respondents with respect to the number of years they had been in practice and the number of years they had held administrative positions. Table A-3 presents data on these distributions.

The data indicate that physician executives tend to have a substantial amount of professional experience; 63 percent of survey respondents indicated that they had been in medical practice for 20 or more years (37.6 percent for 20 to 29 years, 21.1 percent for 30 to 39 years, and 4.3 percent for over 40 years). Only 9 percent had been in practice for less than 10 years, while 27.7 percent had been in practice for 10 to 19 years.

The data also show that the vast majority of respondents have had considerable professional experience in administrative capacities. A total of 52 percent of survey respondents reported having occupied administrative positions for 20 or more years; another 31.8 percent have been administrators for 10 to 19 years (14.7 percent for 10 to 14 years and 17.1 percent for 15 to 19 years). Only 16.3 percent of the survey sample had been in administrative positions for less than 10 years.

Table A-4 presents data on the distribution of senior- and junior-level positions held by survey respondents by stage of career, measured with both respect to number of years in practice and number of years in an administrative capacity. Not surprisingly, it was found that physician executives with higher levels of experience tend to be found in higher seniority positions within organizations. Only 3.8 percent of survey respondents with fewer than 10 years in medical practice reported occupying senior-level administrative positions. Those respondents with 30 to 39 years in medical practice had the highest proportion reported to be in senior-level positions (24.7 percent), followed closely by those with over 40 years in medical practice (22.2 percent).

No respondents with fewer than 5 years administrative experience , and only 6.4 percent of those with 5 to 9 years administrative experience, were found to be in senior-level positions. The percent found in senior-level positions rises directly with increasing amounts of administrative experience, representing 14.4 percent of those with 10 to 14 years experience, 18.6 percent of those with 15 to 19 years experience, and 22.9 percent of those with more than 20 years experience in an administrative capacity.

### Time spent in administrative and clinical activities

Table A-5 presents data on the average percentage of time spent each week by survey respondents on administrative and clinical activities. These data show that, on average, physician executives report spending 65 percent of their professional time on administrative activities and 20.6 percent of their time on clinical activities (the remaining time being spent on activities such as teaching, research, and other professional activities). Senior-level physician executives spend substantially higher proportions of their professional time on administrative activities than do junior-level executives (79 percent and 62 percent, respectively) and lower proportions of time on clinical activities (8.3 percent compared to 23.3 percent for junior-level executives).

The data in Table A-5 also indicate that career progression (with respect to years in both practice and administration) is directly related to amount of professional time typically spent in administrative activities and is inversely related to the amount of time typically spent in clinical activities for physician executives. Those survey respondents with less than 10 years in practice reported spending, on average, 56.2 percent of their professional time doing administrative functions and 27.9 percent of their time in clinical roles. In comparison, physicians with 40 or more years in practice report spending a total of 74.1 percent of their professional time in administrative activities and only 14.3 percent in clinical activities.

The same pattern is observed with regard to the number of years spent in administration. Physicians who have been administrators for 20 years or more report spending 66.9 percent of their professional time in administrative capacities and only 18.9 percent of their time in clinical activities. In contrast, those physicians who have been administrators for less than 5 years report spending 57.6 percent of their time on administration and 28.6 percent of their time on clinical activities.

### Professional mobility and career advancement

One objective of this study was to explore issues of professional mobility for physician executives (i.e., moves among different organizations) and to attempt to relate this mobility of levels to professional advancement (i.e., likelihood of being in a senior-level position). Table A-6 presents information illustrating the relationship between seniority of current position and past professional

*An objective of this study was to explore issues of professional mobility for physician executives and to attempt to relate this mobility of levels to professional advancement.*

mobility among different organizations and different organizational types.

As noted previously, 15.6 percent of the survey sample was found to report that they occupied senior-level executive positions within their health care organizations. In total, of those who had worked in an administrative capacity in only one type of health care organization, 12 percent were in senior-level positions; of those who had worked in more than one type of organization, 20.8 percent were in senior-level positions.

Of those who had worked in only one type of health care organization (e.g., had worked only for hospitals or academic institutions) professional mobility (moves between different organizations) appears to be directly related to career advancement (i.e., being in a senior-level position). Of these physician executives, the highest proportion found to be in senior-level positions (20.5 percent) were those who had worked in four or more separate organizations during their administrative careers.

By contrast, for those physician executives who had moved at some point during their administrative careers across organizational types, professional mobility appears to be inversely related to career advancement. Of those having held positions in more than one type of organization, the highest proportion found to be in senior-level positions (23.4 percent) were for those who had worked in only two separate organizations during their administrative careers. Of those who had worked in four or more different organizations, only 11.1 percent were found to occupy senior-level positions.

## DISCUSSION

The data presented in this paper have provided, for the first time, some basic information about the career progression of physician executives presently working in health care organizations in the United States. A major finding of the analysis was that 60 percent of all physician executives in this sample study reported having worked in only one type of organization and that 57 percent of these respondents report having worked for only one individual organization throughout their administrative careers. These findings suggest a relative profes-

sional stability of physicians working in administrative capacities in health care organizations.

It is not surprising that, by organizational type, the lowest percentage of respondents reporting working for a single organization throughout their administrative careers are those individuals who were working for government agencies at the time the survey was conducted. In comparison, the highest percentage of respondents reporting having worked in an administrative capacity in only one organization are those who are employed by academic institutions.

Although a relative stability was noted in the professional careers of today's physician executives (with regard to the number of organizations typically worked for), the data on the relationship between professional mobility and seniority level suggest, however, that advancement to more senior-level executive positions (as defined for this analysis) may require a willingness to move between organizations and across organizational types. As noted above, for those staying within one type of organization, the highest level of seniority was achieved by those physician executives who have held administrative positions within four separate organizations. Those physician executives who have worked for more than one type of health care organization were more likely to have senior-level positions than were those working in only one type of organization (20.8 percent versus 12 percent).

It should be useful for young clinicians who may be thinking about a career in administration, or about earning a management degree, to know in advance that—at least historically—achieving a position in which the majority of one's professional time is spent on administrative functions (as opposed to clinical duties) may not occur in the first few years following completion of graduate medical education. The extent to which this is true for physicians with recent graduate degrees in management is not known. In addition, with the growth of managed care organizations, these authors suspect that there may be a slight trend toward the employment of physicians with less clinical and administrative experience than in the past. In general, however, top leadership roles in medical organizations cannot be expected to be assigned to inexperienced clinicians or managers.

Regarding how the respondents to this survey reported utilizing their professional time, a sharp reduction was noted in the amount of time spent in clinical activities, with increasing years in practice and in management indicating an ever-increasing move away from clinically related duties as these physician executives advance in their careers. In particular, the data indicate that senior-level physician executives spend less than 10 percent of their professional time engaged in clinical activities and almost 80 percent of their time fulfilling management functions.

•    •    •

This study has presented unique information about the career paths of physician executives in the United States. Such information should prove useful to individuals considering such careers and to the organizations employing them. Additional research on these issues seems warranted. In particular, it would be interesting to examine the career paths of those physicians who have recently attained management degrees, and to explore the expanded career opportunities for physician executives that emerging types of health care organizations (such as managed care systems) may provide.

## REFERENCES

1. Kindig, D.A., and Lastiri, S. "Administrative Medicine: A New Medical Specialty?" *Health Affairs* 5, no. 4 (1986): 146–56.

2. Kindig, D.A., and Lastiri-Quiros, S. "The Changing Managerial Role of Physician Executives." *Journal of Health Administration Education* 7, no. 1 (1989): 33–46.

3. Kindig, D.A., and Dunham, N.C. "How Much Administration is Today's Physician Doing?" *Physician Executive* 17, no. 7 (1991): 3–7.

4. Hillman, A.L., et al. "Managing the Medical–Industrial Complex." *New England Journal of Medicine* 315, no. 8 (1986): 511–13.

5. Kindig, D.A. "Management Education for the Physician Executive: Background and Issues." *Journal of Health Administration Education* 7, no. 4 (1989): 677–89.

6. Kindig, D.A., and Sanborn, A. "Is There a Master's Degree in Your Future?" *Physician Executive* 16, no. 1 (1990): 15—8.

7. Detmer, D., and Noren, J.J. "An Administrative Program for Clinician Executives." *Journal of Medical Education* 56, no. 8 (1981): 640–45.

8. Kindig, D.A. "Administrative Medicine at the University of Wisconsin–Madison." *Journal of Health Administration Education* 7, no. 4 (1989): 734–37.

# APPENDIX

## SURVEY RESPONSES FROM PHYSICIAN EXECUTIVES

### TABLE A-1

### CURRENT TYPE OF ORGANIZATION FOR PHYSICIAN EXECUTIVES

| Current type of organization | Number | % |
|---|---|---|
| Hospitals | 292 | 33.7 |
| Academic institutions | 189 | 21.8 |
| Government agencies | 184 | 21.2 |
| Other organizations | 202 | 23.3 |
| Total | 867 | 100.0 |

### TABLE A-2

### EMPLOYMENT SETTINGS FOR PHYSICIAN EXECUTIVES

| | All administrative positions held within same type of organization | | | | | Administrative positions held in more than one type of organization | | | |
|---|---|---|---|---|---|---|---|---|---|
| | (N) | Organizations worked for | | | | (N) | Organizations worked for | | |
| | | 1 | 2 | 3 | 4+ | | 2 | 3 | 4+ |
| Hospitals | (191) | 56 | 29 | 12 | 3 | (101) | 67 | 25 | 8 |
| Academic institutions | (101) | 70 | 15 | 10 | 5 | (88) | 77 | 19 | 3 |
| Government agencies | (124) | 49 | 27 | 16 | 8 | (60) | 60 | 27 | 13 |
| Other organizations | (100) | 57 | 23 | 9 | 13 | (102) | 71 | 21 | 8 |
| Total | (516) | 57 | 24 | 12 | 7 | (351) | 70 | 22 | 8 |

NOTE: Numbers in parentheses are actual numbers of respondents. Other numbers are percentages of that number, which sum horizontally to 100 percent.

## TABLE A-3

PERCENTAGE DISTRIBUTION OF YEARS IN
MEDICAL PRACTICE* AND YEARS IN
ADMINISTRATION

| Years | % |
|---|---|
| Medical practice | |
| Less than 10 | 9.0 |
| 10 to 19 | 27.7 |
| 20 to 29 | 37.6 |
| 30 to 39 | 21.1 |
| 40 or more | 4.3 |
| Administration | |
| Less than 5 | 5.2 |
| 5 to 9 | 11.1 |
| 10 to 14 | 14.7 |
| 15 to 19 | 17.1 |
| 20 or more | 52.0 |

*Years in medical practice since completing graduate medical
education.

## TABLE A-4

SENIORITY LEVEL OF PRESENT
ADMINISTRATIVE POSITION BY NUMBER OF
YEARS IN MEDICAL PRACTICE AND IN
ADMINISTRATION

| Years | Seniority level (%) | |
|---|---|---|
| | Senior-level positions | Junior-level positions |
| Medical practice | | |
| Less than 10 | 3.8 | 96.2 |
| 10 to 19 | 15.8 | 84.2 |
| 20 to 29 | 18.9 | 81.1 |
| 30 to 39 | 24.7 | 75.3 |
| 40 or more | 22.2 | 77.8 |
| Administration | | |
| Less than 5 | 0.0 | 100.0 |
| 5 to 9 | 6.4 | 93.6 |
| 10 to 14 | 14.4 | 85.6 |
| 15 to 19 | 18.6 | 81.4 |
| 20 or more | 22.9 | 77.1 |
| Total | 15.6 | 84.4 |

## TABLE A-5

AMOUNT OF PROFESSIONAL TIME SPENT IN
ADMINISTRATIVE AND CLINICAL ACTIVITIES

| | Time spent in administration (%) | Time spent in clinical activities (%) |
|---|---|---|
| Seniority level | | |
| Senior positions | 79.0 | 8.3 |
| Years in practice | | |
| Less than 10 | 56.2 | 27.9 |
| 10 to 19 | 64.5 | 22.0 |
| 20 to 29 | 64.2 | 20.2 |
| 30 to 39 | 69.3 | 17.4 |
| 40 or more | 74.1 | 14.3 |
| Years in administration | | |
| Less than 5 | 57.6 | 28.6 |
| 5 to 9 | 60.0 | 23.6 |
| 10 to 14 | 64.1 | 22.0 |
| 15 to 19 | 65.7 | 21.7 |
| 20 or more | 66.9 | 18.5 |
| Total | 65.0 | 20.6 |

**TABLE A-6**

RELATIONSHIP BETWEEN SENIORITY AND ORGANIZATIONAL CHANGE FOR PHYSICIAN
EXECUTIVES

| Number of positions/organizations worked for | Respondents reporting being in senior level (%) | | |
|---|---|---|---|
| | Total | All administrative positions held within same type of organization | Administrative positions held in more than one type of organization |
| 1 | 9.8 | 9.8 | |
| 2 | 20.1 | 13.7 | 23.4 |
| 3 | 15.5 | 14.5 | 16.3 |
| 4 | 16.4 | 20.5 | 11.1 |
| Total | 15.6 | 12.0 | 20.8 |
| (N) | (135/867) | (62/516) | (73/351) |

# Physician managers: Personal characteristics versus institutional demands

Hava Tabenkin,
Stephen J. Zyzanski,
and
Sonia A. Alemagno

*This article presents results of a survey of 169 physician managers and addresses what influences their task performance—organizational demands or personal characteristics?*

*Health Care Manage Rev*, 1989, 14(2), 7–12
© 1989 Aspen Publishers, Inc.

**The complex health care system** in the United States is changing rapidly.[1-4] Some of the consequences of these changes are the development of large medical industrial complexes; a dramatic shift from hospital to ambulatory care; and an increase in independent practice associations (IPAs), preferred provider organizations (PPOs), health maintenance organizations (HMOs), and large multispecialty group practices. At the same time, competition among health care providers is growing, producing a demand to combine quality of care with cost containment. These situations call for effective management, which can best be served by a combination of knowledge and skills of both management and medicine. The issue today is no longer whether there is a role for physicians in management, but rather how to make physicians more effective as partners in the management of medical resources.[5-7] This challenge is being accepted by organizations searching for better and more effective managers while realizing that very few physicians are formally trained in management.[8]

To date, few studies have addressed the problems related specifically to physician managers.[9,10] Many questions need to be addressed such as the following:

- What are the typical personal and managerial characteristics of physican managers?
- How does the organizational structure or context influence their task performance and input into policy?
- Does the unique structure of each organization influence managerial and personal characteristics?

The study presented here addressed these and other questions. The results provide further insights and guidelines for preparing physicians to be effective managers.

**Hava Tabenkin,** *M.D., M.S., is Regional Director of Family Medicine, Yisrael Valley, Israel.*

**Stephen J. Zyzanski,** *Ph.D., is a Professor in the Family Medicine Department of Case Western Reserve University, School of Medicine, Cleveland, Ohio.*

**Sonia A. Alemagno,** *M.A., is an Instructor in the Family Medicine Department of Case Western Reserve University.*

Research for this article was supported in part by the W.M. Keck Research Scholars Fund of the Health Systems Management Center, Case Western Reserve University, Cleveland, Ohio, and by the Jewish Community Federation of Cleveland.

## METHODS

The theoretical premise for this study is based on the Boyatzis model of effective job performance.[11] This model suggests that when the three components of job demands, managerial characteristics, and the organizational environment are in balance, effective action is likely to occur.

To address the research questions within the context of this model, a self-administered, comprehensive mail questionnaire was developed. Questions relating to the nature of tasks and roles performed by physician managers, their personal and managerial characteristics, and the organizational structures in which they work were included.[12] Questionnaire content was derived from the literature on leadership styles and characteristics in the corporate settings and in health care organizations.[13-20] The literature describing the function of executive directors in health care settings also provided insightful material.[21-23] Finally, expert opinion from three senior faculty members of the School of Management, Case Western Reserve University, Cleveland, Ohio, and a pilot study in which twelve physician managers were interviewed also helped to refine the final survey questionnaire.

By means of power analyses for the hypotheses to be tested, a sample of 150 respondents was estimated to be necessary for adequate statistical analysis.[24] Thus, 350 subjects were selected at random from four national sources to obtain the needed sample size based on an expected 50% response rate. These sources were the American Academy of Medical Directors (AAMD), the Primary Care Association of Community Health Centers, the Group Practices Management Association, and the Permanente Medical Group.

## RESULTS

Using the Dillman method for survey design and follow-up,[25] a 53% total response rate was achieved. The highest response rate, 64%, was obtained from members of the AAMD while the lowest, 45%, derived from members of the Primary Care Association of Community Health Centers. Previous research by Dillman suggests that one of the factors contributing to the lower response by members of the Primary Care Association of Community Health Centers was the unavailability of physician managers' names. Also, the overall response rate might have been higher had the questionnaire been less time consuming. Still, given the fact that this was a random sample, a 53% response is a

## TABLE 1

RESPONSE RATE BY SAMPLING SOURCE

| | |
|---|---|
| Primary Care Association of Community Health Centers (N=170) | 45% |
| American Academy of Medical Directors (N=114) | 64% |
| Medical Group Practices Management Association (N=25) | 60% |
| Permanente Medical Group (N=16) | 50% |
| Total sample size | N=325 |
| Total response rate | 53% |

reasonable response rate for this type of study group. Furthermore, without the names, it would have been very difficult to get information on nonrespondents. Thus, the extent of bias represented by the respondents is unknown because descriptive data were not available for nonrespondents. Table 1 summarizes these four sources and their response rates. Out of 172 questionnaires received, 169 were sufficiently complete for further data analysis.

Four major ambulatory–primary care organizations were identified: multispecialty group practices (MGPs) (22%); small primary care group practices (17%); community health care centers (HCCs) (39%); and HMOs—IPA, staff, and group models (22%). Group practices are defined here as medical services offered by three or more physicians formally organized to provide medical care consultation, diagnosis, and treatment through the joint use of equipment and personnel. HMOs are legal entities that provide comprehensive medical care directly (staff models) or arrange for care to an enrolled population through a multispecialty medical group (group model) or IPAs. To examine whether or not physician characteristics differed by type of organization, chi square and analysis of variance tests were performed. The physician characteris-

*The data reveal significant differences between the various organizations in physician manager characteristics.*

tics that differed most by type of practice are presented in Table 2.

The data reveal significant differences between the various organizations in physician manager characteristics. Physician managers in HCCs are significantly younger than those in other organizations. They have also been in practice and in management for significantly fewer years than those in the other groups. Furthermore, physician managers in HCCs are less likely to be board certified.

Physician managers in small primary care practices and HCCs spend significantly more time in patient care and less in management (12 to 15 hours per week versus 20 to 40 hours per week for other physicians). Physician managers in HMOs spend significantly more time in management and less in patient care, with 45% of them not seeing patients at all. A substantial majority of the physician managers in the other organizations continue to see their own patients. Finally, there are signifi-

## TABLE 2

### PHYSICIAN CHARACTERISTICS BY TYPE OF ORGANIZATION

| Characteristics | Organization type | | | |
|---|---|---|---|---|
| | MGP (36) | SGP* (29) | HCC (66) | HMOs (38) |
| Median age[†] | 42 | 46 | 35 | 45 |
| Years in present position[‡] | 2.5 | 4.2 | 2 | 2 |
| Years as physician manager | 4.5 | 5 | 2.5 | 5 |
| Years in practice[†] | 15 | 19 | 8.5 | 17 |
| Hours/week of patient care[†] | 25 | 30 | 32 | 6 |
| Hours/week as physician manager[†] | 20 | 15 | 12 | 40 |
| Male[†] (%) | 92 | 97 | 71 | 95 |
| Board certified[‡] (%) | 92 | 83 | 66 | 92 |
| See their own patients[†] (%) | 89 | 100 | 96 | 55 |

*SGP = Small Group Practice.
[†]p = 0.01
[‡]p = 0.001

## TABLE 3

### DIFFERENCE IN LEVEL OF TRAINING BY TYPE OF ORGANIZATION

| Level of training* | Type of organization | | | |
|---|---|---|---|---|
| | MGP (36) | SGP (29) | HCC (66) | HMOs (38) |
| No training | 17% | 14% | 29% | 8% |
| Some/moderate training | 69% | 72% | 51% | 42% |
| Great deal of training | 14% | 14% | 20% | 50% |
| Totals | 100.0% | 100.0% | 100.0% | 100.0% |

*p = 0.001

cantly more female physician managers in HCCs, 29%, versus only 3% to 8% in the other groups.

Among physician managers in this sample, three levels of training in management were identified. Approximately 19% of the respondents had no training in management; 57% had some to moderate training, which included seminars, informal training, or a graduate course in management. Twenty-four percent had a great deal of training (defined as a graduate degree in management or a degree in progress plus seminars or informal training).

Differences in these three levels of training by type of organization are displayed in Table 3. The results reveal that physician managers in HMOs have significantly more training than physicians in the other three groups. Conversely, those in HCCs reported significantly less training, with 29% reporting no training at all.

Respondents were asked to rate themselves, on a scale of 1 to 10 (low to high), on each of 13 characteristics related to management. These items were subjected to a principal components factor analysis with orthogonal rotation that produced two major factors. The two factors, labeled people- and task-oriented characteristics, along with their respective items and factor loadings, are presented in Table 4. Items are ordered within factors by the strength of their factor loadings. In general, the higher the factor loading, the more important the item is in defining the factor. Factor 1 was interpreted as describing people-oriented characteristics. The two items with the highest factor loadings reflect

## TABLE 4

### MANAGERIAL CHARACTERISTIC FACTORS

| | Loading |
|---|---|
| **People-oriented characteristics** | |
| Ability to delegate | .74 |
| Ability to coordinate | .74 |
| Knowing own limitations | .64 |
| Ability to keep promises | .37 |
| Ability to motivate | .30 |
| **Task-oriented characteristics** | |
| Ability to develop new solutions | .81 |
| Ability to take initiative | .73 |
| Ability to deal with uncertain situations | .69 |
| Ability to take risk | .69 |
| Having self-confidence | .59 |
| Ability to work under stress | .52 |
| Having and using intuition | .50 |
| Ability to motivate | .48 |

the ability of managers to delegate tasks to others and to coordinate, monitor, and follow up the work flow. Factor 1 had an internal consistency reliability (Chronbach's alpha) of 0.85. Factor 2 was interpreted as describing mostly task-oriented characteristics. Key items defining this factor involve the manager's ability to develop new solutions, take initiatives, and deal with uncertain situations. Its alpha reliability was 0.73. These factors reliably describe two important but distinct domains of managerial characteristics. Factor scores were computed by summing the items comprising each factor.

Physician manager self-rating scores on these two factors revealed significant differences between organizations on task-related managerial characteristics. Physician managers in HCCs rated themselves significantly lower on the task-oriented factor in comparison with the other groups. Physician managers in HMOs and primary care practices were found to have the highest task-oriented factor ratings, on the average. Interestingly, there were no significant differences on the people-oriented factor between organizational groups.

Next, 23 specific physician managers' tasks were examined, along with their reported level of involve-

ment in performing the tasks, and their level of input in decision making regarding the tasks. Results revealed that for each of the 23 tasks, a consistently high percent (78% to 100%) of the physician managers in all organizations reported that they were performing these tasks. Between 78% to 98% of the sample also reported having some to a great deal of input in policy making concerning these 23 tasks. Interestingly, the data indicate that only a small percent of physician managers are performing these tasks alone. A factor analysis of the 23 items produced five factors for analysis purposes. Table

## TABLE 5

### PHYSICIAN MANAGER TASK FACTORS

| | Loading |
|---|---|
| **Medical personnel** | |
| Supervising physicians | .80 |
| Advising, motivating physicians | .70 |
| Arbitrating differences between physicians | .50 |
| Recruiting physicians | .45 |
| Negotiating with hospitals on M.D. status | .30 |
| Determining physician salary | .27 |
| **Nonmedical personnel** | |
| Recruiting support staff | .86 |
| Monitoring support staff | .73 |
| **Budget and planning** | |
| Defining the goals and priorities | .69 |
| Planning new services | .48 |
| Managing the budget | .45 |
| Developing new approaches to health care | .44 |
| Determining number/specialties of physicians | .29 |
| Purchasing medical equipment | .12 |
| **Patient and service delivery** | |
| Addressing patient preferences | .64 |
| Assessing needs of population | .59 |
| Contracting with other organizations | .58 |
| Determining physician workloads | .51 |
| **QA** | |
| Monitoring patient care quality | .82 |
| Evaluating physicians | .71 |
| Monitoring other services | .66 |
| Organizing educational programs for physicians | .26 |

5 presents the items and the factor loadings pertaining to medical personnel, nonmedical personnel, and budget and planning, patient and service delivery, and quality assurance (QA). Cronbach alpha reliability coefficients for the factor scores, derived by summing the items comprising each factor, ranged from 0.64 for the medical personnel factor to 0.78 for the budget and planning factor. Patient complaint tasks, although independent of the five factors, were assessed with only one question.

The data reduction value of this factor solution means that a small number of task factor scores can be used to profile a physician manager's involvement in performing tasks within and between organizations. In this sample, physician managers in small group practices and HCCs were found to be significantly more involved in nonmedical personnel tasks and policy decisions at the $p < .001$ level, by analysis of variance. HCC physician managers were significantly less likely to be involved in budgetary and planning activities but significantly more likely to develop and implement policy issues regarding QA than the other group. Overall, managers in MGPs and primary care small group practices were significantly more involved in policy making as found by analysis of variance, $p < .001$.

## DISCUSSION

This study reveals that different primary care organizations have major differences in physician manager levels of responsibility, demographics, level of training, and managerial characteristics.

High self-ratings on managerial characteristics and more extensive formal training were the most significant factors descriptive of high levels of involvement in medical personnel, budget and general policy, and QA issues. These results may add further insight to those of previous studies that have found low levels of involvement by managers in the areas of finance. The data from this study indicate that those physicians with additional training and a high-score profile on key management characteristics are more likely to be involved in budgetary and planning activities.

Another contribution of this study is the development of a 23-item task list, similar to a list developed by Betson and Slater.[26,27] The majority of tasks listed in these works was also included in this study and thus provides opportunities to replicate previous findings. The present study also provides some new insights on the input that physician managers have regarding policy-making decisions on specific tasks. No such previous work was found in the literature. Thus, this study gives greater breadth to existing findings.

Physician managers rated their task-oriented characteristics higher than their people-oriented characteristics. Consistently, no differences were noted among organizations for people-oriented characteristics, whereas task-related characteristics were found to be related to age and type of organization.

•   •   •

These findings suggest the more experience and training in management physicians have, the more competent they feel in management. Thus, organizations need to take formal steps to train young physicians to be better physicians *and* managers. This training needs to recognize that different types of organizational settings will strongly influence the level of involvement and the personal satisfaction of the physician manager. Hence, organizations need to be aware that in addition to required skill levels, creation of the right setting is important for maximizing the personal satisfaction of physician managers and enhancing their ability to contribute significantly to the organization. These data suggest that physician managers would thus have increased confidence in their abilities to perform effectively in multiple areas of health care management, including policy making and finance.

## REFERENCES

1. Starr, P. *The Social Transformation of American Medicine.* New York: Basic Books, 1982.
2. Fuchs, V.R. *Who Shall Live.* New York: Basic Books, 1974.
3. Mayer, T.R., and Mayer, G.G. "HMOs: Origins and Development." *New England Journal of Medicine* 312 (1985): 590–94.
4. Kaluzny, A.D., and Shorteu, S.N. *Health Care Management: A Text in Organization, Theory and Behavior.* New York: Wiley, 1983.
5. Ibid.
6. Percy, B.J. "The Role of the Physician Manager." *Health Management Forum* 5, no. 3 (1984): 48–55.
7. Schenke, R. *The Physician in Management.* Falls Church, Va.: American Academy of Medical Directors, 1980.
8. Sayles, L.R. *Leadership: What Effective Managers Really Do...and How They Do It.* New York: McGraw-Hill, 1979.

9.  Betson, C.L. *Managing the Medical Enterprise: A Study of Physician Managers.* Ann Arbor, Mich.: U.M.I. Research Press, 1986.

10. Tabenkin, H. "Task and Managerial Characteristics of Physician Managers in Primary and Ambulatory Care Organizations." Master's thesis, Case Western Reserve University, 1987.

11. Boyatzis, R.E. *The Competent Manager: A Model for Executive Performance.* New York: Wiley, 1982.

12. Betson, *Managing the Medical Enterprise.*

13. Boyatzis, *The Competent Manager.*

14. Peters, T.J., and Waterman, R.H. *In Search of Excellence.* New York: Harper & Row, 1982.

15. Hersey, P., and Branchard, K.H. "So You Want to Know Your Leadership Style." *Training and Development Journal* 28, no. 2 (February 1974): 22–37.

16. Zenger, J.H. "Leadership: Management's Better Half." *Training* 22, no. 12 (1985): 44–53.

17. Martin, W.B. "Are You a Manager or a Leader?" *Industry Week* 224, no. 5 (March 1985): 93–97.

18. Aluise, J.J. *The Physician as Manager.* Bowie, Md.: The Charles Press, 1980.

19. Kimberly, J.R. "Managerial Innovation of Health Policy: Theoretical Perceptions and Research Implications." *Journal of Health Politics, Policy and Law* 6 (1982): 637–53.

20. Yanda, R.L. *Doctors as Managers of Health Teams.* New York: Amacom Press, 1977.

21. Kuhl, I.K. *The Executive Role in Health Service Delivery Organizations.* Washington, D.C.: Association of University Programs in Health Administration Press, 1986.

22. Slater, C. "The Physician Manager's Role: Results of a Survey." In *The Physician in Management,* edited by R. Schenke. Falls Church, Va.: American Academy of Medical Directors, 1980.

23. Downs, R.L. "The Role of Physician Managers in Larger Multispecialty Groups." *College Review* 1, no. 2 (1984): 83–95.

24. Cohen, J. *Statistical Power Analysis for the Behavioral Sciences.* New York: Academic Press, 1977.

25. Dillman, D.A. *Mail and Telephone Surveys.* New York: Wiley, 1978.

26. Betson, *Managing the Medical Enterprise.*

27. Slater, "The Physician Manager's Role."

# The secret of medical management

James E. Rohrer

*A review of the research on group practices punctures the myth of physician autonomy in hospitals and opens the way for administrators to join in controlling the patient care process.*

*Health Care Manage Rev*, 1989, 14(3), 7–13
© 1989 Aspen Publishers, Inc.

The nature of work in medical care organizations is determined by the mix of patients who must be treated and the mix of services that the organization chooses to offer. The key management problem is to control the quality of patient care and the resources used to produce it. In short, the secret of medical management lies in the control of the patient care process.

Most administrative effort is misdirected, in that it is aimed at supporting the patient care process without helping to control it. Some organizational benefit can be gained from marketing, financing, community relations, strategic planning, purchasing, risk management, organization design, operations research, leadership, and personnel management. However, these activities are secondary to control of the patient care process, which is necessary if the organization is to be efficient and effective.

The purpose of this article is to suggest that administrative effort should be focused on two key interrelated activities: utilization review and quality assessment. First, the myth of physician autonomy, which has deterred administrators from joining with clinical department heads to manage patient care, is critically examined. Second, the history of utilization review and quality assessment is briefly reviewed. Third, the key technical barrier to efficient administrative monitoring of patient care—that is, controlling case mix severity—is explored. Finally, the article offers a strategy for redirecting administrative effort.

## THE MYTH OF PHYSICIAN AUTONOMY

The reasons for the misdirection of administrative activity are obvious. For one, the administrative effort directed at non–patient care functions can, at times, be of enormous benefit to the organization. More importantly, non–patient care functions are arenas of activity that do not encroach on the sacrosanct ground of clinical discretion. All administrators know that they dare not appear to tell physicians how to practice medicine. A myth has arisen that consists of the following argument: Since nonmedical administrators are not able to judge when the use of resources in patient care is unnecessary or when the process of care in individual

James E. Rohrer, *Ph.D., is an Assistant Professor in the Graduate Program in Hospital and Health Administration at the University of Iowa. He currently teaches medical care organization and health policy.*

cases is appropriate, efforts to control the patient care process would lead to revolt by the medical staff. Medical care cannot be delivered without physicians, and each physician demands professional autonomy.

That this is a myth is shown by the fact that it applies only to nonphysician administrators. Certainly when clinical department heads (who are administrators as well as physicians) are present, they do not hesitate to tell their fellow physicians how to practice medicine. In fact, many of them rule over their medical staffs like absolute monarchs, making despotic decisions capriciously and sometimes badly, but almost always getting away with them.

While only a fraction of U.S. hospitals have such dominant clinical department heads, the fact that they exist and manage patient care proves that individual autonomy is not essential to the practice of medicine. Professional autonomy for organized groups of physicians is sufficient.

---

*There are practical reasons why physicians choose to subordinate themselves to a bureaucracy of their own making, among which is the need to increase productivity, quality, and the appropriateness of services.*

---

An expert in organizational behavior might argue that clinical department heads can behave arbitrarily because they derive their authority from being experts in the relevant subject matter. However, their clinical expertise is largely independent of their administrative behavior; their management decisions may be guided by their clinical knowledge, but they are also drawing from other experience. This is to be expected, as management decisions may be directed at administrative as well as clinical problems. Unfortunately, clinical department heads are experts in the clinical subject matter but may be amateurs in administration, in spite of which they make administrative decisions that impinge on the process of patient care.

Despite their usual lack of formal training in administration, clinical department heads are often effective and efficient managers. They glean administrative expertise from experience in their positions. They are often dynamic leaders. The most important determinant of their success, however, is that subordination of individual clinicians to an organized medical staff often

leads to improved performance.[1,2] Analogously, the benefits of organized group practice are real and have been known for some time.

In 1932 the Committee on the Costs of Medical Care (CCMC), chaired by a former president of the American Medical Association, recommended that comprehensive medical services should be provided by hospital-based organized group practices.[3] Although organized medicine repudiated the corporate practice of medicine, the proportion of physicians in group practice increased from 0.9% in 1932 to 46% in 1980.[4] Most group practices are not hospital-based in the sense meant by the CCMC, but they are still more bureaucratized than solo practices. There are practical reasons why physicians choose to subordinate themselves to a bureaucracy of their own making, among which is the need to increase productivity, quality, and the appropriateness of services.

Observing that general practitioners in solo practice operate independently of, and unobserved by their colleagues, Freidson[5] concluded that as physicians band together, they are likely to change the way they practice medicine. The organization of medical practice can be visualized as a continuum ranging from solo practice to "bureaucratic" practice. Bureaucratic practice is group practice in which the characteristics of bureaucracy have emerged. These include the division of labor, systematization of roles and procedures, and hierarchical organization.[6] The advantages of bureaucratization include economies of scale, an increased likelihood of peer review, more frequent consultation, and the substitution of allied health services for physician services.[7] This formulation is analogous to Roemer and Friedman's assertion that the more closely a hospital's medical staff approaches the ideal of the closed staff, where a limited group of physicians has admitting and treatment privileges, the better the performance of the hospital.[8]

Increased bureaucratization can help physicians to be more productive by freeing them from the need to perform tasks other than the exercise of clinical judgment. It may also improve the quality and appropriateness of care,[9] as has been repeatedly demonstrated, both before and after the development of a theory to explain the phenomenon. The following studies, drawn from Donabedian,[10] illustrate the point.

In a 1958 study by Morehead, physicians with hospital appointments were more likely to be judged in Class I (i.e., 76 percent or better compliance with criteria) than were physicians without appointments. Furthermore, the percentage in Class I increased with the number of years of affiliation with the hospital. In the same study, the percentage of physicians in Class I was correlated with the amount of time that physicians devoted to group practice.[11]

In a 1976 study by Payne et al., the percentage of cases that were appropriately admitted to hospitals and had an appropriate length of stay was highest for a prepaid group practice (Kaiser-Permanente), next highest for other multispecialty group practices, and lowest for solo practitioners. Performance index scores were highest for physicians in prepaid group practice, next highest for those in other multispecialty group practices, and lowest for solo practitioners.[12]

In a 1978 study, Payne et al. found that physician performance scores were higher in teaching-hospital outpatient clinics than in primary care office practices for pediatric, adult, and gynecological examinations; for treatment of hypertension, urinary tract infection, heart disease, anemia tonsillitis/pharyngitis, vulvovaginitis; and for appropriate drug use.[13]

In 1979 Riedel and Riedel found that within specialty categories the percentage of criteria adhered to was higher in hospital outpatient departments than in physician offices for the following conditions: hypertension, chest pain, abdominal pain, urinary tract infection, and pharyngitis.[14]

It is clear from these studies that the bureaucratization of medical care is associated with efficiency and quality. In fact, bureaucratization actually causes better performance, because the members of an organized medical practice can jointly offer lower costs and higher quality as well as more specialists and higher levels of medical training, and because administrative procedures exist to control the process of patient care. Fortunately, even ad hoc and ill-considered application of these procedures, in their crudest forms, has some benefit. Even more fortunately, administrative technology exists that can vastly improve management control over patient care. The refinement and judicious use of these mechanisms are the keys to effective medical management.

## THE TECHNOLOGY OF UTILIZATION CONTROL

A complete description of the administrative procedures that can be used to control the services offered in the patient care process is beyond the scope of this article. Instead, this section demonstrates that the technology is both well-developed and underused.

In volume III of the Explorations in Quality Assess-

ment and Monitoring Series,[15] Donabedian illustrates the methods and findings of patient care review studies. That workable review methods have existed for many years is perhaps best proven by citing a 1956 study by Lembcke, that is described by Donabedian.[16] Lembcke presented a scientific method for quality assessment. Valid, reproducible judgments were made

---

*Much of the quality assurance activity in hospitals is pointless.*

---

possible by the following procedures: (1) classification of patients into diagnostic categories; (2) specification of the aspects of care to be judged (e.g., appropriateness of surgery); (3) use of detailed, explicit criteria; (4) verification of basic diagnostic information; and (5) establishment of an acceptable level of compliance in recognition of the fact that no criteria set can fully account for the circumstances of all cases. In the 1956 study Lembcke demonstrated that the number of "criticized" operations on the uterus, ovaries, and fallopian tubes at one hospital declined after the introduction of an auditing process, without affecting the number of justifiable operations.

The Lembcke study demonstrates what can be accomplished with case review. However, it is also true that case review can be a complete waste of time. If there is no reason to believe that the accepted treatment of a particular condition is suboptimal, then an audit will probably result in no improvement. Indeed, this is what frequently happens. In anticipation of a site visit by the Joint Commission on the Accreditation of Healthcare Organizations (Joint Commission), many hospitals have conducted audits of dubious value. The Joint Commission does not require, or even recommend, the investigation of nonproblems, but when a hospital cannot document the review and correction of genuine quality deficiencies, it may attempt to substitute a pointless audit instead. Thus it creates the semblance of compliance with the Joint Commission's criteria without actually having to tamper with the practice of medicine. Such an audit generates the unpleasant aspects of bureaucracy (i.e., committee meetings and paper shuffling) without achieving any improvement in quality or efficiency.

Much of the quality assurance activity in hospitals is as pointless as that described above. One reason for this, already noted earlier, is that genuine quality assurance

(QA) would interfere with the practice of medicine. A second reason is that meaningful problem identification systems, such as a complete system of continuous monitors, have not been in place. A third reason is that the real quality control activity is done informally, within the medical staff, and without the assistance of nonmedical administrators. This should not be interpreted to mean that informal quality control is not rigorous. On the contrary, clinical department heads constantly review the work of their staffs and are not reluctant to bring heavy pressure to bear on miscreants. However, monitoring and control could be accomplished more efficiently if the QA process were to be formalized.

One way to formalize the review process in the interest of increased efficiency is to transform it into the kind of QA program that the Joint Commission intends. This requires developing a problem identification system, central to which is a set of continuous monitors. The technology for such a system is well understood. Professional standards review organizations (PSROs) have screened aggregate data from their inception, as do their descendants, peer review organizations (PROs). The Commission on Professional and Hospital Activities (CPHA), established in 1955, offers a statistical display and analysis service that originally focused on length of stay and professional activities by type of patient, diagnosis, and the nature of any surgical intervention.[17] Some intermediate or end results could also be monitored: death, nosocomial infections, other complications, removal of diseased or normal tissue, transfers to other hospitals or extended care facilities, and discharges with approval or against advice. Tabulations could be produced that summarize activity by department or physician. Indexes could be constructed that indicate the number of tests performed for a particular case or case type.

When this type of information is purchased from an organization that tabulates data for many hospitals, participating facilities can compare their own performance to that of similar hospitals. Indeed, the information value of aggregated data increases dramatically when administrators can make comparisons, either with peer hospitals or with the performance of their own organizations over time.

In short, examples of systems for tabulating and plotting aggregate data have been published for more than a generation, and such systems could have been used to identify potential problems for case review. In many, if not most, cases they were not used, however, because neither the administrative nor the clinical managers understood or felt compelled to learn how to maximize their benefits. Furthermore, such systems can always be criticized because they do not reveal problems in a definitive fashion. For example, a high readmission rate after a particular surgical procedure does not prove that quality deficiencies exist. The high rate could be due to case mix (software that adjusts hospital data for severity has only recently become available) or bad luck.

Despite these uncertainties, profile monitoring is far more efficient than continuous auditing. Furthermore, administrative control over patient care that is directed at correcting clinical inefficiency has been demonstrated to be effective. If this were not true, then hospital utilization would not have declined as hospitals have come under increased pressure to control costs. Hospitals that could not induce physicians to shorten patient stays and avoid debatable admissions are likely to have experienced serious financial problems in recent years.

## THE SEVERITY CONUNDRUM

A system for surveillance of aggregate data can serve as the core of an efficient and effective patient care control system. The value of such a system depends on its screening efficiency—that is, on its ability to detect genuine problems without falsely labelling deviations from the norm as possible problems. Screening efficiency is enhanced by case mix adjustment, because deviations from norms cannot easily be explained away as attributable to the mix of cases. And, as any administrator today knows, aggregate data are far more informative if cases are adjusted for severity.

Severity adjustment is the key technical problem impeding patient care review today. Automated software systems can be purchased that will produce severity-adjusted data for the evaluation of efficiency and effectiveness. However, the decision about which system to buy has baffled many administrators and their clinical advisors. The evaluation of severity adjustment systems is both more complex and, in one sense, less difficult than it first appears.

Unfortunately, the purchasers of the software often do not realize that the construction of a severity index is not just a technical issue, but one that is directly relevant to the objectives of the hospital. What can be obscured by the flashiness of menu-driven report generators are the unstated values that color the assumptions and scaling of the severity-adjusters. This issue is germane to the choice of software products, because it is the patient classification system that converts reams of data into digested or digestible information about quality and efficiency.

The first issue to be confronted is the concept that the severity index will be intended to operationalize. If patient outcomes are being monitored, it is only logical that the severity adjustment be based on factors prior to hospital care that would affect outcomes. However, if utilization rates or other measures of the patient care process are monitored, another basis for severity adjustment may be sought. This point can be illustrated with an example.

---

*To the extent that clinical judgment about the use of hospital resources is open to review, a patient classification system based on the intensity of service use only must be considered to be potentially flawed.*

---

One way to measure severity is to define it as the probability of organ failure, as in the MEDISGRPS system. Each level of severity in MEDISGRPS is, in theory, distinguished from higher and lower levels by the probability that the patient will experience organ failure.[18] Even if the probabilities are accurately assigned, the user should recognize the narrowness of the concept employed by MEDISGRPS. Patients who have a low probability of organ failure but who are handicapped or disfigured would be considered to be successes. Critics might argue that hospitals have a broader sense of responsibility than the prevention of organ failure. In short, any patient classification system must be based on assumptions about organizational purpose as well as on the biological determinants of disease.

Patient standardization systems could also be based on the stage of the disease,[19] the probability of death,[20] ability to function, the intensity of services delivered, or a combination of factors.[21] If a severity index score is based partly on resources used (e.g., placement in intensive care), then the user of the index is implicitly assuming that some decisions about the use of clinical resources are not subject to challenge. While it is true that patients who are admitted to an intensive care unit (ICU) are clinically comparable and that their patterns of resource use are more similar to each other than to those of patients not admitted to the ICU, a resource-based classification system can still be criticized to the extent that admission to the ICU is influenced by factors

other than patient needs—for example, practice style. Users of the system can legitimately ignore such criticisms if they have defined the purpose of the hospital to be the provision of support services to clinicians. However, such a system could never be used to evaluate fully the quality of or need for ICU care. To the extent that clinical judgment about the use of hospital resources is open to review, a patient classification system based on the intensity of service use only must be considered to be potentially flawed.

As difficult as these issues are, they represent only one aspect of the value-laden problems with patient classification. Fortunately, administrators need not resolve all of these ethical problems before they implement a severity-adjusted patient care monitoring system. In a perfect world, a specialized severity adjustment system would be used for each indicator that is routinely monitored. Each severity index would be tailored to the mission of the hospital by extending the strategic planning process to include discussion of how the organization measures its own performance. However, such perfection is probably not essential. Most severity adjustment systems rank patients in roughly the same order.

The action-oriented administrator would be justified in selecting a severity adjustment system on the basis of criteria other than validity, with the understanding that it will be necessary to "trade up" every five or ten years. The selection might be made on the basis of price, or of the number of other hospitals that are using the same system and can therefore provide comparable data. On the other hand, perhaps a system should be selected that will operate with the clinical information that is already automated at the purchasing hospital. Any adjustment for severity, after all, will improve the screening efficiency of the monitoring system.

## REDIRECTING ADMINISTRATIVE EFFORT

Monitoring and controlling the patient care process are the keys to effective management of medical organizations. The common perception that administrators cannot involve themselves in patient care can be seen to be a myth when it is recognized that the autonomy of individual physicians is routinely subordinated to the organized medical staff. Furthermore, opportunities exist to improve the management of patient care by replacing informal monitoring with existing technology. The most accurate, and politic, way to describe this activity is as the provision of efficient and effective assistance to clinical department heads, and not as administrative interference with professional judgment.

It must be remembered that clinical department heads are also administrators. Management of the patient care process must be accomplished with and through them, just as managing a research organization must be accomplished through senior scientists. Cooperation may not always be achievable; however, the medical staff and hospital administrators have common interests that should serve as the basis of a working relationship.

Not all hospitals are large enough to have clinical department heads. However, this does not imply that they cannot increase control over the patient care process. The medical staff may become organized in the short run, with help from the hospital administrator. Strategic decisions can be made that may increase the degree of medical staff organization in the long run. For example, health maintenance organizations (HMOs) may be established or physicians' practices purchased.

Ways to recruit, train, integrate, empower, provide data to, and reimburse physicians for meaningful participation in the institutional management of patient care—in short, to increase the degree of organization of the medical staff—should be developed and disseminated. However, the analysis of patient care data for management control need not wait. Some benefit can be achieved even at low levels of medical staff organization; indeed, the act of analyzing the data constitutes an increase in medical staff organization. For example, if staff physicians are informed that data analysis suggests that a wide diversity of opinions exists regarding the indications for a common surgical procedure, then the ensuing discussion could lead to consensus on practice standards, or at least to greater uniformity in practice. Feedback on clinical variations has been advocated for several years as a means of changing physician behavior.[22]

The technology for managing patient care is found in utilization review and quality assessment systems. If hospital administrators are to use this technology more effectively than they have in the past, they will have to convince medical staff leaders that these administrative procedures assist rather than impede them. They will have to use efficient systems for screening aggregate data and integrate physician leadership much more meaningfully with hospital management. Such systems will require the automation of as much clinical information as possible.

Truly sophisticated management of the medical care process must await integration of off-site practices with hospital operations, development of a coherent strategy for collection and use of accurate and relevant data, and development of national practice standards that can be applied with all of the authority of medical science. However, smaller steps need not await these developments. Management of medical care can become more effective now if existing techniques are brought into wider use.

Revitalizing quality assurance/utilization review systems will inevitably involve conflict. With finesse, the administrator may be able to contain that conflict within the arena where it can best be managed—that is, among clinical department heads and their staffs. It would, of course, be far easier to avoid the QA issue and concentrate on managing the administrative side of the hospital, such as payroll, purchasing, dietetics, housekeeping, marketing, and other activities that indirectly support patient care, However, the medical care organization that is able to grapple directly with managing patient care will have far more control over its production process. Managed properly, the care process will display examplary efficiency and effectiveness.

## REFERENCES

1. Wolinsky, E.D., and Marder, W.D. *The Organization of Medical Practice and the Practice of Medicine.* Ann Arbor: Health Administration Press, 1985.
2. Eisenberg, J. and Kabcenell, A. "Organized Practice and the Quality of Medical Care." *Inquiry* 25, no. 1 (1988): 78–89.
3. Committee on the Costs of Medical Care. *Medical Care for the American People: The Final Report of the Committee.* Chicago: University of Chicago Press, 1932.
4. Roemer, M.I. *An Introduction to the U.S. Health Care System.* 2d ed. New York: Springer Publishing Company, 1986.
5. Freidson, E. *Profession of Medicine: A Study of the Sociology of Applied Knowledge.* New York: Harper & Row, 1970.
6. Ibid.
7. Wolinsky, F. "Why Physicians Choose Different Types of Practice Settings." *Health Services Research* 17 (1982): 399–419.
8. Roemer, M., and Friedman, J.W. *Doctors in Hospitals.* Baltimore: Johns Hopkins Press, 1971.
9. Eisenberg and Kabcenell, "Organized Practice."
10. Donabedian, A. *The Methods and Findings of Quality Assessment and Monitoring.* Explorations in Quality Assessment and Monitoring Series, vol. 3. Ann Arbor: Health Administration Press, 1985.
11. Ibid.

12. Ibid.
13. Ibid.
14. Ibid.
15. Donabedian, *The Methods and Findings of Quality Assessment and Monitoring.*
16. Ibid.
17. Donabedian, A. *A Guide to Medical Care Administration. Volume II: Appraisal.* Washington, D.C.: American Public Health Association, 1969.
18. Brewster, A. Presentation at University of Iowa Hospitals and Clinics, fall 1986.
19. Louis, D.Z., and Gonnella, J.S. "Disease Staging: Applications for Utilization Review and Quality Assurance." *Quality Assurance and Utilization Review* 1 (February 1986): 13–18.
20. Knaus, W.A., et al. "APACHE II: A Severity of Disease Classification System." *Critical Care Medicine* 13(1985):818–829.
21. Horn, S.D. "Measuring Severity: How Sick Is Sick? How Well Is Well?" *Healthcare Financial Management* (October 1986):21–32.
22. Wennberg, J., and Gittelsohn, A. "Health Care Delivery in Maine. I: Patterns of Use in Common Surgical Procedures." *Journal of the Maine Medical Association* 66 (1975):123–139, 149.

# Impact of IPAs on fee-for-service medical groups

John J. Aluise,
Thomas R. Konrad,
and
Bates Buckner

*Individual practice association (IPA) is the newest and most rapidly growing HMO model. Despite potential benefits, IPAs have experienced a variety of difficulties. A case study analysis of community practices in North Carolina revealed satisfactory results as well as concerns.*

In the past fifteen years, prepaid health plans, especially health maintenance organizations (HMOs), have made a dramatic impact on traditional patterns of medical practice. According to the latest HMO census report, 27.7 million people, approximately 13% of the U.S. population, are enrolled in one of 654 HMOs. From 1981 to 1986, the HMO industry has enjoyed a remarkable annual growth rate of 20% in enrollment and nearly 50% in the number of plans.[1] Until recent years when the individual practice associations (IPAs) were established, the group and staff models were the dominant types of HMO systems. Currently IPAs have over 17.5 million people enrolled—63% of all HMO members. Since federal guidelines do not distinguish between IPAs and network models, they will be treated as one entity throughout this paper.

## IPAs

The unique feature of an IPA plan, and perhaps a reason for its becoming the leading form of HMO, is the capability of practicing physicians to continue to work independently, providing medical care to fee-for-service patients as well as to those patients enrolled in the IPA-HMO. According to a federally sponsored publication,[2] advantages for fee-for-service medical groups affiliating themselves with IPAs are as follows: (1) preserve or expand the group's patient base in a competitive market, (2) improve cash position, (3) expand control over health care delivery, (4) reduce paperwork, (5) reduce bad debts, (6) profit from cost containment, (7) enhance efficiency of fee-for-service practice, (8) improve ability to budget, and (9) gain market exposure through sales effort of HMO. Another advantage of the IPA-HMO is that it can serve as a marketing function for primary care physicians, thus becoming an ongoing source of new patients and increased revenues. IPAs are also considered desirable from the con-

**John J. Aluise,** *Ph.D., is an Assistant Professor of Family Medicine, School of Medicine, University of North Carolina, Chapel Hill, North Carolina.*

**Thomas R. Konrad,** *Ph.D., is Director of the Program on Health Professions and Health Care Organizations, Health Services Research Center, University of North Carolina, Chapel Hill, North Carolina.*

**Bates Buckner,** *B.S., is a Graduate Research Assistant, Department of Health Policy and Administration, School of Public Health, University of North Carolina, Chapel Hill, North Carolina.*

*Health Care Manage Rev,* 1989, 14(1), 55–63

sumers' perspective because they include numerous delivery sites and the choice of a personal physician from a panel of participating providers. However, according to one IPA executive, it takes at least two years before a physician fully embraces the HMO, understands its operating principles, and realizes what it can do for his or her practice.[3] This time frame may even be longer if the IPA does not have an effective screening process for selection of participating physicians.

The IPA plan typically requires the primary care physician to function as a case manager, sometimes referred to as the gatekeeper. Physicians who perform the case manager role serve as the patient's primary physician and refer the patient to specialist services, as needed, as a condition of third party payment.[4] This role is viewed as essential to the HMO principles of utilization control and cost containment because the success of prepaid plans is based on the extent to which primary physicians limit unnecessary referrals, admissions, and expensive diagnostic and surgical procedures.[5]

Critics of IPAs mention that cost containment efforts will result in lowering the quality of care and that the doctor–patient relationship will be compromised by restricting the patients' choice of physician and by limiting physicians' decision-making authority.[6,7] Some of the controversy surrounding IPAs is attributed to the case manager role required of primary care physicians. Consulting physicians have voiced fears that primary physicians, as case managers, will exert monopolistic control over access to important medical services.[8] Other difficulties that have been described include: (1) the potential for adversarial relationships between primary physicians and patients, and between primary care physicians and consultants, (2) the probability for ethical and professional conflicts when physicians' decisions differ from insurer's benefits, (3) the requirement for additional administrative work to comply with authorization procedures, and (4) confusion when practices affiliate with more than one IPA.[9–11]

## RESEARCH ON HMOs

Most of the reported research on HMOs has involved the staff and group models that are operated almost exclusively as prepaid group practices with the physicians working on salary or under exclusive contracts with the HMO. According to Wolinsky's review of nine studies of HMO performance, HMOs lower the rate of hospitalization, reduce the average cost of medical care,

offer a range of health benefits, minimize unnecessary surgery, and curb overutilization of high-cost tests and procedures inherent in the fee-for-service system.[12] In Ellsbury's compilation of information on current trends in the HMO field, she identified a set of characteristics common to successful HMOs.[13] They include adequate patient access, consumer and provider grievance procedure, coordination of care, management information system, physician involvement in financial management and risk sharing, emphasis on group practices, and effective medical and administrative leadership. Ellsbury concluded that if fee-for-service practices are to effectively integrate prepaid patients into their organizations, they should expand their provider group to include nurse practitioners or physician's assistants and develop administrative mechanisms within the practice to monitor physician utilization and to coordinate the authorization process for referrals and use of high-cost procedures.

In Hurley's review of case management in managed care systems, he analyzed the multiple roles of primary care physicians in managed care systems and designed a behavioral model of the physician as case manager.[14] According to Hurley's research, case management incorporates several key elements: (1) limitations on the freedom of choice of a provider, (2) an attempt to modify patient utilization patterns by managing or coordinating service delivery, and (3) financial incentives and risk sharing to alter physician behavior and/ or encourage formation of new entities. Case management has become an integral feature of IPA-HMOs. The primary care physician receives a capitated fee per patient per month and is designated as the patient's personal physician, that is, provides comprehensive medical services and coordinates the patient's use of other medical services. Access to other providers must be approved by the personal physician before payment can be authorized. These stipulations are coupled with shared financial risk by the primary physician, the intention being to limit utilization of specialty care and high-cost procedures unless it can be substantiated as medically essential.

Hurley concluded his analysis of case management with a theoretical model of the physician as case manager. He identified four major roles: (1) healer–care giver, advocate, confidante; (2) expert–clinician, therapist, risk manager; (3) coordinator–guide, broker, educator; and (4) rationer–authorizer, resource allocator, auditor. The primary physician's degree of financial risk and commitment to case management responsibilities determine how much these four functions are performed.

The information available about the features, benefits, and difficulties of group and staff HMOs provides the conceptual framework for analyzing the IPA model of prepayment. Since IPAs have engendered a considerable amount of criticism, particularly by the medical community, a base of information specifically about IPAs was considered an important contribution to the health administration literature.

## IPAs IN NORTH CAROLINA

During the past five years, HMOs have established a foothold in the North Carolina health care market. As of November 1986, enrollment in HMOs within the state reached nearly 234,000, with over 80% of the enrollees in IPA plans.[15] Since HMOs, particularly the IPA model, represent a major departure from traditional methods of health care reimbursement, a study was undertaken to determine the effects of a "mixed" model of fee-for-service and prepayment plans within a community

practice. The case study approach was chosen to provide researchers with in-depth knowledge about such issues as the effect of prepayment on practice productivity, the office management system, working relationships between patients and consultants, and professional satisfaction of primary physicians and their office personnel. This investigative approach provides a mechanism for identifying relevant features and variables when studying emergent or unique organizational systems. Case studies also allow for accumulation of information over time to formulate a prospective analysis of historical, financial, and organizational factors.[16-18]

Eleven fee-for-service practices with IPA contracts agreed to participate in the study. Criteria for forming the study group included geographical dispersion in the state, two or more family physicians, and two or more years affiliation with one or more IPA plans. Three practices were located in Charlotte, North Carolina, four in Greensboro, two in Durham, one in Raleigh, and one in Chapel Hill. The combined IPA enrollment of these eleven practices was 22,500, which

**TABLE 1**

ORGANIZATIONAL DATA FOR ELEVEN PRACTICE SITES*

| Category of information | Practice sites | | | | | | | | | | |
|---|---|---|---|---|---|---|---|---|---|---|---|
| | 1 | 2 | 3 | 4 | 5 | 6 | 7 | 8 | 9 | 10 | 11 |
| Years in practice | 2 | 10 | 16 | 6 | 7 | 11 | 2 | 10 | 5 | 6 | 11 |
| Years affiliated with IPA | 2 | 3 | 2 | 3 | 3 | 3 | 2 | 4 | 2 | 2 | 4 |
| Family physicians (FTEs)† | 4 | 2 | 4 | 3 | 2 | 4 | 2 | 3 | 5 | 3 | 9 |
| Family nurse practitioners/ physician assistants | 1 | 1 | | | | 3 | | 1 | | | |
| Total primary care providers | 5 | 3 | 4 | 3 | 2 | 7 | 2 | 4 | 5 | 3 | 9 |
| Supervisors | 1 | 2 | 1 | 1 | 1 | 2 | | | 1 | 2 | 4 |
| Business staff | 3 | 3 | 3 | 2 | 2 | 10 | 2 | 5 | 8 | 8 | 17 |
| Nursing staff | 3 | 3 | 5 | 3 | 2 | 5 | 2 | 4 | 5 | 4 | 9 |
| Laboratory/X-ray | 1 | 1 | | 1 | | 2 | | | | | 6 |
| Total office staff | 8 | 9 | 9 | 7 | 5 | 19 | 4 | 9 | 14 | 14 | 36 |

*As of August 1987.
†FTE—full time equivalent.

represents 15% of the total IPA enrollment in the state. During a two-month period, each practice was visited twice. Practice managers and at least one physician in each practice were interviewed. Financial statements and practice productivity reports for the latest 12-month period were reviewed. All physicians and office staff were asked to complete a two-page questionnaire on their opinions about the effect of the IPA plan on the practice and their personal work. Thirty-one of the 41 physicians (76%) and 87 of the 134 office personnel (65%) returned completed questionnaires. Most of the office staff who did not respond to the survey indicated that they had not been with the practice long enough to feel they could answer the questions. Table 1 presents organizational information about each practice.

Findings discussed below are based on the information from the eleven community practices, all of whom are in the first years of integrating prepaid plans into their established fee-for-service practice system. The following sections on productivity, practice management, working relations, and professional satisfaction offer a preliminary analysis of IPA plans from the perspective of the community practice.

The impact of IPA plans on these practices will be studied prospectively. A second phase of the study will include additional practice sites within the state and in another state and also surveys of consultants and patients to assess their attitudes about the impact of IPAs.

## Productivity analysis

HMOs promote an increase in patient enrollments and, through a capitation payment per patient per month, a commensurate share of revenue to the affiliated practice. According to information displayed in Table 2, ten of the eleven practices produced a percentage of revenue from the two leading prepaid plans, referred to as Plan A and Plan B, in excess of the percentage of prepaid patients to the total patient volume. For example, Practice 4 had 2,000 prepaid patients from Plan B, representing 40% of total patient volume. Prepaid revenue from Plan B to Practice 4 was $20,000 per month, 49% of the monthly receipts. Only Practice 11 had slightly less revenue from prepaid plans than its corresponding share of patient volume—24% prepaid patients versus 20% prepaid revenue. Comparing IPA

---

**TABLE 2**

PRODUCTIVITY STATISTICS TOTAL PRACTICE AND IPA PLANS

| Practice sites | Active patients | IPA enrollees* Plan A | Plan B | IPA practice revenue/ month (000) | Revenue/ month (000)[†] Plan A | Plan B | Office visits/ month | IPA office visits/month[‡] Plan A | Plan B |
|---|---|---|---|---|---|---|---|---|---|
| 1 | 5,000 | 810 (16) | 300 (6) | $51.9 | $3.8 (7) | $8.7 (17) | 1,600 | 280 (17) | 85 (5) |
| 2 | 10,000 | | 600 (6) | $58.0 | | $6.9 (12) | 810 | | 145 (18) |
| 3 | 15,000 | | 400 (3) | $50.2 | | $4.5 (9) | 1,120 | | 100 (9) |
| 4 | 5,000 | | 2,000 (40) | $40.6 | | $20.0 (49) | 1,400 | | 440 (31) |
| 5 | 4,500 | | 1,200 (27) | $27.5 | | $9.6 (35) | 710 | | 260 (37) |
| 6 | 16,000 | | 1,750 (11) | $89.2 | | $1.51 (7) | 3.360 | | 620 (20) |
| 7 | 4,000 | 720 (18) | 325 (8) | $25.4 | $7.6 (30) | $4.0 (16) | 710 | 235 (33) | 90 (3) |
| 8 | 9,000 | 1,600 (18) | 850 (9) | $68.8 | $27.4 (40) | $11.4 (17) | | | |
| 9 | 15,000 | 845 (6) | 855 (6) | $89.5 | $8.2 (9) | $9.1 (10) | 1,900 | 200 (10) | 220 (12) |
| 10 | 12,000 | 850 (7) | 760 (6) | $74.9 | $9.6 (13) | $8.7 (11) | 2,300 | 210 (9) | 195 (8) |
| 11 | 34,000 | 3,825 (11) | 4,470 (13) | $361.5 | $27.0 (8) | $42.0 (12) | 5,300 | 730 (14) | 1,160 (21) |

*Numbers in parentheses = % of total practice.
[†]Numbers in parentheses = % of total revenue.
[‡]Numbers in parentheses = % of total office visits.

revenue with the number of office visits by prepaid patients reveals that most practices maintained a close approximation between revenue and office visits. The only site that had a much higher percentage of prepaid office visits than IPA revenue was Practice 11 with 20% revenue versus 35% prepaid patient office visits. Since utilization of services is normally higher in the first years of a prepaid plan, it appears that the eleven practices achieved a reasonable rate of financial return from their affiliation with IPAs while experiencing the expected rate of utilization.

However, during interviews with practice managers, two financial problems were uncovered that do not appear on the practice financial statements. The first was additional administrative burdens that the practice incurred as a result of affiliation with prepaid plans. Additional time was being spent by both office personnel and physicians to educate patients, complete paperwork, communicate with consultants, and resolve questions arising from inadequate support from the administrative offices of the prepaid plans. Most practices had to incur the cost of hiring at least one additional clerical staff person to handle HMO work. In response to a question about office expenses, 97% of the physicians indicated that costs have increased either slightly or considerably due to prepaid plans. Although the administrative work of physicians and their staff has not been systematically documented, anecdotal evidence suggests that a nominal fee of $1.50 to $3.00 per enrollee per month added to the capitation rate would cover additional case management responsibilities.[19] A second financial concern was the money placed in reserve, a portion of which would be returned if the practice was "cost effective." The method and timing for dispersing these funds was not clearly communicated to the practices, and the managers of several practices expressed the opinion that they did not receive their fair share of these reserve funds.

### Practice management

Clearly, life after affiliation with an HMO will not be business as usual. Unfortunately, in the case study sites, this was largely learned after the fact. Practice managers and physicians openly admitted they had little idea what they were getting into when they signed their initial HMO contracts. The majority of physicians surveyed indicated that their primary reasons for joining the IPAs were the fear of losing established patients, a desire to increase patient volume and revenue, and

(because other physicians were joining) a desire not to be left behind. The opportunity to lower health care costs and to provide comprehensive medical services to a predetermined patient population for a fixed fee were not motivating factors. Thus, when the prepaid patients presented with demands for complete physical examinations, appointments at the patients' convenience, and referrals to patients' personally chosen specialists

---

*Clearly, life after affiliation with an HMO will not be business as usual.*

---

or psychotherapists, family physicians found themselves in the uncomfortable position of saying no to patients they may never have seen before. The increase in patient volume, most of which occurred very soon after new patients were enrolled, required that practices quickly develop alternative methods for providing access to their practice. Four of the practices hired family nurse practitioners or physician's assistants to provide routine primary care, conduct preliminary screening examinations, and participate in the management of nonacute and chronic medical problems. Several practices delegated greater responsibility to nurses to handle initial telephone calls from patients so they could determine the urgency of patients' medical needs and decide how quickly, if at all, patients needed to be seen. Educating newly enrolled patients about registration and authorization processes of the IPA and responding to inquiries from specialists about the payment mechanisms consumed a much larger than expected percentage of staff and physician time. At least one physician in each practice was designated as the liaison with the HMO, which involved evening meetings and additional administrative tasks. Practices also adapted their computer systems so they could compare prepaid for fee-for-service revenues and utilization.

Practice managers complained that, following the initial sign up period, management of the prepaid patients was complicated by the IPA plans' inadequate service of the practices. The management information supplied by the IPA plans was viewed as difficult to interpret and as providing too little information for physicians and managers to evaluate the performance of the prepaid plan compared to the fee-for-service component of the practice. Calls to the IPA office about patient registration, payment and authorization procedures, and other questions pertinent to the affiliation reportedly resulted in either unresponsive or poorly informed communications with the IPA staff. Despite the changes that many practices instituted to facilitate the increase in patient volume and the adjustment to the IPA procedures, it was apparent that the administration of the IPA plans was not working in consort with affiliated practices to smooth out the administrative difficulties.

### Working relations and professional satisfaction

Though the practices enjoyed an increase in patient enrollment and in some instances a new source of young families, practice managers and many of the physicians were concerned that the prepaid plans fostered an adversarial relationship (to a greater degree) between the practice and its HMO patients and (to a lesser degree) between the practice and consulting physicians. When patients chose a prepaid plan, most did not fully understand the requirements of authorization for specialty and ancillary services and many did not have a previous relationship with the practice. Thus, the initial contact between patient and practice may occur with a request for referral or with an appointment to be seen immediately for a comprehensive physical examination, complete with laboratory tests and X -rays. Family physicians in the case study often reported that they felt like they were on the defensive in their very first encounter with HMO patients. Problems also were reported when specialists performed additional services or procedures or preferred to manage patients differently than family physicians had originally instructed. Family physicians indicated that they were uncomfortable confronting specialists about both clinical judgments and financial arrangements.

Practice managers and business clerks also reported frequent communication breakdowns between the practice and the IPA regarding number and type of services covered, payment to specialists, and other procedures unique to each plan. These difficulties were compounded in practices with two or more prepaid plans.

Physicians reported that working relations within the practice and the morale of physicians and office staff have suffered since joining the IPAs. Prior to working with the IPA plans, nearly 90% of the family physicians rated their working relations with patients as either good or excellent. These same categories of satisfaction by physicians dropped to 41% after affiliation with the

### TABLE 3

#### FAMILY PHYSICIANS' PROFESSIONAL SATISFACTION

| Professional satisfaction factors | Respondents—somewhat or very satisfied (%) | |
|---|---|---|
| | Before IPA | After IPA |
| Professional autonomy | 92 | 37 |
| Respect from patients | 96 | 46 |
| Quality of care provided | 96 | 67 |
| Amount of paperwork required | 79 | 7 |
| Relations with colleagues in other specialties | 88 | 55 |
| Opportunity to practice medicine the way you prefer | 88 | 28 |

prepaid plans. Table 3 presents a summary of physicians' professional satisfaction ratings before and after affiliating with IPA plans.

The perceptions by office personnel were similar to those of physicians. Since affiliating with IPA plans, office staff reported dramatic declines in physician and staff morale, physician–patient relations, and staff–patient relations. When asked to rate their overall satisfaction with their practice's affiliation with prepaid plans, only 38% of office personnel responded somewhat satisfied or very satisfied. The leading complaints by office staff were (1) the lack of information provided to patients about their prepaid health plan, which resulted in an inordinate amount of time spent educating patients, and (2) confusion regarding the authorization procedures.

### Comparison of two IPA plans

All eleven practices in the study participated in one of the two major IPA plans, and six were also affiliated with a second IPA plan. Based on interviews and survey responses, it was possible to draw a comparison of the two leading IPA plans, which will be referred to as Plan A and Plan B.

## Plan A

Two distinguishing features of Plan A are the inclusion of specialists as members of the approved provider group and the additional payment to primary care physicians for certain laboratory tests and clinical procedures. Participating practices considered the large number of state employees enrolled in Plan A as an advantage because many of these enrollees were young healthy adults and families with small children. Financially, most practices have benefited from the revenue from Plan A's capitation and additional payments from fee-for-service procedures and the reserve funds. One practice did report that Plan A reneged on a large percentage of the payment to the practice from the hospital reserve fund. The practice manager surmised that the reason may have been because of the financial burden Plan A incurred from the acquisition of a local HMO. The major critique of Plan A is that its parent organization is primarily an indemnity insurance organization and the IPA is a relatively small feature of the system. Problems frequently mentioned were (1) the lack of administrative support, (2) misleading marketing and educational programs, and (3) a nonexistent management information system. These difficulties were compounded when Plan A's enrollment increased over 400% from April 1986 to November 1986, primarily due to the selection of Plan A by over 86,000 state and local government employees.[20] Another difficulty that resulted from Plan A's affiliation with medical and surgical specialists is that patients who had previous relationships with these specialists assumed they could continue receiving care from them without anything more than tacit approval by the primary physician. It also appears that many specialists who affiliated with Plan A also felt that their association meant that they would have open access to patients and the freedom to treat patients as they saw fit. Generally, the practices affiliated with Plan A in this study were satisfied with the capitation and additional reimbursement for primary care providers and the large number of state employees it had enrolled. However, there was a consensus that more attention needs to be given to the administrative mechanisms to service the affiliated practices.

## Plan B

Plan B incorporates the precepts of the case manager role to a much greater extent than does Plan A. Practice managers and participating physicians frequently commented that Plan B was very conscientious in initial efforts to educate patients and to support their affiliated community practices. Administrative personnel and the regional medical director were knowledgeable and accessible, factors that were less evident with Plan A. Plan B also identified "preferred providers" who offered quality services at reasonable fees; primary care physicians received the names and fees of these specialists and were encouraged to use them if appropriate. Capitation rates from Plan B were competitive with Plan A, but Plan B did not provide additional reimbursement for selected tests and procedures as did Plan A. Management information reports comparing productivity and utilization data of the affiliated practices were provided regularly. Initially, monthly meetings were held for all participating physicians to discuss the impact of prepaid plans on the practices and to further explain Plan B's operating procedures. Recently these meetings have been occurring less frequently.

The major concern regarding Plan B stems from a merger with another national HMO. The national HMO's preference appears to be network model IPA. The network arrangement would require a commitment by the affiliated practice for at least 2,500 enrollees to provide primary medical services and coordinate all other aspects of health care, including payment to specialists. Following the merger, Plan B officials approached their affiliated practices to promote this expanded version of their prepaid contract. If a small practice could not service that large a number of enrollees, one or two practices could join together. The financial incentive for shifting into the network model would be that the capitation payment would be raised to cover not only primary care services but also referrals and other medical expenses, exclusive of hospital charges. Estimates were that the increase would be approximately double the average of $10 per member per month capitation rate. The primary care physicians would contract with and reimburse specialists and other health care services. As one physician described this arrangement, "We will become a mini-insurance franchise for Plan B." Problems anticipated include additional administrative work, much higher financial risk, and the potential of conflicts between primary care physicians and specialists when coordinating services and negotiating fees. The network contract requires that the practice (1) maintain a regular utilization and quality of care review process and (2) administer the coordination of benefits procedures. According to one practice administrator, the management responsibilities and the office procedures necessary to function as an IPA network would require major changes in the practice management system. One of the two practices that is disaffiliating with Plan B stated that the new proposal was the reason they chose to terminate their IPA contract. They were not interested in expanding their prepaid patient volume and subsequently increasing administrative work. As the case study investigation continues, the consequences of practices that disaffiliate with IPA plans will be incorporated into this analysis.

## DISCUSSION

The successful implementation of IPAs is still under scrutiny. The most satisfactory results have occurred when a plan had an effective, well-respected medical director and when the delivery of primary and specialty care was managed by a primary care physician who bore some of the financial risk for utilization of services. As in any form of HMO, an IPA is only as good as the quality of its providers and their commitment to the goals of the prepaid system.[21]

IPAs with a larger number of participating providers, similar to those in North Carolina, put added stress on the management of the prepaid delivery system. Control of referrals and utilization of services become more difficult as the panel of providers increases.[22] The practice management system, including physicians and office personnel, may not be adequately prepared to meet the expectations that patients have for medical services on a prepaid basis.[23,24] Family physicians may be unaccustomed to, or unwilling to coordinate, the full range of patients' medical care, including the payment

---

*The most satisfactory results have occurred when a plan had an effective, well-respected medical director.*

---

to subspecialists.[25,26] The authors' initial findings from the case study investigation support these contentions. As several physicians and practice managers commented, the administrators and medical directors of the IPA plan spent a great deal of time marketing their new method of health care reimbursement to employers and physicians, but the IPA plans seem less enthusiastic when it comes to "service after the sale."

Despite the lamentations of a few physicians in the case study who commented, "I'm a physician, not an insurance agent" and "We hope this HMO business is just a transition phase of medicine," several of the family physicians interviewed seem ready to take their place in the contemporary environment of the medical marketplace. As one stated, "This is what I was trained for—providing comprehensive care and coordinating the other medical services that my patients require." He went on to say, "I now have a much better idea of what specialists do when I send them patients, and, even more importantly, how much they charge." Another physician respondent said, "Don't be afraid to negotiate; HMOs need family physicians. The bottom line is the doctor–patient relationship."

A final question posed to the physicians in the survey was, "What advice would you offer to others who are considering an affiliation with an IPA?" The following points summarize their comments and suggestions:

- Review the contract carefully. Seek advice from others who have recently rejoined an IPA. Learn the rules and discuss them with all physicians in the practice.
- Set up a financial management system within the practice to monitor fee-for-service charges for prepaid patients, including number and type of services performed.
- Obtain a guarantee for primary care services offered to prepaid patients based on the collection rate of the practice.
- Require the prepaid plans to provide a quarterly report of the financial status of the practice's prepaid enrollment, including reserve accounts.
- Carefully review the marketing information of the IPA plan and obtain the names of the companies to whom they are offering their plans.
- Limit prepaid enrollment to 25% of the practice. Limit number of plans within the practice to a manageable number, probably two or three.
- Establish cost containment and utilization review procedures within the practice and apply them to both fee-for-service and prepaid patients.
- Hire a qualified practice manager who can work closely with the IPA administration.

•    •    •

IPAs are at a more rudimentary stage of development than group and staff model HMOs; therefore, a common denominator for the success of the IPAs is the base of physician support. In addition, IPAs with the best chance for success are those with (1) good management and information systems, (2) access to the medical delivery system through primary care physicians who assume general management responsibilities for the patient's care, (3) physician payment based on a standardized reimbursement system, (4) mechanisms for risk sharing by participating physicians, (5) well-established procedures for preauthorization of hospitalization and referrals, and (6) arrangements for utilization and peer review. Continuing investigation of the IPA developments in North Carolina will be necessary to determine how many of these success factors come to fruition.

*Further information about the research method, including data gathering instruments and physician and staff questionnaires, are available upon request from John J. Aluise, Ph.D., Assistant Professor, Department of Family Medicine, Campus Box 7595, University of North Carolina, Chapel Hill, North Carolina 27599-7595.*

## REFERENCES

1. *National HMO Census Report,* Excelsior, Minn.: InterStudy, 1986.
2. U.S. Department of Health and Human Services. *Guide for Fee-for-Service Medical Groups on Affiliating with HMOs.* Technical Assistance Monograph. Office of Health Maintenance Organizations, No. 240-81-0046. Washington D.C: Government Printing Office, 1983.
3. U.S. Department of Health and Human Services. *Determinants of HMO Success.* Office Health Maintenance Organizations, No. BHMORD 240-83-0095. Washington, D.C.: Government Printing Office, 1986.
4. Sommers, A. "And Who Shall Be the Gatekeeper? The Role of Primary Physician in the Health Care Delivery System." *Inquiry* 20 (1984): 301–13.
5. Luft, H. *Health Maintenance Organizations, Dimensions of Performance.* New York: Wiley, 1981.
6. Freund, D., and Allen, K. "Factors Affecting Physicians' Choice to Practice in a Fee-for-Service vs Individual Practice Association." *Medical Care* 23 (1985): 700–809.
7. L. Harris and Associates. *Medical Practice in the 1980's. Physicians Look at Their Changing Careers.* Menlo Park, Calif.: L. Harris and Associates, Kaiser Foundation, 1980.
8. Shouldice, R. "Should Fee-for-Service Group Practices Develop a Prepaid Component?" *Medical Group Management* 28, no. 1 (1981): 54–59.
9. L. Harris and Associates, "*Medical Practice.*"
10. Shouldice, "Should Fee-for-Service Group Practices."
11. Wolinsky, F. "The Performance of Health Maintenance Organizations, an Analytic Review." *Milbank Memorial Fund Quarterly* 58 (1980): 537–87.
12. Ibid.
13. Ellsbury, K. *A Guide for Primary Care Physicians on HMOs.* Seattle: University of Washington, Department of Family Medicine, unpublished report, 1985.
14. Hurley, R. "Toward a Behavioral Model of the Physician as Case Manager." *Social Science Medicine* 23, no. 1 (1986): 75–82.
15. North Carolina Foundation for Alternative Health Plans, Department of Human Resources. *An Overview of the Status of Health Maintenance Organizations in North Carolina.* Raleigh, N.C., 1986.
16. Patton, M. *Qualitative Evaluation Methods.* Beverly Hills, Calif.: Sage, 1983.
17. Barton, A. *Organizational Measurement and Its Bearing on the Study of College Environments.* Princeton, N.J.: College Entrance Exam Board, 1969.
18. Manheim, H. *Sociological Research.* Homewood, Ill.: Dorsey, 1977.
19. Hurley, R. "The Status of Medicaid Competition Demonstrations." *Health Care Financing Review* 8, no. 2 (Winter 1986): 65–76.
20. North Carolina Foundation for Alternative Health Plans, *An Overview.*
21. Kingston, J. "The Influence of Competition by Prepaid Group Practice on the Development and Management of an Individual Practice Association-Health Maintenance Organization." In *Proceedings of the 30th Annual Group Health Institute.* Washington, D.C.: Group Health Association, 1980, pp. 280–90.
22. Ibid.
23. Luft, *Health Maintenance Organizations.*
24. Burke, R. "The Pros and Cons of Independent Practice Associations." *Ohio State Medical Journal* 75 (1979): 318–19.
25. Ellsbury, K. "Gatekeeping—Clinical and Administrative Issues." *Western Journal of Medicine* 145, no. 2 (1986): 254–57.
26. Davidson, R. "Primary Care Physician Satisfaction with Case Management." *Western Journal of Medicine* 145, no. 2 (1986): 251–53.

Part V

# ORGANIZATION and MANAGEMENT ISSUES IN MANAGED CARE

# Determinants of HMO success: The case of Complete Health

Linda S. Widra
and
Myron D. Fottler

*The health maintenance organization (HMO) industry has experienced a variety of difficulties and criticisms in recent years. Various hybrid models have been proposed to alleviate these problems. This article presents an in-depth case study of factors associated with the success of one such hybrid: an individual practice association (IPA)-model HMO affiliated with an academic health center. The major success factors identified include the plan design/structure, the strategic orientation/practices, and the stakeholder management orientation practices.*

*Health Care Manage Rev,* 1992, 17(2), 33–44
© 1992 Aspen Publishers, Inc.

**Intensifying concerns** over health care costs have compelled a growing integration of previously separate delivery and financing systems. In response to these changing imperatives, alternative delivery systems advocating managed care have assumed a more visible presence in health care but have failed (thus far) to provide a panacea to the cost/quality/access dilemma.[1]

Indeed, as experience with these systems has grown, the so-called "pure" forms have met increased criticism from physicians, the business community, third party payors, Congress, federal regulators, hospital executives, labor unions, and patients for a wide variety of real or alleged deficiencies. Among the most significant of the deficiencies cited are low quality, poor management, interference with physician autonomy, inability to contain costs, lack of access for the poor or the elderly, and restraint of trade.[2-11] Such problems persist despite double-digit percentage growth in membership throughout the 1980s to 32 million or 13 percent of the U.S. population.[12]

Evidence of a slackening of previously spectacular growth rates in health maintenance organization (HMO) enrollment is emerging. In 1987, the number of Americans enrolled in HMOs increased by the smallest percentage in five years. Moreover, the number of HMOs going bankrupt increased sharply from 5 or 6 in 1986 to 30 in 1987. The "shakeup" and a "shakeout" of the HMO industry that began in the mid 1980s continues to the present as a result of increased competition in the industry as well as the problems mentioned above.[10]

The development of hybrid models that capture the positive features of different forms of managed-care systems and minimize deficiencies has been predicted.[13] This article showcases one such hybrid, a corporate model IPA-HMO affiliated with an academic health center in the Southeast. Although still a relatively young plan, the experience of this model to date suggests that it

**Linda S. Widra,** *Ph.D., is Vice President, Nursing, Wilson N. Jones Memorial Hospital, Sherman, Texas.*

**Myron D. Fottler,** *Ph.D., is Professor and Director of the doctoral program in Administration—Health Services, School of Business and Department of Health Services Administration, School of Health-Related Professions, University of Alabama at Birmingham, Birmingham, Alabama.*

The authors would like to thank Carol Fottler, Prisilla Roberts, and Dr. Michael Morrisey of the University of Alabama at Birmingham for their perceptive comments on earlier drafts of this paper. In addition, the authors acknowledge the cooperation and helpfulness of the staff of Complete Health, Inc., without which this article could not have been written. Finally, the authors thank Joan Mazzolini of the *Birmingham Post-Herald* for providing access to her file of information on Complete Health.

may represent a more palatable option to both providers and consumers of health care, that it satisfactorily serves the diverse needs and incentives of major health care purchasers, and that it has responsively blended corporate attributes of efficiency, economy, and commitment to quality.

This is the first article to examine a hybrid model HMO that was based on multiple success factors drawn from previous industry experience or recorded in the HMO literature.[14] It is the particular combination of success factors (rather than isolated unique features), which have been incorporated into a proprietary structure and framed within an academic health center affiliation, that differentiates this HMO from more traditional models. In addition to identifying factors associated with the plan's early success, we will also point out some challenges and concerns.

## EVOLUTION OF AN INNOVATION

Complete Health, an IPA-model HMO with a federally qualified subsidiary, was founded in 1986 under the sponsorship and financial backing of the University of Alabama Health Services Foundation (UAHSF) and a group of businessmen in Birmingham, Alabama. The UAHSF is a medical group practice organization whose physician members are affiliated with the University of Alabama Medical Center, University of Alabama at Birmingham (UAB). The Foundation is the only group of physicians associated with a public medical school that owns a for-profit HMO.[15]

Dr. John W. Kirklin of UAB initially shared his desires for an HMO that had an academic medical center as a centerpiece with a local Birmingham entrepreneur, William W. Featheringill. Featheringill researched various managed-care systems nationally, developed the Complete Health managed-care model, and raised venture capital from his own resources and other prominent Birmingham businesspeople and companies to fund Complete Health. Of the initial capitalization, 51 percent was provided by the Medical Advancement Foundation (a subsidiary of the UAHSF), and 49 percent was provided by a group of local investors organized by Birmingham-based Private Capital Corporation.

When Complete Health entered the market in March 1986, there were a number of other HMOs in operation or just beginning operation in the Birmingham area. Since 1986, Complete Health has expanded from the Birmingham market, becoming a statewide HMO with operations throughout Alabama. With approximately 100,000 members, it is presently larger than its three largest competitors combined. It turned profitable in the third quarter of 1988 and has remained profitable since.[16]

From a base of two people who started the company in 1986, Complete Health now employs 375 people and has contracts with 2,316 HMO provider physicians and 47 HMO provider hospitals. The company has a 99 percent retention rate for previously enrolled members and a 99.5 percent provider retention rate.[16] It has begun expansion into Louisiana and has plans underway to expand into Florida, Georgia, Tennessee, Mississippi, and Arkansas. Eventually, it plans to serve the entire Southeast.

Currently, only six other public universities or private physicians' groups affiliated with such universities own or participate in a joint venture in HMOs. Compared to these university HMOs, Complete Health in Birmingham is the second oldest and the largest, possessing an enrollment three times larger than that of any other HMO owned by a public medical school or its private physicians. Furthermore, of the HMOs nationwide owned by public medical schools or their physicians, Complete Health is the only one that is active statewide.[15]

Several incentives prompted active interest in this alternative delivery concept on the part of the Health Services Foundation and University administrative officials. First, both groups were becoming increasingly concerned with the erosion of the patient referral base brought about by the arrival of HMOs that were affiliated only with community hospitals. Owning an HMO would allow UAB physicians to direct enrollees to UAB-affiliated physicians, clinics, and the University Hospital. Up to that point, the medical center physicians had seen other HMOs formed in which they were not allowed to participate. Without their own HMO, they anticipated a further erosion of their patient base.

There was also a significant interest in delineating the role of the academic health center in an HMO. Since a basic philosophy driving the academic health center is the preparation of qualified medical practitioners and since the future of health care delivery is likely to be dominated by managed-care systems, the appropriate-

*HMO affiliation was viewed as a mechanism whereby the academic health center could look more closely at itself, its competitive potential, and its capacity to deliver quality health care more efficiently.*

ness of HMO affiliation was obvious. Moreover, HMO affiliation was viewed as a mechanism whereby the academic health center could look more closely at itself, its competitive potential, and its capacity to deliver quality health care more efficiently.

Enrollment figures generally have surpassed expectations. After attracting nearly 13,000 enrollees during its first year of operation, Complete Health completed its fifth year of operations with an enrollment of 100,000. Table 1 indicates Complete Health has experienced initial enrollment growth that surpasses that of other successful national HMOs at the same stage even though the others are located in areas of much greater population density.

Complete Health also possesses the largest current HMO enrollment and enrollment growth rate in Alabama. It is noteworthy that this level of enrollment was achieved in spite of substantial competition. During the time period encompassed by Complete Health's immediate start-up phase, 10 other HMOs, 8 of which served the Birmingham area, were actively competing for new enrollees in Alabama.[17]

In general, statewide development has paralleled that of the local level. Market plans define major regions that comprise a statewide network linked by small feeder cities. In order to assuage any concerns related to control by Birmingham, expansion plans call for the establishment of regional medical directors and medical advisory committees as well as local credentialing and acceptance of physician providers.

---

## TABLE 1

### FIFTH-YEAR ENROLLMENT IN COMPLETE HEALTH AND IN OTHER SUCCESSFUL HMOs

| HMO plan (state) | Year established | Fifth-year enrollment |
|---|---|---|
| Maxicare (California) | 1974 | 25,249 |
| Lifeguard (California) | 1979 | 48,040 |
| Harvard Community Health Plan (Massachusetts) | 1969 | 50,000 |
| Complete Health (Alabama) | 1986 | 100,000* |

*Enrollment as of November 1990.

Sources: Peter D. Fox and Lea Ann Heinen, *Determinants of HMO Success* (Ann Arbor: Health Administration Press, 1987), pp. 68, 152, 194 and Complete Health enrollment data, November, 1990.

## SUCCESS DETERMINANTS

Table 2 summarizes the factors influential in the early success of this HMO. This table was developed after extensive interviews with administrators, physicians, and university officials familiar with the operation of Complete Health. It compares a typical IPA-form HMO to Complete Health on the basis of the plan structure/design, strategic orientation/practices, and stakeholder management orientation/practices.

### Plan design/structure

The Complete Health model was designed with input generated from industry consultants, a comprehensive managed-care literature review, and operational experiences collected from across the nation. As a result of these preliminary efforts, Complete Health was able to avoid many of the major missteps in start-up and development that have plagued many other managed-care systems. The key model ingredient and core strength is flexibility, as expressed in a continuous process of endeavoring to meet changing parameters of consumer preference and market acceptability.

The academic medical center affiliation has created incentives for a corporate structure with considerable independence of medical and administrative components. Unlike other HMOs where the medical director is simply another administrative officer accountable to the chief executive officer (CEO), medical policy and medical practice in Complete Health is physician directed (i.e., the medical aspect of managed care is managed and controlled by physicians). Complete Health has been described as possessing a high "tolerance level" among physician providers due to the administrative independence exercised by physicians as well as the monitoring of physician practice patterns by peers rather than by nonphysicians.

Complete Health's medical directors work closely with a 17-member Medical Advisory Committee composed of panel directors from each participating hospital, representing both primary care physicians and representatives of various specialties. This committee meets bimonthly to discuss new problems and recommend policy related to such issues as credentialing, utilization control, and benefit structure. It reports to the Board of Directors, half of whose members are physicians.

Complete Health was established as a for-profit enterprise whose sponsorship and financial backing contribute toward the perception of staying power in the industry. This proprietary status carries the potential for

---

**TABLE 2**

---

A COMPARISON OF COMPLETE HEALTH AND A TYPICAL IPA-HMO

|  | Typical IPA | Complete Health |
|---|---|---|
| **Plan design/structure** | | |
| 1. National research prior to plan design | No | Yes |
| 2. Medical center affiliation | No | Yes |
| 3. Physician control of medical practice | Varies | High |
| 4. Adequate capitalization | Varies | Yes |
| 5. Key stakeholder equity interest | Low | High |
| 6. Risk-sharing among physicians | Varies | Yes |
| 7. Modification of plan design/structure | Occasional | Continual |
| **Strategic orientation/practices** | | |
| 8. Early market entry | Varies | Yes |
| 9. Entrepreneurial orientation | Low | High |
| 10. Experienced management team | Varies | Yes |
| 11. Emphasis on both cost containment and service quality | Low | High |
| 12. Market/service orientation | Varies | High |
| 13. Customized provider agreements | Few | Many |
| 14. Customized service packages | Few | Many |
| 15. Diversification | Varies | High |
| **Stakeholder orientation/practices** | | |
| 16. Identification and management of key stakeholders | Haphazard | Systematic |
| 17. Physician selection by affiliated physicians | Sometimes | Always |
| 18. Physician evaluation of physician practice patterns | Partial | Complete |
| 19. Responsiveness to stakeholder preferences | Varies | High |
| 20. Individual experience rating for employers | Sometimes | Always |
| 21. Education/communication/feedback to all key stakeholders | Limited | Extensive |
| 22. Responsiveness to key stakeholder problems and information requests | Low | High |
| 23. Patient freedom of choice regarding providers | Partial | Total |

---

enhanced capital access via equity financing, for instilling greater cost consciousness, and for offering more competitive employer incentives.[18,19] Consequently, Complete Health has had both the perception and the reality of adequate capitalization (unlike many of its competitors). Most members of the Board of Directors and top management are major equity shareholders in Complete Health. The Board also represents major stakeholders, including physicians associated with Health Services Foundation and the major investors.

Complete Health is a privately held company and intends to stay that way. According to Featheringill:

We are now solidly profitable and when you become solidly profitable, your need for equity capital diminishes. I feel that the only real justification for taking a company public is liquidity and, more so, to raise money. I think if you are a public company, the CEO is going to spend 20 to 25 percent of his time talking to analysts and brokers and worshiping at the altar of the god of the quarterly earnings statement. Your focus becomes extremely short-ranged. I really think that Complete Health, this entire endeavor, is going to be a better company if we can make long-term decisions.[20(p.23)]

At Complete Health, the central force driving the risk-sharing mechanism is peer group pressure. That is, the

---

*At Complete Health, the central force driving the risk-sharing mechanism is peer group pressure.*

---

key ingredient for reshaping inefficient practice patterns into more cost-effective ones lies in the pressure imposed by some physicians upon their deviant peers. Acting upon this philosophy, Complete Health organizes its physician providers into hospital panels and furnishes them with utilization and referral data to enable objective appraisal of panel member performance.

The effectiveness of intrapanel peer review—and peer pressure—is substantially fueled by economic incentives incorporated into risk-sharing contractual provisions. In general, Complete Health physicians receive professional compensation on a fee-for-service basis, similar to the financial arrangements described in other IPA-based systems.[14] All physician payments are subject to a 15 percent withhold, however, which represents the degree of economic risk to which the physician is exposed. Following periodic fund analysis and adjustment, eligible surpluses are distributed—first at the panel level and subsequently at the level of the individual physician member.

Thus, over-utilizers experience not only personal financial repercussions of their practice patterns but also exert a negative economic impact upon fellow panel members. Panel intolerance of the excesses of one or more individual members is a powerful mechanism in modifying physician behavior in the direction of greater compliance with standard utilization parameters. When indicated on the basis of objective data related to physician practice patterns, the provider withhold can be adjusted incrementally.

Finally, the most important aspect of the plan design/ structure is its flexibility and responsiveness to changed conditions. Even though the plan design/structure was developed based upon research concerning the best practices of the mid-1980s, it is understood that the industry is rapidly changing. Consequently, nothing is "carved in stone." All relationships and agreements are subject to change and negotiation. Refinement of all aspects of the model is an ongoing process.

### Strategic orientation/practices

At the time Complete Health entered the Birmingham HMO market in 1986, there was only one established HMO. Even though HMOs were well developed in other parts of the country, they were a relatively new entity in Alabama in 1986. Although several other HMOs were begun in the state in 1985–1986, the company did have the advantage of early market entry with few large, well-established competitors.

Unlike most HMOs that have been founded by established insurance companies or other corporations as a way to exploit a growth market and make money, Com-

plete Health was begun by an entrepreneur. Featheringill is a venture capitalist who has started up four other successful companies outside of health services. In 1990, he won the John S. Jemison Venture Award, a local award given by the Birmingham Chamber of Commerce to a local entrepreneur, for his development of Complete Health.

According to Featheringill:

> The start-up of any company is very risky . . . . The key to success in starting up a company is the management team. In my opinion, the managers have to be hands-on doers with a sense of great energy. Not everyone can fit into a start-up management team . . . . This is a very dangerous and complicated business to get into. You can easily lose a lot of money if you do not know what you are doing . . . . Start-up companies are very loose with no well-defined structure. There are just a jillion things to do. It is a very difficult thing to do. The basic key is recruiting people with the talent to do the job.[21(p.B-7)]

The quality of the management team has been a fundamental basis upon which the company's initial success has been based. After an initially high turnover rate among executive personnel, Featheringill has been able to build a group of managers who are both experienced and respected in the field of managed care. For example, the senior vice president for medical affairs founded the Tampa Bay Health Plan; the vice president for marketing had several years of experience in managed care with American Medical International (AMI); and the senior vice president for operations was previously senior vice president for operations at Physicians Health Plan in Minneapolis.

Porter believes successful companies should *either* emphasize low costs as a basis for competitive advantage *or* differentiate their services or products based on quality or other attributes.[22] Complete Health, however, has a corporate orientation that emphasizes *both* cost containment *and* service quality. According to Featheringill:

> When an industry becomes hot, there is often a lot more venture capital and a lot less expertise. They key to continued success has been keeping costs down while providing quality care. Other HMOs fail because they do not adhere to that basic principle.[21(p.B-7)]

A market/service orientation permeates the entire organization. Complete Health has sought to provide an alternative delivery system characterized by the ability of enrollees to enjoy broad selection, to retain established physician–patient relationships, and to otherwise avoid restrictions that may adversely affect patient satisfaction and perceived quality of care. Periodic consumer satisfaction questionnaires have consistently revealed high levels of satisfaction with the Plan, and the re-enrollment rate is in excess of 99 percent. Only one account has been lost and less than 0.5 percent of Complete Health physicians have ceased participation. By comparison, a recent study of 1,553 enrollees in three Minneapolis/St. Paul HMOs showed an annual disenrollment rate of 5.4 percent.[23]

While most HMOs give "lip-service" to a service or customer orientation, many give first priority to generating operating income; Complete Health gives *first* priority to customer service and this philosophy permeates the entire organization. In some HMOs, there are communication and bureaucratic barriers when the inevitable problems arise. The result is delay and frustration for the customer and potential loss of business for the HMO in the long run. At Complete Health the philosophy is "Tell us what we can do to fix it" and "Let's do whatever it takes to solve the problem."

Consequently, when Complete Health markets both the quality of technical care available through its affiliated physicians and institutions, it also markets the quality of its own service in meeting provider or consumer needs. The goal is to make sure that the marketing of technical and service quality is based upon substance rather than image.

Increasingly, major purchasers of health services have shed their traditional role as silent payors and are aggressively functioning as powerful architects of the health care delivery and financing system. Complete Health has endeavored to anticipate the needs and incentives of employers by emphasizing flexibility in benefit design. Unlike competitors who adopt a product-oriented approach in trying to sell a particular benefit package, Complete Health emphasizes greater interaction with employers in order to tailor a benefit package to meet specific employer objectives, such as cost sharing, utilization control, and the avoidance of adverse selection.

It is through this customization of benefit structures that Complete Health has been able to achieve a dominant market share in Birmingham and Alabama. Rather than offer a single benefit package and employ community rating as traditional HMO models have done, Complete Health offers multiple plan options and experience rates each employee group individually. This approach enables more accurate assessment of premiums based upon health care utilization experience, specific employee group demographics, and appropriate assignment to weighted risk categories.

Finally, Complete Health has a strong orientation toward related diversifications that build upon its existing strengths in information systems, claims processing, and utilization review. In addition to its HMO business, it has expanded into such areas as health-facility management and administration of insurance and flexible health plans. The company developed a proprietary software system for utilization review that has become state-of-the-art in the industry. This system is now being used by 50 HMO operations nationwide including Aetna, Blue Cross and Blue Shield of Texas and Florida, and Mutual of Omaha.

In 1989, Complete Health replaced Blue Cross and Blue Shield as the administrator for the Alabama Public Education Employees Health Insurance Plan (PEEHIP) through a statewide network. The Alabama Health Network (AHN) is a preferred provider organization (PPO) servicing 116,000 members.[24] Product or service lines currently available through Complete Health include the HMO, the Alabama Health Network PPO, Dental HMO, flexible benefits administration, and a Medicare supplement called Senior Partners.

### Stakeholder orientation/practices

One recent article has identified inadequate identification, assessment, and management of key stakeholders as the major problem facing HMOs in the United States.[25] Stakeholders are those individuals, groups, or organizations who (a) have a stake in the decisions and actions of the organization, (b) are affected by its strategies and policies, and (c) may attempt to influence those decisions and actions.[26] Stakeholder groups, when identified, are usually varied in terms of the stakes involved and the relationship of the stakeholder to the organization. Thus, stakeholder management requires the development and implementation of a comprehensive management plan that reflects the relative importance of various stakeholders in achieving the organization's strategic objectives.[27]

Four key HMO stakeholders identified by Fox and Heinen[14] and Topping and Fottler[25] are affiliated physicians, nonaffiliated physicians, employers, and plan enrollees. While many other HMOs have been somewhat negligent in identifying, assessing, and managing their key stakeholders, Complete Health has been systematic in its identification, assessment, and management of its key stakeholders. Prior to establishment of the HMO, the founders identified physicians, employers, and enrollees as the key stakeholders and several others as less significant, but still important. The latter included state government regulatory bodies and the media.

Physician selection for HMO participation often constitutes an exercise in convenience rather than a systematic process. Fledgling HMOs may typically accept any and all interested physicians in order to expeditiously establish a provider network. Such an approach may be met with subsequent regret, as problems surface in key areas of plan compliance and inefficient practice patterns. At Complete Health, more concerted efforts were made to recruit high-quality, cost-efficient physicians from the beginning. Additionally, in line with its academic medical center ties, recruiting preference is given to providers who are "friends" of UAB with respect to their patient referral history when Complete Health enters a local market.

Physician selection typically commences with identification of those physicians in a particular area who are regarded by the professional community as clinically respected and politically important. Such information is obtained through market representatives skilled in assessing the medical climate in a particular area, as well as through the UAB physician network that, through its tertiary-care activities, may have considerable knowledge of the physician base in a referral area. The criterion for "quality" is the opinion of the physician's peers in the local area. Once this physician nucleus has been successfully recruited and educated about how the system works, Complete Health personnel actively solicit their input in guiding the selection of additional physicians and panel members. The value of the contributions of this nucleus of physicians derives from their awareness that they are assisting in the selection of physicians with whom they will be sharing financial risks, a powerful stimulus for conscientious selection.

Initial physician selection in the Birmingham area resulted in a complementary balance of academic health center physicians and community providers. The greater collaboration and collegiality fostered by Complete Health affiliation have contributed toward the bridging of historical schisms that have characterized these physician populations.

Reflective of the philosophy that physicians should manage physicians, panels of participating physicians are organized at each provider hospital, with a primary-care physician from each panel functioning as the panel director. The panel director reports directly to the plan medical director and assists thereby in the chain of medical communication.

Monitoring of utilization patterns within each panel enables physicians to exert pressure on their peers as necessary to ensure that the panel in its entirety is functioning within utilization guidelines. This structuring of physician relationships has been generally effective in promoting compliance with economic objectives and in minimizing interventions in medical practice by nonphysician personnel. Nonfinancial sanctions, in the form of peer pressure and formal admonishments, are generally imposed initially within the panel and by physician peers. With adequate substantiating utilization experience, Complete Health has (with Medical Advisory Committee backing) imposed financial sanctions in the form of 35 percent withholds upon several physician over-utilizers. Despite the financial sanctions, the major constraint on utilization continues to be peer pressure in the form of moral suasion and other nonfinancial sanctions.

Patient utilization is managed rather than merely reviewed. Annually budgeted utilization is determined by Plan experience, the availability of alternatives to expensive inpatient care, and actuarial analysis. While the elements of utilization management described herein are not totally unique to Complete Health, it can reasonably be asserted that they represent the best current practice in the managed-care industry.

Of the three major components affecting utilization—patient, hospital, and physician—control mechanisms largely focus upon physicians and the efficiency of their practice patterns. Physician contributions are particularly beneficial in evaluating quality of care, the medical necessity of services rendered, and in establishing norms for diagnostic and therapeutic practice. Each physician receives a detailed profile of personal utilization data as well as his or her standing in the physician panel and in the Plan as a whole. Such information is used to monitor performance, to investigate deviations from projected utilization, and to justify the imposition of sanctions when indicated.

Another important component of utilization management is the performance of daily concurrent review. More commonly found is the assignment of a standard length of stay with review occurring shortly before its expiration. The obvious advantages to be gained from concurrent review performed on a daily basis are reception of more timely information regarding patient status and the enhanced potential for early discharge. Experience at Complete Health has shown that in many cases patients can be safely discharged earlier and followed by home visit for a day or two.

While the Complete Health utilization experience compares favorably with that of local competitors in both managed-care and indemnity systems, the current inpatient utilization level is approximately 361 days per 1,000 enrollees per year. Sufficient information now exists in the Complete Health's utilization history database to identify deviations in practice patterns and to assume a more restrictive position where indicated. Consequently, the plan has experienced reductions in its inpatient hospital utilization each year since its inception and expects to continue to do so in the future.

Efforts are currently underway to introduce proven protocols designed to reshape utilization parameters without adversely affecting quality and clinical outcomes. While it is desirable that this be done without creating the perception of system interference with the practice of medicine, a tightening of payment controls

---

*Academic health center physicians, in particular, may experience internal conflict between the profitability motives inherent in their ownership interests in the HMO and their professional motives to provide state-of-the-art care.*

---

inevitably carries this risk. Academic health center physicians, in particular, may experience internal conflict between the profitability motives inherent in their ownership interests in the HMO and their professional motives to provide state-of-the-art care.

Customization of benefit packages and individual experience rating for employers have already been discussed in the previous section. In addition, ongoing communications (education programs for managing employer stakeholders) are also important. There is an emphasis on informed involvement, communication, and participation.

Complete Health maintains and strengthens relationships with employers through periodic social activities and information-sharing meetings. These have been effective in building harmonious relationships between Complete Health and its actual and prospective employer purchasers. In addition, special events, such as seminars featuring nationally prominent speakers, are offered for benefit managers. A newsletter with information about the plan is sent to employers on a regular basis. All of these activities emphasize the relative priority placed upon direct communication and interaction rather than advertising per se.

Many alternative delivery systems aggressively promote their product and, once the formal contractual arrangement is secured, tend to assume a more passive role toward communication and education. Complete Health has recognized that proper utilization of the plan is central to its economic viability. Proper utilization, in turn, depends on educated and informed plan participants. Consequently, periodic publications in the form of provider and member newsletters serve to communicate in-

formation regarding Complete Health to all involved. Additionally, the Complete Health Hotline allows enrollees, employers, and providers to communicate directly with Complete Health representatives if they have questions or problems.

A major enrollee dissatisfier has been HMO restriction of freedom of choice of provider.[14] In addition to the negotiation of contractual arrangements at competitive discounts with nearly half of the providers in the Birmingham area, Complete Health offers a unique nonparticipating provider option. This feature allows referred enrollees to use specialist physicians who are not members of Complete Health and to have 80 percent of the charges specified in the Maximum Fee Schedule covered. While experience has revealed that this nonparticipating provider option constitutes only 1.5 percent of all referrals, it does provide more flexibility and freedom of choice than does the typical HMO.

## Other selected outcome indicators

As already noted, Complete Health has shown substantial *early* success in terms of physician satisfaction, enrollee satisfaction, and enrollment growth. The former two criteria are indicated by retention rates of over 99 percent while the enrollment growth is documented in Table 1.

As is true for most start-up companies, the economic returns have been more tenuous. Table 3 indicates profits and losses at Complete Health during the five-year period 1986–1990. The first three years showed losses. The 1989 fiscal year (FY) was the first profitable year. The 1990 fiscal year, which ended March 31, 1991, showed a

---

**TABLE 3**

ANNUAL COMPLETE HEALTH PROFITS AND LOSSES, 1986–1990

| First year* | Profit or Loss, $ |
|---|---|
| 1986 | − 1,400,000 |
| 1987 | − 2,000,000 |
| 1988 | − 813,000 |
| 1989 | + 1,700,000 |
| 1990 | + 5,392,000 |

*Each fiscal year ends on March 31 of the following year. Thus, the 1990 fiscal year ended on March 31, 1991.

Sources: Complete Health and Alabama Department of Insurance.

**TABLE 4**

A COMPARISON OF SELECTED COMPLETE HEALTH OUTCOME INDICATORS WITH THOSE OF OTHER HMOs NATIONALLY

| Outcome indicator | Complete Health | Comparison to other HMOs | | | | | |
|---|---|---|---|---|---|---|---|
| | | All HMOs | IPAs | For profit | 4–7 years | 100,000+ enrollees | East central region |
| 1. Operating profit margin (operating reverence operating expenses – total revenue) | +0.04 | –0.04 | –0.06 | –0.06 | –0.05 | –0.01 | –0.03 |
| 2. Net return on revenue (net income – total revenue) | +0.03 | –0.04 | –0.05 | –0.06 | –0.04 | –0.01 | –0.03 |
| 3. Net return on assets (net income – total assets) | +0.13 | –0.15 | –0.19 | –0.19 | –0.16 | –0.05 | –0.11 |
| 4. Net return on equity (net income – total net worth) | +0.75 | –1.20 | –1.72 | –1.48 | –1.27 | –0.67 | –0.62 |
| 5. Current ratio (current assets – current liabilities) | 1.20 | 0.96 | 0.95 | 0.98 | 0.94 | 0.92 | 0.92 |
| 6. Debt to equity ratio (total long-term liabilities – total net worth) | 0.56 | 0.17 | 0.05 | 0.03 | 0.02 | 0.64 | 0.18 |
| 7. Administrative expense ratio (administrative expenses – operating revenue) | 0.14 | 0.15 | 0.16 | 0.16 | 0.14 | 0.12 | 0.13 |
| 8. Health care expense ratio (total medical and hospital expenses – operating revenue) | 0.82 | 0.92 | 0.92 | 0.92 | 0.92 | 0.92 | 0.92 |
| 9. Inpatient hospital utilization (number of inpatient hospital days per 1,000 enrollees) | 361 | 433 | 431 | 428 | 413 | 446 | 445 |

Sources: Complete Health financial and utilization ratios are calculated from the income statement, balance sheet, and other data provided by Complete Health for the 1990 fiscal year ending March 31, 1991. Data for various categories of HMOs nationally are based on information provided by 332 plans as reported in D. Hodges, K. Camerlo, and M. Gold, *HMO Industry Profile Volume 2: Utilization Patterns, 1988* (Washington, D.C.: Group Health Association of America, September 1990), p.37 and S.J. Palsbo and M.R. Gold, *HMO Industry Profile Volume 3: Financial Performance, 1988* (Washington, D.C.: Group Health Association of America, June 1990), pp. 40–49.

significant increase in profits from $1.7 million (FY 89) to $5.4 million.

Table 4 shows a comparison of a number of outcome indicators for Complete Health as compared to national mean averages for HMOs and particular subcategories of HMOs with characteristics shared by Complete Health (i.e., type of HMO, size, and geographic region). These comparative data for 1988 are the most recent available at the time this article was written. The Complete Health information is calculated from the income statement, balance sheet, and other information provided by Complete Health for the 1990 fiscal year.

Comparisons indicate that while Complete Health made money in 1990, the average HMO and all relevant subcategories of HMOs lost money in 1988. The first four outcome indicators are various measures of profitability. Each shows positive returns for Complete Health as compared to negative mean returns for other HMOs. The greatest difference was in the net return on equity where Complete Health showed returns of 0.75 compared to –1.20 for the average HMO.

Items 5 and 6 show liquidity and capital structure. The current ratio for Complete Health (1.20) is significantly higher than that of the typical HMO (0.96). This indicates greater liquidity. The higher debt to equity ratio for Complete Health (0.56) indicates they rely more on long-term debt than does the average HMO (0.17); however, they are near the average of 0.64 reported by HMOs with 100,000+ enrollees.

Items 7, 8, and 9 analyze the expense structure in more detail. The administrative expense ratio is approximately average for all HMOs and the various subcategories. However, both the health care expense ratio and inpatient hospital days per 1,000 enrollees are lower for Complete Health, than the average for other HMOs or other HMO subcategories. The lower hospital days per 1,000 enrollees (361) may be one explanation for the lower health care expense ratio. As noted in Table 4, the figure is below average as compared to the mean for all HMOs (433) as well as the mean for the various HMO subcategories. It is also possible that Complete Health enrollees have fewer ambulatory visits per year than enrollees in other HMOs, although these data were not available.

The 361 inpatient hospital days per 1,000 enrollees is below regional and national average. Moreover, it declined from 370 in 1989. Nevertheless, this figure is still considerably greater than desired by plan administrators. Some of the better managed-care plans in Minneapolis and Seattle are experiencing inpatient hospital utilization rates of about 250 days per 1,000 enrollees. A partial explanation may be found in the relative inexperience with managed-care plans in the South as compared to other parts of the nation where HMOs have been well established for many years. Until recently physician practice patterns were practically untouched by the constraining influence of managed-care concepts.

## IMPLICATIONS

In its brief history, Complete Health has emerged as a managed-care leader in its particular markets. Its symbiotic affiliation with an academic health center has constituted a springboard to credibility and early success. Organizationally structured to enhance the independence of the business and the medical components of its operations, Complete Health has grown rapidly through the provision of a broad range of services in a purchaser-oriented, responsive, and innovative manner. It has successfully implemented blended strategies of differentiation based on the high technical quality of an academic health center as well as its own high service quality combined with cost containment.

The long-term goal is for Complete Health to become the leading HMO and health insurance manager in the Southeast. The company has experienced early success

in terms of physician satisfaction, enrollees' satisfaction, and enrollment growth. It is not a national leader in the areas of utilization control and economic returns but is showing consistent improvements in both. At this point, the long-term goals appear to be both challenging and attainable.

Historically, the establishment of formal affiliations between HMOs and academic medical centers has been controversial. There may be potential conflict between the imperative of the HMO to control costs and the traditional philosophy of the medical center to provide the most technologically sophisticated level of care available.[28] Nevertheless, this case study of Complete Health indicates that successful linkages can be developed due to the mutuality of benefits enjoyed by each.

HMO affiliation provides the medical center with referral of patients who otherwise would be unlikely to access their services. Participating community physicians and their patient enrollees might be induced to "try" the medical center services. If the experience is satisfactory, these community physicians might be induced to refer their non-HMO patients as well. Moreover, the greater emphasis on referrals from community primary-care physicians creates a more balanced case mix with an associated improvement in the overall reimbursement mix.[29]

From the plan viewpoint, affiliation with an academic medical center may stimulate physician affiliation and consumer enrollment due to consumer/provider perceptions concerning the scope and quality of services available at the medical center.[30] This provides a vital marketing advantage in competing with HMOs not affiliated with a medical center.

It is impossible to empirically *prove* that the development of Complete Health has benefited the medical center, although all parties agree that it has *probably* stimulated clinic visits and inpatient hospital days. Obviously, one would have to know what would have happened to patient demand in the absence of Complete Health to empirically demonstrate its impact. Between 1986 and 1990 enrollees showed a rough stability in clinic visits, a significant increase in admissions to University Hospital, and a less significant increase in patient days at University Hospital. The latter was related to a declining average length of hospital stay over this time period. University officials believe that clinic visits and inpatient hospital days might have declined in the absence of Complete Health.

Whether the initial success experienced by Complete Health can be sustained indefinitely is unclear. The organization is presently in the start-up phase, which is typified by creativity and innovation. There are several dangers to the organization at this stage.[31] First, the organization may expand too fast, spread itself too thin, and run out of capital. Second, expansion may require the development of new administrative structures and processes that may lead to bureaucracy and a reduction in entrepreneurship and innovation. As new and different physicians in different parts of the state and region are brought into the Plan, it may become more difficult to modify their practice patterns under the existing structure. There may eventually develop a tradeoff between the present practice of physicians managing physicians and the necessity for cost containment to remain competitive. Third, as a number of competitors in a given market increases, so too does the disenrollment rate.[23] Increasing competition may increase disenrollment.

Complete Health currently faces two other challenges where the outcomes are uncertain. First, physician utilization patterns are becoming more efficient, but very slowly. As noted, hospitalization rates are still too high. This may be due to the fact that university-based physicians practice medicine at University Hospital at the same time they are affiliated with Complete Health. Incentives to admit their patients to the hospital may still be strong. Yet the Plan is "treading lightly" in terms of modifying practice patterns, because it fears being accused of "interfering with the practice of medicine" or (worse yet) "reducing the quality of patient care." As in the case of all managed-care programs, Complete Health is trying to achieve a delicate balance between keeping physicians and patients satisfied on one hand and achieving cost containment so that the Plan is competitive in the market on the other hand.

Second, the pressure for cost containment has caused the Plan to maintain low overhead in terms of administrative and professional staff. Many have been working 50 to 70 hours per week over long periods of time. As the enrollment has grown, so too have employee workloads, stress levels, and—relatedly—staff turnover. At some point in the future, this situation could adversely affect the quality of service to physicians and enrollees. A plan for employee career development and managerial succession may need to be developed.

•   •   •

While ultimate exportation of the Complete Health model to other academic health centers is envisioned, refinement of the model is an ongoing process. What we have provided here is "a snapshot of a moving train." The Complete Health experience to date suggests that

this alternative delivery concept may be revitalized through creation of more flexible and market-sensitive modeling. The establishment of formal linkages between an HMO and an academic health center can be a mutually beneficial endeavor when concerted efforts are made to capitalize on the distinctive contributions and strengths of each.

While none of the success factors discussed in this article is totally unique to Complete Health, their *combination* in an IPA-model HMO affiliated with an academic health center *is* unique. Even in situations where there is not a formal linkage between an HMO and an academic medical center, many of the success factors associated with Complete Health's initial success may be applicable. All health care settings need to do a better job in creating incentives, encouraging entrepreneurial activity and a long-run orientation, developing a market/service orientation, customizing service packages, building upon strengths, and managing key stakeholders.

## REFERENCES

1. Lawrence, D. "Learning from HMOs." *Health Management Quarterly* 7, no. 3 (1990): 12–15.
2. Atkinson, B. "Competition Turns the Promising Alliances of Physicians, HMOs into Courtroom Battles." *Modern Healthcare* 17, no. 13 (1987): 68.
3. Droste, T. "HMOs: Employers Shed Casual Attitudes, Contracts." *Hospitals* 62, no. 12 (1988): 60–61.
4. Hirschorn, M.W. "Some Doctors Assail Quality of Treatment Provided by HMOs." *Wall Street Journal* 208, no. 54 (September 16, 1986): 1.
5. McCormick, B. "Labor Union Plays Hardball with HMO." *Hospitals* 61, no. 14 (1987): 40.
6. Norman, J.R. "Can Insurers Nurse Their HMOs Back to Health?" *Business Week* (January 16, 1989): 80–81.
7. Powills, S. "HMOs: Quality Comes Under GM's Watchful Eye." *Hospitals* 60, no. 14 (1986): 40.
8. Thomas, M.C. "St. Louis Doctors Declare War on Prepaid Care." *Medical Economics* 63, no. 24 (1986): 46–50.
9. Thomas, M.C. "Trouble in the Heartland of HMOs." *Medical Economics* 64, no. 5 (1987): 48–51.
10. Traska, M.R. "HMOs: A Shakeup (and Shakeout) on the Horizon." *Hospitals* 60, no. 3 (1986): 40–45.
11. Traska, M.R. "Upset Minnesota HMO MDs Consider Unionizing." *Hospitals* 61, no. 9 (1987): 52.
12. Gruber, L.R., Shadle, M., and Polich, C.L. "From Movement to Industry: The Growth of HMOs." *Health Affairs* 7, no. 3 (1988): 197–208.
13. Gabel, J., et al. "The Commercial Health Insurance Industry in Transition." *Health Affairs* 6, no. 3 (1987): 46–60.
14. Fox, P.D., and Heinan, L. *Determinants of HMO Success.* Ann Arbor, Mich.: Health Administration Press Perspectives, 1987.

15.  Hansen, J.B., and Blalock, B. "The Health Services Foundation: UAB's Private Heart of Gold." *The Birmingham News* (November 20), 1988: 1A, 18A.

16.  Complete Health Information Summary, November 1990: 1.

17.  American Medical Care and Review Association. *Directory of Health Maintenance Organizations.* Bethesda, Md.: American Medical Care and Review Association, 1988.

18.  Dunn, K., and Shields, G. "For-Profit Status Creates New Financing Opportunities." *Healthcare Financial Management* 14, no. 12 (1984): 36–46.

19.  Ermann, D. "Health Maintenance Organizations: The Future of the For-Profit Plan." *Journal of Ambulatory Care Management* 9, no. 2 (1986): 72–84.

20.  Durrett, M.A. "Complete Health's Rebust Growth." *Business Alabama Monthly* 4, no. 3 (1990): 23.

21.  Rupinski, P. "Founder Watches HMO Grow: Complete Health Rides Demand for Low Costs." *Birmingham Post-Herald* (January 25, 1991): B-7.

22.  Porter, M.E. *Competitive Advantage: Creating and Sustaining Superior Performance.* New York, N.Y.: Free Press, 1985.

23.  Long, S.H., Settle, R.F., and Wrightson, C.W. "Employee Premiums, Availability of Alternative Plans, and HMO Disenrollment." *Medical Care* 26, no. 10 (1988): 927–38.

24.  McDonald, W.H. "Is Complete Health on a Roll?" *The Alabama MD* 25, no. 32 (1989): 1–4.

25.  Topping, S., and Fottler, M.D. "Improved Stakeholder Management: The Key to Revitalization of the HMO Movement." *Medical Care Review* 47, no. 3 (1990): 365–93.

26.  Fottler, M.D. "Health Care Organizational Performance: Present and Future Research." *1987 Yearly Review of Management of the Journal of Management* 13, no. 2 (1987): 179–203.

27.  Blair, J.D., and Fottler, M.D. *Challenges in Health Care Management: Strategic Perspectives for Managing Key Stakeholders.* San Francisco, Calif.: Jossey-Bass, 1990.

28.  Pawlson, L.G., and Kaufman, R.P. "HMOs and the Academic Medical Center: A Reassessment." *Health Care Management Review* 7, no. 3 (1982): 77–80.

29.  Inglehart, J.K. "Moment of Truth for the Teaching Hospital." *New England Journal of Medicine* 307, no. 3 (1982): 132–36.

30.  Fink, D.S. "Developing Marketing Strategies for University Teaching Hospitals." *Journal of Medical Education* 55, no. 4 (1980): 574–79.

31.  Fottler, M.D., and Smith, H.L. "The Organizational Life Cycle and Strategic Human Resources Management." In *Strategic Management of Human Resources in Health Services Organizations*, edited by M.D. Fottler, S.R. Hernandez, and C.L. Joiner. New York, N.Y.: Wiley, 1988.

# An assessment of employers' experiences with HMOs: Factors that make a difference

Arthur L. Dolinsky
and
Richard K. Caputo

*This study investigated those factors that influenced employers' experiences with health maintenance organizations (HMOs). It examined a national cross-sectional sample of chief executive officers (CEOs) and benefits managers. Findings revealed that different administrative issues such as the volume of paperwork, confusion about benefits, and educating employees about HMO benefits were of primary importance in affecting management's experiences with HMOs. Differences were found between CEOs' and benefits managers' responses.*

Increasingly, employers have become managerial intermediaries between their employees and health maintenance organizations (HMOs). Benefits managers introduce and explain HMO benefits to their employees, and organizational staff perform many administrative tasks including the processing of HMO forms and billing. In order to ensure a successful relationship between HMOs and companies, a strong managerial partnership between both is necessary.[1]

Though HMOs have existed for over half a century, only recently have they gained acceptance as an alternative health care system. In 1970, roughly three million people were enrolled in HMOs. By 1988, 31 million were enrolled, a tenfold increase, with a continued increase expected into the 1990s.[2] Such growth contributes to increased employer managerial responsibilities, such as more HMOs from which to choose, more options within and between plans to scrutinize, and multiple reimbursement procedures to follow.

Despite this growth and the crucial roles employers play in ensuring the success of HMOs, little is known about management's experiences in dealing with HMOs. In particular little is known about those factors that contribute to a strong managerial partnership between HMOs and employers.

The purpose of the present study was to examine the extent to which different problems need to be addressed to ensure a beneficial working relationship between the HMOs and employers. The study employed data from a national cross-sectional sample of senior executives and corporate benefits managers, drawn from the 1984 Kaiser Foundation national health care survey.[3] It assessed those factors which contributed to a positive managerial experience with HMOs.

## REVIEW OF THE LITERATURE

Different factors have been highlighted conceptually as affecting the extent to which employers have favorable experiences with HMOs. In spite of their assumed importance, management's experiences with HMOs have received little empirical attention.

Atlas and Corcoran highlighted employers' concerns about administrative burdens, in part resulting from recent government legislation. In addition, they pointed

---

**Arthur L. Dolinsky,** *Ph.D., is an Associate Professor, College of Business, Fairleigh Dickinson University.*

**Richard K. Caputo, Ph.D.,** *is Assistant Professor, School of Social Work, University of Pennsylvania.*

*Health Care Management Rev,* 1991, 16(1), 25–31

to HMO costs, quality of care, and fiscal stability.[4] Others also cited similar problems employers may encounter with HMOs.[5]

A primary motive for employers choosing HMOs has been the prospect of reduced health care costs. In the United States, health care costs have increased faster than the rate of inflation—at an unprecedented rate since the 1970s. For example, the mean health care expense per capita was $238 in 1970 and rose to $499 in 1977.[6] Not surprisingly, such increased costs have been incurred by employers providing health care coverage for their employees. In 1981, for example, medical costs at Honeywell Inc. approached 40 percent of its profits. And Honeywell had company. Medical services were the second largest cost (after salaries) of doing business for service companies, and they were the third largest cost (after materials and salaries) of doing business for manufacturers.

In general, employers seek to balance costs with quality goods and services they receive. The same holds for health care services. A primary objective of using HMO services is cost containment; however, employers are also concerned about quality of care. Although employers lack precise measures of the quality of care that HMOs provide, they nonetheless monitor disenrollment patterns and conduct employee satisfaction surveys of HMO use.[7] Indeed, employers' concern about the quality of care is likely to expand in the future in light of the increased competitiveness of the health care market and, hence, concrete measures become that much more necessary.[8]

Employers' concerns regarding the fiscal stability of HMOs have changed in recent times. Previously, when HMOs were a relatively new entrant into the health care system, employers' concerns stemmed from the uncertainty of the public's acceptance of HMOs as a viable alternative to the fee-for-service system. Currently, however, the concerns stem from the competitive structure of the HMO industry. In June 1981 there were 243 HMOs. At the end of 1984 there were 337 HMOs. Now there are over 600.

In 1988 mergers, acquisitions, and closings accounted for a decline in 34 HMOs.[9]

A plethora of government legislation has potentially contributed to employers' reluctance to encourage employee membership and has stymied employer–HMO relationships. Delays in early federal regulations concerning the dual choice provision of HMO legislation, for example, resulted in the demise of Sound Health Association (SHA), the first federally qualified HMO.[10] Subsequent to the initial 1973 HMO Act, a

*Both legislative changes and the intermediary managerial role that employers play may contribute to potential employer administrative burdens. Multiple plans, for example, are a major source of administrative difficulty.*

number of amendments have made employers somewhat more receptive to HMOs, but they nonetheless claim that the industry has outgrown federal oversight in light of new marketplace demands.[5,11]

Both legislative changes and the intermediary managerial role that employers play may contribute to potential employer administrative burdens. Multiple plans, for example, are a major source of administrative difficulty. They require additional organizational resources to understand and communicate differences to prospective employee members.[11] Furthermore, employers that contract with several HMOs face multiple reimbursement procedures and different forms. Other sources of administrative difficulty include paperwork and time required for processing HMO forms and billings, monitoring employee satisfaction with contracted HMOs, and negotiating appropriate strategies to determine premiums.[12]

In addition to the above concerns, other factors may impede the relationship between employers and HMOs. These include concern about health care provisions for transferred and traveling employees, the potential for adverse selection, and union resistance to HMOs. This study examines the extent to which different factors and concerns contribute to the favorable relationship between HMOs and employers. Furthermore, it explores differences between the perceptions of benefits managers and CEOs.

## DATA AND METHODS

This study uses data drawn from the 1984 Kaiser Foundation national health care survey.[3] Those data were comprised of four nationally representative samples: HMO members, a cross section of the United States public, corporate employers, and physicians. This particular study examines only the corporate employers.

The corporate sample contained 403 respondents, which included 200 benefits managers and 203 senior executives.In light of the study's objective of determining those factors contributing to a favorable experience with HMOs, we excluded 103 respondents employed in firms that did not offer employees an HMO option. Missing values on certain variables further reduced the sample size to 214. Of these, 123 were benefits managers and 91 were CEOs.

Members of the sample were questioned about their organization's overall experience in working with HMOs. In addition they were asked whether the firm as a whole considered a number of different issues as potential problems when offering and managing HMO benefits. Included were concerns such as the confusion and administrative difficulties caused by differences in benefits offered by HMOs, financial stability of HMOs, government involvement with HMOs, and a lack of financial incentives to employers. See the box entitled "Factors Influencing Employers' Experiences with HMOs" for an enumeration of the complete set of potential problems.

Management's experience with HMOs was measured by respondents' indicating whether their organization's overall experience with HMOs had been very favorable, somewhat favorable, somewhat unfavorable, or

very unfavorable. Roughly 90 percent of the sample indicated that their organization's experience was either very favorable or somewhat favorable. This finding parallels the skewed level of satisfaction with HMOs reported by current HMO members. On the whole, those who continue with HMOs tend to be satisfied. Due to this skewed distribution, we dichotomized management's experience as either very favorable or less favorable. With respect to the different potential problems, respondents were asked whether the company considers each to be a serious problem, a problem but not serious, or not a problem. We dichotomized these responses as either a problem or not. We used bivariate analyses, whereby two-by-two contingency tables were constructed, to assess the relationship between management's overall experience with HMOs and each of the different potential problems.

## RESULTS

On the whole, roughly 75 percent of the sample reported having had a less-than-very-favorable experience with their respective HMOs. As Table 1 indicates, 73 percent of benefits managers and 79 percent of CEOs indicated a less-than-very-favorable experience.

With respect to the potential problems organizations face when offering and managing HMO benefits, most frequently reported was financial stability of HMOs. In contrast, the least reported problem was union resistance to HMOs. All others fell between these. CEOs most frequently reported both confusion and administrative difficulties caused by differences in benefits offered by different HMOs and concern about health care provisions for transferred and traveling employees. Least frequently, they reported union resistance to HMOs. Benefits managers most frequently reported financial stability; least frequently, union resistance to HMOs.

Table 2 summarizes the extent to which each of the different potential problem areas affect an organization's experience with HMOs.

### Factors affecting the relationship between employees and HMOs

Results for the overall sample indicate that the most important determinant of how favorable an experience organizations have with HMOs is whether or not they face HMO administrative difficulties. In particular, two such difficulties, confusion regarding different benefits among HMOs and the time and paperwork required for

---

**Factors Influencing Employers' Experiences with HMOs**

- Administration:
  Paperwork and time required for processing HMO forms and billings
  Confusion and administrative difficulties caused by differences in benefits offered by different HMOs
  Time and effort required to educate employees
- Financial stability: Concern about the financial stability of HMOs
- Quality of care: Concern about the quality of health care offered by HMOs
- Cost containment: A lack of financial incentives to employers
- Government involvement with HMOs
- Other:
  Lack of experience with HMOs
  The cost to employees
  Employee resistance to HMOs
  Concern about health care provisions for transferred and traveling employees
  Union resistance to HMOs
  Potential for adverse selection, if large numbers of employees were to join HMOs

## TABLE 1

PERCENTAGES OF RESPONDENTS INDICATING A LESS THAN VERY FAVORABLE OVERALL EXPERIENCE WITH HMOs AND THOSE EXPERIENCING DIFFICULTIES WITH DIFFERENT PROBLEM AREAS

|  | Total sample N = 214 | Benefit managers N = 123 | CEOs N = 91 |
|---|---|---|---|
| Overall experience with HMOs | 75 | 73 | 79 |
| Potential problem areas: |  |  |  |
| A. Administration: |  |  |  |
| Paperwork | 32 | 33 | 32 |
| Confusion | 55 | 53 | 59 |
| Time and effort | 53 | 54 | 53 |
| B. Financial stability | 61 | 66 | 56 |
| C. Quality of care | 54 | 52 | 57 |
| D. Cost containment | 42 | 44 | 40 |
| E. Government involvement | 35 | 35 | 36 |
| F. Other: |  |  |  |
| Lack of experience | 45 | 41 | 53 |
| Cost to employees | 44 | 48 | 40 |
| Employee resistance | 43 | 41 | 47 |
| Concern for transferred | 60 | 62 | 59 |
| Union resistance | 28 | 28 | 28 |
| Adverse selection | 52 | 56 | 48 |

processing HMO forms and billings, were significant ($x^2 = 8.81$ and $x^2 = 4.17$, respectively). Sixty-one percent of those respondents who reported a less-than-very-favorable experience with HMOs indicated that the variety of benefits was a problem in contrast to 38 percent of those who reported having a very favorable experience with HMOs. With respect to time and paperwork required to process HMO forms, the respective percentages were 36 and 21.

A related administrative problem area, time and effort to educate employees, was also found to be significant in determining an organization's experiences with HMOs ($x^2 = 4.58$). Nearly 60 percent of those reporting a less-than-very-favorable experience with HMOs indicated that time and effort to educate employees was a problem, in contrast to only 40 percent of those who reported having a very favorable experience with HMOs.

A second factor that may impede the relationship between employers and HMOs concerns cost containment. Results indicated that a perceived lack of financial incentives to employers also was found to be sig-

nificant in determining an organization's experiences with HMOs ($x^2 = 2.72$). Forty-six percent of those reporting a less-than-very-favorable experience with HMOs indicated that cost containment was a problem, in contrast to 33 percent of those who reported having a very favorable experience with HMOs.

### Differences between viewpoints of benefit managers and CEOs

In the overall sample, there were no significant results regarding quality, fiscal stability, and government involvement. When we consider benefits managers and CEOs separately, however, differences regarding these problem areas emerge.

For benefits managers both quality and government involvement were significantly related to an organization's experience with HMOs ($x^2 = 2.89$ and $x^2 = 3.75$, respectively), while fiscal stability approached significance ($x^2 = 2.56$). Fifty-seven percent of those reporting a less-than-very-favorable experience with

## TABLE 2

THE RELATIONSHIP BETWEEN PERCEIVED PROBLEM AREAS AND ORGANIZATIONS' EXPERIENCES WITH HMOs: OVERALL SAMPLE, BENEFITS MANAGERS, AND CEOs

|  | Overall | Benefits managers (Chi-square values) | CEOs |
|---|---|---|---|
| A. Administration: |  |  |  |
| Paperwork | 4.17† | 2.72* | 1.54 |
| Confusion | 8.81‡ | 6.89‡ | 1.42 |
| Time and effort | 4.58† | 3.69* | 1.09 |
| B. Financial stability | 1.02 | 2.56 | .033 |
| C. Quality of care | .144 | 2.89* | 2.58 |
| D. Cost containment | 2.72* | 3.39* | .145 |
| E. Government involvement | 2.21 | 3.75* | .003 |
| F. Other: |  |  |  |
| Lack of experience | .336 | .344 | .001 |
| Cost to employees | 2.64 | 2.43 | .640 |
| Employee resistance | .139 | .017 | .279 |
| Concern for transferred | .018 | .065 | .021 |
| Union resistance | .042 | .003 | .060 |
| Adverse selection | 2.03 | 1.06 | 1.27 |

*Significant at or below .10.
†Significant at or below .05.
‡Significant at or below .01.

Results for the overall sample indicate that the
*most important determinant of how favorable*
*an experience organizations have with HMOs*
*is whether or not they face HMO*
*administrative difficulties.*

HMOs indicated that quality was a problem, in contrast
to 39 percent of those who reported having a very
favorable experience with HMOs. With respect to government involvement, 40 percent of those reporting a
less-than-very-favorable experience with HMOs
claimed it was a problem, compared to 21 percent of
those who reported having a very favorable experience
with HMOs. Regarding financial stability, the relative
proportions were roughly on the magnitude of four to
three. It also should be noted that those problem areas
(administrative and related problems and costs) which
emerged as significant determinants of an organization's
experiences with HMOs for the overall sample also
were found to be present when only considering benefits managers.

Lastly, results obtained when considering the CEO
subsample need to be addressed. Overall, none of the
problem areas were found to be significant determinants as to whether or not the CEO's organizations had
favorable experiences with HMOs. The only problem
area that approached significance was quality of care.
Paradoxically, the result was in the opposite direction.
Seventy-three percent of those CEOs who claimed that
organizational experience with HMOs was very favorable indicated that quality of care was a problem, compared to 52 percent who reported a less-than-very-
favorable experience with HMOs.

## DISCUSSION

This study highlighted the importance of a number of
different perceived problem areas that determine an
organization's experience with HMOs. Problem areas
highlighted in the literature included administrative-
related issues, quality of care, financial stability, costs,
and government involvement. In addition, other problem areas included union resistance to HMOs and

concern about health care provisions for transferred
and traveling employees.

### Administrative issues

The overall results indicated that the different administrative issues and costs were significant in determining whether or not organizations had very favorable
experiences when dealing with HMOs. Of these, administrative issues were the most significant. When
only benefits managers were considered, however,
quality of care and government involvement were additionally found to be significant and financial stability
of HMOs approached significance. Thus, when the
sample is limited to the benefits managers, those issues
highlighted in the literature as determining an
organization's experience with HMOs were empirically supported. With respect to other problem areas,
they were found to be of limited importance in determining whether or not an organization had a favorable
experience with HMOs. Regarding CEOs, none of the
problem areas were found to significantly determine
the nature of an organization's experience with HMOs.

The results suggest several managerial strategies that
can improve employers' experiences when working
with HMOs. The most pressing issues are of an administrative nature. To overcome these difficulties, HMOs
must find ways to reduce the paperwork and time
required for processing forms and billings, to reduce
the time and effort required to educate employees, and
to minimize confusion associated with a variety of
benefits they offer.

To minimize paperwork, HMOs may want to standardize and streamline their forms wherever possible.
Such a strategy of standardization across HMOs would
not only benefit employers, but would give HMOs a
competitive edge on traditional fee-for-service health
care providers. HMOs can also relieve employers of the
responsibility of paperwork by doing it themselves. For
large organizations with many HMO enrollees, it also
might be feasible to place an HMO employee there to
assist in such administrative tasks.

To reduce confusion and administrative difficulties
about benefits, employers can offer only one HMO with
limited options. Employers may reduce the number of
plans they offer, but they would do so at the cost of
restricting employee choice. This option, however, is
not desirable, since employees tend to prefer choice
among benefits. More realistically, HMOs need to balance variety and manageability of different options. To
identify an optimal balance, HMOs may want to survey

potential enrollees regarding the desirability of different combinations of options and at the same time determine the extent to which these increased combinations entail additional administrative problems. In addition, dissemination of information about benefits should be done as clearly and concisely as possible, keeping in mind the role of the benefits manager and the employees' particular concerns.

To reduce the time and effort employers spend on educating their employees about different options within and between HMO plans, HMOs may want to encourage employers to host workshops and information-sharing sessions between HMO representatives and client employees. Furthermore, this strategy and others cited above will not only create better working relationships between the HMOs and their clients, but will promote a sense of trust which is crucial when providing health care services and maintaining clients.

### Fiscal stability, cost, and quality of care

Moving away from direct administrative problem areas, fiscal stability, cost, and quality of care also influenced employer experiences with HMOs. It is imperative that HMOs demonstrate competency and efficiency in each of these three areas. For example, HMOs should routinely provide employers with recently audited financial reports, such as those going to state insurance departments or other state regulatory bodies.[13] They should develop indicators other than length of hospital stay in demonstrating their ability to reduce health care costs. Likewise, as employers become increasingly concerned about quality of care, HMOs should implement review processes that will at least consider the structure of quality-assurance activities, outcomes of care, and patient perceptions of quality.[8] Once these issues are satisfactorily addressed, HMOs can then better attract employers and more realistically establish a sound partnership in promoting and providing services to employers and their employees.

### Government involvement

A final problem area affecting an organization's experience with HMOs revolves around government involvement. Individual HMOs have limited control in this area. It is imperative that HMOs demonstrate that they can successfully regulate themselves in the areas of quality, such as services, costs, and fiscal stability. Toward this effort, HMOs might consider establishing a standards-producing structure, perhaps modeled after the American Medical Association. They might also consider adopting models of review that already exist for hospitals, conducted by the Joint Commission for the Accreditation of Health Care Organizations, or for ambulatory care, conducted by the Accreditation Association for Ambulatory Health Care. These and other private sector review alternatives if developed and adopted should mitigate government involvement and thereby facilitate better working relations between employers and HMOs.

### CEO perceptions

Finally, CEOs did not identify any potential problem areas which distinguished whether their organization experienced a very favorable or other type of relationship with HMOs. This finding raises questions in light of the exhaustive list of problem areas and in light of benefits managers' responses. Additionally, those CEOs who reported very favorable experiences with HMOs also stated that quality of care was a problem, while those who reported less-than-very-favorable experiences said that quality of care was not a problem. Such findings suggest that CEOs may be too far removed from the on-going daily dynamics between HMOs and their organizations. In light of the increased portion of profits that health care costs consume, it is imperative that CEOs become more conscientiously and actively involved in health care and HMO matters.

•　　•　　•

This study investigated those factors that influenced employers' experiences with HMOs. It examined a national cross-sectional sample of CEOs and benefits managers. Findings revealed that different administrative issues such as the volume of paperwork, confusion about benefits, and educating employees about HMO benefits were of primary importance in affecting management's experiences with HMOs. Other factors found to be important included cost, quality of care, financial stability, and government involvement. Differences were found between CEOs and benefits managers. For benefits managers, all factors cited above were found to be important in determining their organization's experience with HMOs. In contrast, for CEOs, no factors were found to be significantly related to their organization's experience with HMOs.

Overall, the findings suggest that individual HMOs should focus on these factors to strengthen their relationships with employers. With regard to government involvement, HMOs should focus on industry-wide, self-regulating mechanisms. Future research should focus on the relative roles CEOs and benefits managers play in an organization's interactions with HMOs. To what extent are CEOs far removed from the everyday dynamics between their organizations and HMOs? Furthermore, what organizational alternatives can be developed to enhance the relationship between employers and HMOs?

## REFERENCES

1. Spencer, E.D. "Buying Health Care in the New Era of Medicine: A Business Perspective." *Compensation & Benefits Management* (Winter 1988): 107–12.
2. Stein, R.S., Linn, M.W., Edelstein, J., and Stein, E.M. "Elderly Patients' Satisfaction with Care under HMO Versus Private Systems." *Southern Medical Journal* 82 (January 1989): 3–8.
3. Harris, L. and Associates. *Health Maintenance Organizations in the United States, 1984.* Menlo Park, Calif.: Kaiser Family Foundation, 1984.
4. Atlas, R.F., and Corcoran, M.E. "HMO Evaluation and Action Strategies for Employers." *Journal of Compensation and Benefits* (March–April 1989): 253–57.
5. Peres, A. "Is the HMO Act Good for Employers?" *Business and Health* (February 1988): 8–13.
6. U.S. Department of Health and Human Services. National Health Care Expenditures Study, "A Summary of Expenditures and Sources of Payment for Personal Health Services" from the National Medical Care Expenditure Survey. Washington, D.C.: U.S. Government Printing Office, 1987.
7. Feldman, S., Fritz, D., and Stanfield, C. "Using Employee Satisfaction to Choose HMOs." *Business and Health* (February 1988): 17–20.
8. Luft, H.S. "HMOs and the Quality of Care." *Inquiry* 25 (Spring 1988): 147–56.
9. Traska, M.R. "What Every Employer Needs to Know about HMOs." *Business & Health* (June 1989): 18–29.
10. MacStravic, R.E.S. "The Demise of an HMO: A Marketing Perspective." *Journal of Health Care Marketing* 4 (Fall 1982): 9–16.
11. Fox, P.D. "The Future of HMOs." *Compensation & Benefits Management* (Winter 1989): 101–06.
12. Cave, D.G. "HMO Community Rating by Class: Employers and HMOs Need to Collect Health Status Information." *Employee Benefits Journal* (March 1989): 17–25.
13. Goldman, R.L., Shoen, C.B., and Koop, W.C. "Financial Evaluation of HMOs and PPOs." *Health Marketing Quarterly* 5, no. 3/4 (1988): 89–100.

# Management information systems: Their role in the marketing activities of HMOs

David B. Aronow

*HMOs are particularly dependent on their information resources in providing cost-effective, high quality, accessible care. Understanding the role of MIS in HMO marketing activities may guide administrators in evaluating information systems applications within their organizations.*

*Health Care Manage Rev*, 1988, 13(4), 59–64
© 1988 Aspen Publishers, Inc.

**Successful management** of health maintenance organizations (HMOs) requires continual, careful balancing of the provision and utilization of limited health care resources in order to offer cost-effective, high quality, accessible care to enrolled members. Only through the understanding and use of accurate, comprehensive, and timely financial, clinical, and operational information has this been possible.[1,2]

In the current competitive and cost-containing environment, the HMO, with its relatively fixed-revenue stream and inherently risk-filled expense budget, is additionally dependent on its information resources for strategic decision making to maintain, if not expand, its market share.[3-6]

This article reviews the role played by management information systems (MIS) in the current marketing activities adopted by HMOs. After a brief discussion of MIS in HMOs in general, five areas of MIS application to HMO marketing are described. The article closes with analysis of MIS characteristics of particular value to HMO marketing and a look at health care information systems of the future. It is hoped that this concise and timely review of the role of MIS in marketing activities will help HMO administrators evaluate the breadth of information systems applications within their organizations.

The term marketing is used in this article in accordance with Kotler's definition of marketing for health service organizations: "the analysis, planning, implementation and control of carefully formulated programs designed to bring about voluntary exchange of values with target markets for the purpose of achieving organizational objectives."[7] As such, the target markets for HMOs include practitioners to provide health care, employers to offer HMO membership, individuals and families to choose membership, hospitals and other providers to contract for services, and public and private sources of capital. However, marketing efforts toward health care practitioners and providers will not be discussed in this article.

**David B. Aronow**, *M.D., M.P.H., is a fellow in Medical Informatics at Massachusetts General Hospital and the Harvard School of Public Health. He has redirected his career to health administration from the practice of emergency medicine.*

## MIS IN HMOs

MIS may be defined as "an organized set of processes that provides information to managers to support the operations and decision-making within an organization."[8] Although HMOs have been in operation for 60 years, not until the 1950s were attempts made to develop computerized MIS to analyze utilization of services.[9] In the 1970s, interest grew both in clinical record keeping and financial applications.[10,11] By the early 1980s, experiential standards and guidelines from the Office of Health Maintenance Organizations (OHMO) provided bases for discussion of HMO MIS as sets of three, four, or five interdependent modules oriented toward the several broad areas of HMO planning, operations, and control activities.[12-16]

Five HMO industry surveys have been conducted to assess MIS use, problems, costs, and priorities.[17] The results of only two have been published.[18-20] Compared with hospital MIS, the HMO MIS industry was found to be less mature, with a broader variety of vendors and greater use of in-house computing support. HMOs were found to have fewer financial functions and more clinical functions automated as compared to hospitals.

## HMO MIS APPLICATIONS TO MARKETING

Every cataloging of HMO information system functions includes entries that support marketing functions. However, only recently has marketing explicitly been discussed in the HMO literature as an important MIS function.[21-24] In the 1983 Revision of Volume I of the OHMO MIS handbook, the term "marketing" is inconspicuously mentioned, without elaboration, as one of a long list of MIS roles.[25] Even the "comprehensive" 1984 Arthur D. Little, Inc., survey of HMO MIS does not include marketing activities explicitly in the reported MIS functions.[26,27]

HMO marketing activities may be grouped into five areas: (1) market analysis, (2) benefit package development, (3) sales of the package, (4) strategic marketing and planning, and (5) performance monitoring. These areas are, of course, closely interrelated, and are completely dependent upon the other financial, operational, and clinical functions of the HMO.

### Market analysis

The marketing department of an HMO has the responsibility of identifying and recruiting both employers and employees in congruence with the HMO's goals and objectives. To do this, the department needs to research the demographic, health status, and utilization records of each potential target group as well as the health benefit programs of each significant employer. Using data for similar groups from its own experience, industry reports, and secondary data sources such as census information and the Department of Labor, the department can use its MIS to describe the group, project utilization, and estimate of the financial consequences of pursuing the group.[28-30] This review will guide the HMO in deciding which markets to enter, and is of particular importance in evaluating markets such as entitlement program enrollees or government employees.[31]

With similar analysis of current and prospective individual and family members, MIS can help assess the particular needs and interests of the membership, as well as assist in developing enrollment targets.[32,33]

### Benefit package development

As it conducts its market analysis and needs assessment, the marketing department can recommend to management specific benefits to emphasize, benefits to bundle together, or service modifications to consider. These might include promotion of periodic physician examinations,[34] opening of an urgent care center to control emergency department utilization,[35] and developing video/data hookups to more isolated centers to permit nonphysician practitioners to obtain consultations.[36] Be the concern product, promotion, place, or price, MIS has a role in every phase of the marketer's design of the benefit package.

The most important recently identified MIS-dependent benefit to market may be the quality of care (QoC) an HMO provides. There is a rich literature concerned with the relation of QoC to MIS, but as yet little has been published linking MIS and QoC to marketing. In 1985, Patients' Choice, Inc., (PCI) reported its new MIS-based quality assurance (QA) program. PCI did not discuss how it was marketing the program, but was direct about its motivation: "With the medical community entering the competitive business marketplace, it is essential that sound business and financial principles be merged into the medical delivery system."[37] In 1986, Harvard Community Health Plan, Inc., was more explicit, promoting its QoC program in its member newsletter.[38] However, as Michenzi and Miller note in their discussion of HMO response to competition, "Reminding members that the HMO services are first rate is not sufficient; the price members are willing to pay for such services must also be considered."[39]

## Sales of the package

Promotion, publicity, advertising, and consumer education are all necessary to sell the HMO benefit package to prospective enrollees. Each of these activities is an intensive user of personnel, time, and money resources, and all can be made more efficient with the record-keeping, word-processing, and scheduling assistance MIS can provide. MIS can also help demonstrate an HMO's advantages to employer–clients. Simulations based on similarly composed employee groups can be run to show health care cost savings,[40] and efficiency studies of the HMO itself can be reviewed with employers.[41]

Shalowitz and Shalowitz present an additional benefit to promote sales—the potential for monitoring occupationally related diseases. With attention to confidentiality issues, a worker's clinical experience can be reviewed by industry or process to identify unusual problems, aid in the isolation of causes, and monitor treatment and corrective occupational activities.[42]

## Strategic marketing and planning

Strategic marketing activities based on MIS include simulation and forecasting, decision support, and the provision of information to the financial community. The latter activity is the selling of the organization in order to raise capital,[43] while the others are aspects of developing and implementing a strategic plan.

Simulating service patterns and forecasting enrollment and utilization, and using the information developed for and by other marketing activities, are the bases for rate setting, revenue budgeting, expense budgeting, risk assignment, and staffing. These functions use the MIS spreadsheet capabilities to answer questions of "what happens if."[44–48]

---

*Simulating service patterns and forecasting enrollment and utilization, and using the information developed for and by other marketing activities, are the bases for rate setting, revenue budgeting, expense budgeting, risk assignment, and staffing.*

---

MIS's capability as a decision support system is also essential.[49,50] Plotnick, for example, discusses two dimensions of information needs in HMOs: definition of the critical areas of operation to be controlled, and the standards by which these areas are measured. The critical areas correspond to the organization's objectives, and are labeled critical because optimal performance is essential for the survival of the HMO. The areas are defined, standards (or targets) for performance are set, and measurement techniques are established based on the MIS's decision support functions during the strategic planning process.[51]

## Performance monitoring

It is in performance monitoring that MIS have their greatest regular impact for HMOs. Once performance criteria have been defined, there must be ongoing monitoring and reporting of penetration and utilization indicators, as well as maintenance of enrollment, encouragement of growth, and analysis of disenrollment.

Several authors discuss the need for, and the suggested make-up of, regular reports detailing utilization and cost patterns by enrolled group.[52,53] This information, coupled with group penetration data and disenrollment analysis, can guide decisions concerning investment of further marketing resources in specific groups, as well as the profitability of specific member groups.[54,55]

Mueller and Comer, in their analysis of MIS objectives and presentation of recommendations for small HMOs, also suggest maintaining a database catalog of all groups in the market area with employee demographics, description of the nature of the work, and specifics of the health insurance programs offered.[56] Performance of employers themselves can also be monitored for timeliness of premium payment.[57]

Finally, performance information provides the feedback necessary to evaluate forecasts, allow budgeting, and validate the strategic planning process discussed above.[58,59] Summarizing how an HMO marketing department can measure success, Michenzi and Miller state that the "measure of success is anchored in the department's ability to use available information to determine whether projections of member usage were indeed within an acceptable range. The key is to determine whether use of services was estimated correctly and whether the services were used appropriately by the medical profession."[60] Both service use projection and measurement, and the comparison of the two, are MIS dependent.

## MIS CHARACTERISTICS IMPORTANT TO MARKETING

Two characteristics of MIS are particularly important to HMO marketing activities: integration and flexibility. Integration of functions is necessary to provide the multifaceted information discussed above. Flexibility is necessary to allow the marketer to address the needs of his or her variety of targets, including management.

In 1984, Hews noted that "Many HMOs have fairly sophisticated information systems, yet lack integrated information from several sources of systems. Such integration (combinations of financial, clinical, and operational information) could facilitate many decisions managers are called upon to make."[61] Other authors have addressed the same issue[62,63] and vendors are attempting to address the issue.[64] However, the extent of the problem is unclear—function integration was not studied in the 1984 HMO MIS survey.[65]

Information systems flexibility is also discussed in the literature.[66-68] Two areas of concern are identified: system flexibility to interact with other automated and manual information systems, and user friendliness/plasticity. An interesting report of the difficult evolution of an integrated and flexible MIS, the Harvard Community Health Plan, is provided by Miller.[69]

• • •

MIS are essential to the marketing activities of HMOs. In market analysis, benefit package development, promotion, performance monitoring, forecasting, and strategic market planning, the MIS can provide the HMO with the competitive edge it needs in today's health care marketplace. HMOs will see more computing, more reliance on MIS, more clinician use of MIS, and more integrated, flexible MIS.

Amid some controversy, experts suggest that as HMOs, hospitals, and other health care delivery sites become more integrated and interdependent, their information systems will interconnect and eventually merge, simultaneous with the consolidation of vendor industries.[70-73] This trend is summarized by Grams et al: Health care information systems "will provide sophisticated financial, management, and medical/clinical information and decision support systems for the health care delivery systems. This will require inte-

grated and shared data bases, standard communications networks, input/output devices that are appropriate in their design and location for the user, and cost effective computing power."[74]

## REFERENCES

1. Rock, A.S. "An Information System for HMOs: Designed From the Ground Up." *Computers in Healthcare* 4, no. 10 (1983): 46–49.
2. Hews, M.L. "Establishing a Strategy for Information Resources in an HMO." In *1984 Group Health Institute Proceedings.* Washington, D.C.: Group Health Association of America, 1984, pp. 332–41.
3. Ibid.
4. Lefort, P.F. "Healthcare Information Systems: Creating the Competitive Edge." *Healthcare Financial Management* 39, no. 6 (1985): 33–34, 36, 38, 40.
5. Shalowitz, J., and Shalowitz, M. "Use of a Data Base System for HMO Management." In *MEDCOMP '82 Proceedings.* Los Angeles: IEEE Computer Society, 1982, pp. 154–57
6. Steinwachs, D.M. "Ambulatory Care Management Information Systems: Future Directions." *Journal of Ambulatory Care Management* 8, no. 2 (1985): 84–94.
7. Rubright, R., and MacDonald, D. *Marketing Health and Human Services.* Rockville, Md.: Aspen Publishers, 1981, pp. 2–3.
8. Kroeber, D.W., and Watson, H.J. *Computer-Based Information Systems: A Management Approach, Second Edition.* New York: MacMillan, 1987, p. 7.
9. Steinwachs, "Ambulatory Care Management Information Systems: Future Directions."
10. Kuhn, I.M., et al. "Automated Ambulatory Medical Record Systems in the U.S." In *Information Systems for Patient Care*, edited by B.I. Blum. New York: Springer-Verlag, 1984.
11. Miller, J.A. "Managing Systems in an HMO—the Harvard Plan Experience." In *Group and IPA HMOs.* Rockville, Md.: Aspen Publishers, 1981, pp. 215–26.
12. Birch and Davis Associates, Inc. *The Design, Selection, and Implementation of a Management Information System for Health Maintenance Organizations Volume 1.* Washington, D.C.: U.S. Department of Health and Human Services, 1980.
13. Miller, "Managing Systems in an HMO—the Harvard Plan Experience."
14. Plotnick, D. "Computer Applications for Management Planning and Control: Industry Standards in a Health Maintenance Organization." *Journal of Ambulatory Care Management* 8, no. 3 (1985): 67–77.

15. Rock, "An Information System for HMOs: Designed From the Ground Up."
16. Shalowitz and Shalowitz, "Use of a Data Base System for HMO Management."
17. Drazen, E.L., and Moore, N.L. "Use of Computerized Information Systems in U.S. Health Maintenance Organizations and Hospitals." *Computer Methods and Progress in Biomedicine* 22 (1986): 105–10.
18. Birch and Davis Associates, Inc. *The Design, Selection, and Implementation of a Management Information System for Health Maintenance Organizations Volume II.* Washington, D.C.: U.S. Department of Health and Human Services, 1980.
19. Drazen and Moore, "Use of Computerized Information Systems in U.S. Health Maintenance Organizations and Hospitals."
20. Greenblatt, E.S., Moore, N.L., and Drazen, E.L. "Results of HMO Information Systems Survey: Current Status, Future Needs." In *1985 Group Health Institute Proceedings.* Washington, D.C.: Group Health Association of America, 1985, pp. 341–47.
21. Mueller, K.J., and Comer, J.C. "A Management Information System for Small HMOs." *Medical Group Management* 32, no. 6 (1985): 26–28, 32.
22. Plotnick, "Computer Applications for Management Planning and Control: Industry Standards in a Health Maintenance Organization."
23. Rock, "An Information System for HMOs: Designed From the Ground Up."
24. Shalowitz and Shalowitz, "Use of a Data Base System for HMO Management," 155–157.
25. Birch and Davis Associates, Inc. *The Design, Selection, and Implementation of a Management Information System for Health Maintenance Organizations Volume I Revised.* Washington, D.C.: U.S. Department of Health and Human Services, 1983.
26. Drazen and Moore, "Use of Computerized Information Systems in U.S. Health Maintenance Organizations and Hospitals."
27. Greenblatt, Moore, and Drazen, "Results of HMO Information Systems Survey: Current Status, Future Needs."
28. Michenzi, A.R., and Miller, P.M. "HMOs: Competition, Pricing, and Profits." *Topics in Health Record Management* 6, no. 4 (1986): 46–57.
29. Mueller and Comer, "A Management Information System for Small HMOs."
30. Shalowitz and Shalowitz, "Use of a Data Base System for HMO Management."
31. Plotnick, "Computer Applications for Management Planning and Control: Industry Standards in a Health Maintenance Organization."
32. Ibid.
33. Shalowitz and Shalowitz, "Use of a Data Base System for HMO Management."
34. Ibid.
35. Plotnick, "Computer Applications for Management Planning and Control: Industry Standards in a Health Maintenance Organization."
36. Lefort, "Healthcare Information Systems: Creating the Competitive Edge."
37. Marshall, G., and Kirkman-Liff, B.L. "Rapid and Comprehensive Quality Assurance: Cost-Effectiveness of an Online System." In *1985 Group Health Institute Proceedings.* Washington, D.C.: Group Health Association of America, 1985, p. 366.
38. "Everybody Keeps Talking About Quality, But We're Actually Setting the Standards." *Harvard Health Newsletter* 16, no. 4 (1986): 1, 3, 6, 7.
39. Michenzi and Miller, "HMOs: Competition, Pricing, and Profits," 55.
40. Shalowitz and Shalowitz, "Use of a Data Base System for HMO Management."
41. Michenzi and Miller, "HMOs: Competition, Pricing, and Profits."
42. Shalowitz and Shalowitz, "Use of a Data Base System for HMO Management," 157.
43. Michenzi and Miller, "HMOs: Competition, Pricing, and Profits."
44. Lefort, "Healthcare Information Systems: Creating the Competitive Edge."
45. Michenzi and Miller, "HMOs: Competition, Pricing, and Profits."
46. Mueller and Comer, "A Management Information System for Small HMOs."
47. Plotnick, "Computer Applications for Management Planning and Control: Industry Standards in a Health Maintenance Organization."
48. Shalowitz and Shalowitz, "Use of a Data Base System for HMO Management."
49. Lefort, "Healthcare Information Systems: Creating the Competitive Edge."
50. Steinwachs, "Ambulatory Care Management Information Systems: Future Directions."
51. Plotnick, "Computer Applications for Management Planning and Control: Industry Standards in a Health Maintenance Organization."
52. Mueller and Comer, "A Management Information System for Small HMOs."
53. Shalowitz and Shalowitz, "Use of a Data Base System for HMO Management."
54. Michenzi and Miller, "HMOs: Competition, Pricing, and Profits."
55. Shalowitz and Shalowitz, "Use of a Data Base System for HMO Management."
56. Mueller and Comer, "A Management Information System for Small HMOs."
57. Shalowitz and Shalowitz, "Use of a Data Base System for HMO Management."

58. Michenzi and Miller, "HMOs: Competition, Pricing, and Profits."

59. Plotnick, "Computer Applications for Management Planning and Control: Industry Standards in a Health Maintenance Organization."

60. Michenzi and Miller, "HMOs: Competition, Pricing, and Profits," 55.

61. Hews, "Establishing a Strategy for Information Resources in an HMO," 332.

62. Grams, S., et al. "Panel: Trends in Health Care Information Systems." In *Proceedings of the Eighth Annual Symposium on Computer Applications in Medical Care*, edited by G.S. Cohen. Los Angeles: IEEE Computer Society, 1984.

63. Lefort, "Healthcare Information Systems: Creating the Competitive Edge."

64. Rock, "An Information System for HMOs: Designed From the Ground Up."

65. Greenblatt, Moore, and Drazen, "Results of HMO Information Systems Survey: Current Status, Future Needs."

66. Hews, "Establishing a Strategy for Information Resources in an HMO."

67. Igou, K.D. "Roundtable: HMO Information Systems." *Computers in Healthcare* 7, no. 6 (1986): 53–54.

68. Lefort, "Healthcare Information Systems: Creating the Competitive Edge."

69. Miller, "Managing Systems in an HMO—the Harvard Plan Experience."

70. Drazen and Moore, "Use of Computerized Information Systems in U.S. Health Maintenance Organizations and Hospitals."

71. Grams, et al., "Panel: Trends in Health Care Information Systems."

72. Igou, "Roundtable: HMO Information Systems."

73. Jadach, T. "HMOs in the Evolving Healthcare Industry." *Computers in Healthcare* 6, no. 11 (1985): 31, 34, 36.

74. Grams, et al., "Panel: Trends in Health Care Information Systems," 142.

# Controlling disenrollment in health maintenance organizations

Daniel G. Shimshak,
Maureen C. DeFuria,
John J. DiGiorgio,
and
Jacob Getson

*With increasing competition, health maintenance organizations (HMOs) are struggling to maintain their enrollment levels. As a result, growing interest has emerged in studies of disenrollment, including factors associated with disenrollment and its implications for the HMO manager, as well as approaches for measuring and monitoring disenrollment.*

*Health Care Manage Rev*, 1988, 13(1), 47–55

**Much of the marketing literature** on health maintenance organizations (HMOs) is concerned with enrollment. This is not surprising considering the development of many new HMOs and the efforts to increase their market share. However, growth is measured by the difference between new enrollment and disenrollment. Even when marketing potential is good, controlling disenrollment becomes an important concern for overall growth.

High disenrollment rates can result in several adverse effects. They inhibit plan growth and have direct implications for the stability of the plan. Disenrollment leads to reduced income and creates prospective budgeting and planning problems. Finally, in order for the benefits of managed health care to be fully realized, people have to stay enrolled in an HMO for a period of time.

Luft[1] suggests that the success of HMOs depends on maintaining patient satisfaction, and satisfaction is a behavioral predictor of disenrollment. Enrollees typically have the periodic option of changing plans, and one would expect them to exercise that option to find the plan they like best. Over time a plan that is consistently disliked by its enrollees can expect to lose membership and develop a bad public image.

HMO success also depends on controlling expenses, which are greatly affected by disenrollment. Not only do new enrollees go through a learning experience in adapting to a new HMO, but also adverse selection may occur where new members join with a backlog of medical care needs, resulting in a higher demand for services. This belief that HMO members have greater medical care needs is the subject of considerable debate. Some evidence indicates that new members tend to use more services than existing members, a phenomenon that would prove costly to an HMO with a high rate of disenrollment.[2]

**Daniel G. Shimshak,** *Ph.D., is an Associate Professor and Chairman of the Management Sciences Department at the University of Massachusetts, Boston.*

**Maureen C. DeFuria,** *M.S., is a Manager and Acting Director in the Systems and Operations Division of Blue Cross and Blue Shield of Massachusetts in Boston.*

**John J. DiGiorgio,** *M.P.S., is the Director of Systems and Operations for the Yankee Alliance HealthCare Corporation in Andover, Massachusetts.*

**Jacob Getson,** *M.A., is a Senior Vice President for U.S. Healthcare, Inc., in Weston, Massachusetts.*

Disenrollment is classified as involuntary and voluntary. Involuntary or mandatory disenrollment is the consequence of geographic relocation, a change in employment status, or loss of insurance privileges (e.g., Medicaid ineligibility). Voluntary disenrollment is a conscious decision to leave an HMO. In the absence of empirical data, one might associate voluntary disenrollment with dissatisfaction and mandatory disenrollment strictly with changes in status. However, studies indicate a more complex situation. This article discusses the concept of disenrollment, including factors associated with disenrollment and its implications for the HMO manager. Several measures to control disenrollment and an approach to monitoring disenrollment are presented.

## DISENROLLMENT PREDICTORS

Most of the literature written on disenrollment describes disenrollment patterns within particular prepaid group practices and examines the factors related to its occurrence. Early studies considered sociodemographic characteristics. Disenrollment was found to be highest for younger women[3] who were members of smaller families.[4] A general pattern of high attrition in the first year of membership, with rapid slackening thereafter, was observed.[5]

More powerful in predicting disenrollment behavior were utilization variables. Disenrollees were found to have low utilization rates and no firm physician-patient relationship.[6,7] Greater utilization by remaining members supports the adverse selection issue described in the risk-vulnerability theory of enrollment choice.[3] In addition, several studies of the greatly debated start-up issue found that for disenrollees, as for continuous enrollees, utilization decreases with increasing duration of membership.[9-13]

Many studies considered dissatisfaction and disenrollment. Disenrollees were substantially more dissatisfied with various facets of the HMO than those who remained in the plan. In considering reasons for leaving, dissatisfaction with various aspects of medical service, such as the perceived quality of care, was reported most frequently.[14] Mechanic, Weiss, and Cleary found that having fewer physical health problems, facing inadequate access to services, and having difficulty in establishing a stable relationship with a particular physician who is available when wanted substantially account for the decision to disenroll.[15]

Hennelly and Boxerman[16] thoroughly investigated determinants of disenrollment. They considered the relationship between disenrollment, dissatisfaction, and out-of-plan use of covered services and found that dissatisfaction was the most important predictor of disenrollment. After that, age of the subscriber was predictive with younger subscribers more likely to resign from the plan. Furthermore, if these families had nonplan family members or additional insurance coverage, the temptation to disenroll was intensified. Interestingly, out-of-plan visits were inversely related to disenrollment. Contrary to the notion that out-of-plan use led to disenrollment, families who used only plan services were more likely to disenroll than were users of outside services. The investigators later found that while causes of both voluntary and mandatory disenrollment were different, three important factors appeared as correlates of both resignation types: dissatisfaction, insurance alternatives, and sociodemographic descriptors.[17]

## MANAGERIAL IMPLICATIONS

Studies have shown the complexity of the disenrollment phenomenon and have stressed the need for the HMO manager to respond to those factors associated with disenrollment.[18] For example, results show that older groups have a higher probability of remaining with the plan than younger groups. If the plan is unable to offset this retention pattern by enrolling more young people, it will, in the long run, accrue an older population. This in turn would act as a weighting factor to raise the general utilization level of the plan. Marketing efforts are needed to offset this effect. Furthermore, the lack of use of services by disenrollees suggests that management should continually contact and remind nonusers of the HMO's readiness to serve.

Dissatisfaction with the plan, particularly with the costs of care, the quality of care (use of nonphysician practitioners), and inaccessibility of services (length of waiting), significantly influences the decision to leave. These attitudes can be altered by effective management practices such as offering low-cost plans, developing quality assurance programs, and adjusting staffing patterns and practices.

Boxerman and Hennelly[19,20] suggest that the factors associated with disenrollment can be grouped into two categories: factors outside the manager's control and factors over which the manager has some control. The first category considers the existence of alternative health insurance coverage and sociodemographic factors. Most employed persons receive health insurance as an employee benefit. As a result, families with multiple workers are likely to have overlapping coverage. It was observed that the presence of multiple coverage or nonplan family members, presumably covered by some form of insurance, served as a disincentive to continuing membership. In addition, sociodemographic characteristics of members have been found to be related to disenrollment. These are variables over which the HMO manager has little direct control. The manager can monitor and evaluate the enrollee population with a well-designed management information system to capture data on alternative health insurance coverage and sociodemographic variables. Such a system would allow administrators to easily obtain a profile of their membership, to monitor enrollment behavior, and to forecast probable numbers and types of disenrollees. The HMO manager does have some control over the second category of variables involved with providing services that satisfy enrollees. One strategy involves offering low-cost premium options to attract and keep persons who are unhappy with the costs of care. A second area of concern should be with the professional staff. Administrators should carefully deal with the often conflicting problems of limiting the use of nonphysician providers and reducing long appointment waiting times. At the same time, these problems must be resolved in a cost-effective manner so that the cost and quality of care are not jeopardized. Although under the control of the manager, these attitudinal problems are not easily resolved.

## MEASURES OF DISENROLLMENT

Disenrollment statistics are often inflated as a result of administrative procedures that may count a transfer from one type of coverage to another as a disenrollment. Moreover, disenrollment rates reflect the geographical location of the HMO, the changing employment situation in the area, the impact of premium policies, and the HMO's competition with other health care providers. Thus it is difficult to generalize from one context to another.[21] However, measuring, tracking, and reacting to changes in disenrollment are important functions of an HMO manager who is concerned with the future of the plan.

Several disenrollment statistics based on different measuring techniques have been reported. All can be calculated for a given time period as well as on a year-to-date basis.

*Disenrollment rate.* This measure expresses disenrollment in a given time period as a percentage of the total enrollment. While there are various ways of representing total enrollment, the most commonly used method in the literature defines it as the total membership at the end of the given time period plus the number of disenrollees. This is calculated as follows:

$$\text{Disenrollment rate} = \frac{\begin{array}{c}\text{No. of disenrollees}\\\text{during time period}\end{array}}{\begin{array}{c}\text{No. of members at}\\\text{end of time period}\\+ \text{ no. of disenrollees}\\\text{during time period}\end{array}}$$

*Annualized disenrollment per 1,000.* Similar to other HMO measures, this measure expresses disenrollment as a function of the number of member-months. It is annualized and determined on the basis of 1,000 members rather than on a per member basis. This measure is equal to the number of disenrolled members divided by the number of member-months multiplied by 12 to get an annualized figure, and then multiplied by 1,000 to get a rate per 1,000 members. The member-month figure includes those incurred by disenrollees prior to leaving the HMO. This measure is calculated as follows:

$$\begin{array}{c}\text{Annualized}\\\text{disenrollment}\\\text{per 1,000}\end{array} = \frac{\begin{array}{c}\text{No. of disenrollees during}\\\text{time period x 12,000}\end{array}}{\begin{array}{c}\text{No. of member-months}\\\text{for time period}\end{array}}$$

*Additions to terminations ratio.* Unlike the two previous measures that represent the magnitude of disenrollment, this ratio expresses the net effect of disenrollment on membership in a given time period. If the ratio is equal to one, there is no net gain in total membership. Values greater than one occur when the number of new members is larger than the number of disenrollees, so that total membership increases. Values less than one occur when total membership decreases, due to there being more disenrollees than new members. This measure is calculated as follows:

$$\begin{array}{c}\text{Additions to}\\\text{terminations ratio}\end{array} = \frac{\begin{array}{c}\text{No. of members added}\\\text{during time period}\end{array}}{\begin{array}{c}\text{No. of disenrollees}\\\text{during time period}\end{array}}$$

*Problems must be resolved in a cost-effective manner so that the cost and quality of care are not jeopardized.*

Varying disenrollment rates are reported in the literature. Luft presents the results of several studies and reports most annual disenrollment rates in the single digits.[22] However, there were a number of important exceptions in which high rates occurred. Some surprising results are reported by Wollstadt, Shapiro, and Bice in the study of a program used by Medicaid beneficiaries. Over two years they found the average annual rate for all disenrollees to be 42 percent while that for voluntary disenrollees was 23 percent. These figures were found by taking the ratio of the number of disenrollees to the total enrollment (including those who disenrolled).[23] Mechanic, Weiss, and Cleary studied a staff model HMO serving several counties in a large metropolitan area and reported an annual disenrollment rate of approximately 20 percent, reflecting a 14 percent voluntary disenrollment rate.[24] Annual turnover rates of 10 percent to 15 percent are common, with some figures even higher.[25] Such turnover is a potential threat to the growth and financial viability of these health plans.

It is not unusual to find that both types of disenrollment, voluntary and mandatory, are seasonal in nature. Open enrollment periods among associated employer groups provide workers with the opportunity to voluntarily change their levels of insurance coverage or type of plan. As a result, often the highest voluntary disenrollment rates have been observed during the first or fourth quarters when contract negotiations (open enrollment) for many employer groups take place. Similarly, mandatory disenrollment has a repetitive pattern. Often the highest mandatory disenrollment rates occur in the third quarter, a time of high job mobility and transient behavior, while the lowest rates occur in the first and fourth quarters since job changes tend to be minimized every year during the winter.

## MONITORING DISENROLLMENT

It is necessary to monitor disenrollment to ensure that it is at an acceptable level. This monitoring can be done by recording and evaluating over time. If the disenrollment measure is acceptable, no action is taken; if the measure is not acceptable, corrective action is instituted. The steps required to effectively control disenrollment include determining measure, comparing measure to standard, evaluating measure, taking corrective action if necessary, and evaluating corrective action.

A particular disenrollment measure must be selected for analysis. In addition, there must be a performance standard to evaluate the measurements. This should be determined by the HMO administrator on the basis of expertise or historical disenrollment performance and will often reflect the level of disenrollment being sought.

A definition of out of control must be established. Even a disenrollment process that is functioning as it should will not yield measures that conform exactly to a standard, simply because of the natural or random variations that are inherent in all processes. In other words, a certain amount of variation between actual disenrollment and the predetermined performance standard is inevitable. The main task of the control process is to distinguish between random and nonrandom variability. A process that exhibits only random variability is said to be in control. Nonrandom or excessive variability is due to assignable causes and the process is considered to be out of control.

In the event that the disenrollment measure is judged to be out of control, corrective action must be taken. This involves uncovering the cause of the nonrandom variability (e.g., premium increase, reduction

## FIGURE 1

SAMPLE CONTROL CHART FOR
DISENROLLMENT MEASURE

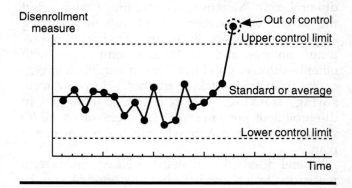

in benefits, increased competition) and instituting action to bring disenrollment back in control. To ensure that corrective action is effective, it is necessary to closely monitor disenrollment for a sufficient period of time. Corrective action should eliminate the problem.

Disenrollment can be monitored using control charts that serve as a record (see Figure 1). The control chart approach involves setting upper and lower control limits for individual disenrollment measures based on a predetermined performance standard. These limits define the range of random variability. Disenrollment is measured over time and plotted on the chart. Values that fall within the control limits suggest, but do not prove, that disenrollment is in control (i.e., variations are random), while one or more values on or outside of the control limits suggest that disenrollment is out of control (i.e., variations are nonrandom). In addition, when unnatural patterns of variation are present, even though the points are within the limits, disenrollment is out of control. A more detailed discussion of the theory and method of control charting can be found in the Appendix.

As an example, the data in Table 1 have been taken from the Division of Insurance Quarterly Statements filed by a Massachusetts HMO from 1981 through 1985. Membership data are reported along with the

## TABLE 1

ANALYSIS OF DISENROLLMENT DATA FOR A SAMPLE MASSACHUSETTS HMO FROM 1981–1985

| Quarter | Additions | Terminations | Total membership | Member-months | Disenrollment rate (%) | Annualized disenrollment per 1,000 | Additions to terminations ratio |
|---|---|---|---|---|---|---|---|
| 1981 | | | | | | | |
| 1 | 1,245 | 267 | 5,636 | 15,226 | 4.5 | 210 | 4.66 |
| 2 | 1,341 | 424 | 6,553 | 17,848 | 6.1 | 285 | 3.16 |
| 3 | 1,350 | 535 | 7,368 | 21,355 | 6.8 | 301 | 2.52 |
| 4 | 1,659 | 376 | 8,651 | 23,332 | 4.2 | 193 | 4.41 |
| 1982 | | | | | | | |
| 1 | 1,627 | 448 | 9,830 | 27,125 | 4.4 | 198 | 3.63 |
| 2 | 1,647 | 518 | 10,959 | 30,225 | 4.5 | 206 | 3.18 |
| 3 | 3,276 | 531 | 13,704 | 37,991 | 3.7 | 168 | 6.17 |
| 4 | 4,127 | 809 | 17,022 | 47,050 | 4.5 | 206 | 5.10 |
| 1983 | | | | | | | |
| 1 | 5,389 | 986 | 20,578 | 57,791 | 4.6 | 205 | 5.47 |
| 2 | 2,955 | 1,122 | 22,411 | 64,149 | 4.8 | 210 | 2.63 |
| 3 | 3,777 | 1,330 | 24,858 | 71,412 | 5.1 | 223 | 2.84 |
| 4 | 3,123 | 1,647 | 26,334 | 76,122 | 5.9 | 260 | 1.90 |
| 1984 | | | | | | | |
| 1 | 4,511 | 1,801 | 29,044 | 82,631 | 5.8 | 262 | 2.50 |
| 2 | 3,787 | 1,795 | 31,036 | 88,893 | 5.5 | 242 | 2.11 |
| 3 | 2,117 | 2,097 | 31,056 | 91,975 | 6.3 | 274 | 1.01 |
| 4 | 3,052 | 1,761 | 32,347 | 95,640 | 5.2 | 221 | 1.73 |
| 1985 | | | | | | | |
| 1 | 3,803 | 2,339 | 33,811 | 100,760 | 6.5 | 279 | 1.63 |
| 2 | 3,978 | 2,883 | 34,906 | 103,489 | 7.6 | 334 | 1.38 |
| 3 | 3,600 | 2,787 | 35,719 | 106,282 | 7.2 | 315 | 1.29 |
| 4 | 3,759 | 2,552 | 36,926 | 109,283 | 6.5 | 280 | 1.47 |

calculations of the three disenrollment measures. A control chart for the disenrollment rate has been developed using the mean disenrollment rate as the performance standard (see Figure 2). This standard reflects historical performance alone. All points fall within the control limits, implying that the disenrollment process is in control.

## FIGURE 2

### CONTROL CHART FOR DISENROLLMENT RATE FOR A SAMPLE MASSACHUSETTS HMO

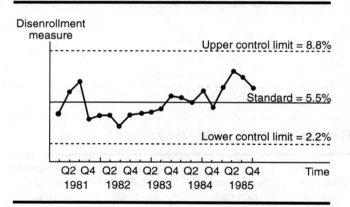

•  •  •

Disenrollment has become a topic of considerable interest to HMO administrators since the period of rapid initial growth has passed and federal government subsidies have diminished. Many HMO plans have reached their projected enrollment and are trying to maintain existing levels. Thus it is hardly surprising to witness the shift from interest in analysis of HMO marketing to studies of member satisfaction and factors associated with disenrollment.[26]

Although the manager will never be able to eliminate disenrollment, it can be managed through effective monitoring followed by careful planning and policy modification. Managers need to maintain information on their members, including demographic data, socioeconomic data, and the presence of other health insurance. The causes for member disenrollment should also be gathered for study. Managers can demonstrate a sincere interest in members' attitudes through periodic assessment. This can take the form of an interview or a membership survey. The study of disenrollment data will serve to

indicate when corrective action is necessary. In addition, such data will be useful in forecasting disenrollment patterns.

Disenrollment is inevitable. Some people will try an HMO and voluntarily leave it while others will leave for mandatory reasons. Regardless of the reason, the costs of high rates of disenrollment make effective management activities a necessity.

## REFERENCES

1. Luft, H.S. *Health Maintenance Organizations: Dimensions of Performance.* New York: Wiley, 1981.
2. Griffith, M.J., and Baloff, N. "Membership Duration and Utilization Rates in a Prepaid Group Practice." *Medical Care* 19 (1981): 1194–1210.
3. Wollstadt, L.J., Shapiro, S., and Bice, T.W. "Disenrollment from a Prepaid Group Practice: An Actuarial and Demographic Description." *Inquiry* 15 (June 1978): 142–50.
4. Wesinger, R.P., and Sorensen, A.A. "Demographic Characteristics and Prior Utilization Experience of HMO Disenrollees Compared with Total Membership." *Medical Care* 20 (1982): 1188–96.
5. Forthofer, R.N., Glasser, J.H., and Light, N. "Life Table Analysis of Membership in an HMO Retention." *Journal of Community Health* 5 (Fall 1979): 46–53.
6. Wersinger and Sorensen, "Demographic Characteristics."
7. Gold, W.E. "Predicting HMO Disenrollment Behavior: Results of a Study of Demographic and Behavioral Characteristics of HMO Members." In *Finance and Marketing in the Nation's Group Practice HMOs.* Washington, D.C.: 31st Annual Group Health Institute, June 1981, pp. 175–81.
8. Lewis, K. "Comparison of Use by Enrolled and Recently Disenrolled Populations in a Health Maintenance Organization." *Health Service Research* 19 (April 1984):1–22.
9. Yesalis, C.E., and Bonnet, P.D. "The Effect of Duration of Membership in a Prepaid Group Health Plan on the Utilization of Services." *Medical Care* 14 (1976):1024–36.
10. Mullooly, J.P., and Freeborn, D.K. "The Effect of Length of Membership upon the Utilization of Ambulatory Care Services." *Medical Care* 17 (1979): 922–36.
11. Griffith and Baloff, "Membership Duration."
12. Griffith, M.J., Baloff, N., and Spitznagel E.L. "Utilization Patterns of Health Maintenance Organization Disenrollees." *Medical Care* 22 (1984): 827–34.
13. Stiefel, M.C., Gardelius, D.A., and Hayami D.E. "Selection Bias: A Comparison of Inpatient Utilization, Demographics, and Premiums for HMO 'Leavers,' 'Stayers,' and 'Joiners.'" In *HMOs in a New Era of Health Benefits.*

Philadelphia: 34th Annual Group Health Institute, June 1984, pp. 235–52.

14. Sorensen, A.A., and Wersinger, R.P. "Factors Influencing Disenrollment from an HMO." *Medical Care* 19 (1981): 766–73.

15. Mechanic, D., Weiss, N., and Cleary, P.D. "The Growth of HMOs: Issues of Enrollment and Disenrollment." *Medical Care* 21 (1983): 338–47.

16. Hennelly, V.D., and Boxerman, S.B. "Out-of-Plan Use and Disenrollment: Outgrowths of Dissatisfaction with a Prepaid Group Plan." *Medical Care* 21(1983): 348–59.

17. Hennelly, V.D., and Boxerman, S.B. "Disenrollment from a Prepaid Group Plan." *Medical* Care 21 (1983): 1154–67.

18. Zapka, J.G., Stanek, E.J., and Raitt, J. "HMO Disenrollment—Who Leaves and Why?—Operational Considerations." In *New Health Care Systems: HMOs and Beyond.* Minneapolis: 36th Annual Group Health Institute, June 1986, pp. 558–71.

19. Boxerman, S.B., and Hennelly, V.D. "Determinants of Disenrollment: Implications for HMO Managers." *Journal of Ambulatory Care Management* 6 (May 1983): 12–23.

20. Hennelly, V.D., and Boxerman, S.B. "Managing Disenrollment in HMOs." In *HMOs in the Mainstream: Sustaining Growth and Quality.* Dallas: 33rd Annual Group Health Institute, June 1983, pp. 250–57.

21. Mechanic, Weiss, and Cleary, "The Growth of HMOs."

22. Luft, *Health Maintenance Organizations.*

23. Wollstadt, Shapiro, and Bice, "Disenrollment from a Prepaid Group Practice."

24. Mechanic, Weiss, and Cleary, "The Growth of HMOs."

25. Hennelly and Boxerman, "Out-of-Plan Use."

26. Sorensen and Wersinger, "Factors Influencing Disenrollment."

# A model for understanding benefit segmentation in preventive health care

Joby John
and
George Miaoulis

*The marketing of traditional health care services, such as hospital and physician services, has matured with the integration of research from the medical sociology discipline and the marketing literature. In this article, we present a model to illustrate how an understanding of predispositions to health care behavior, integrated with benefit segmentation analysis, can contribute to more focused and effective marketing strategies for health-related products and services.*

*Health Care Manage Rev*, 1992, 17(2), 21–32
© 1992 Aspen Publishers, Inc.

One of the most pervasive changes in American society in the past three decades has been a shift from cure-oriented to preventive-oriented health care. Although the focus and intensity of this trend has changed since its beginnings in the 1960s, the orientation toward preventive health care will continue to have a major impact on food and drug sales, leisure markets, apparel industry, and publishing in the 1990s. The marketing of traditional health care services such as hospital services has matured during the past decade with the integration of research from the medical sociology discipline and the marketing literature (e.g., patient satisfaction research). Similarly, more effective marketing strategies for health care packaged goods can be developed by integrating the knowledgebase available in the "health care disciplines."

In this article, we demonstrate how an understanding of predispositions to health behavior (borrowed from the health care disciplines) can contribute to more effective and focused marketing strategies for nontraditional health care goods and services. Marketing strategies for health care goods, health-concerned goods/services, and health-related goods/services can be based on the "Health Belief Model" and an analysis of consumer's attitudes, beliefs, and benefits sought from preventive health behavior. As an illustration, we integrate the Health Belief Model with benefit segmentation analysis to present a model of the potential segments in the preventive health care market.

We will first introduce the Health Belief Model, followed by a discussion of the appropriateness of benefit segmentation analysis in the preventive health behavior environment. Then, the results of an *exploratory* benefit segmentation study of preventive health beliefs and benefits will be discussed and we will propose the marketing strategy implications for health care products in the preventive health care market. These propositions for determining the attractiveness of each segment are based on the exploratory benefit segmentation study and are, therefore, preliminary in nature. Further evaluation of actual behaviors regarding the consumption of the various health care products would be needed to confirm these propositions.

**Joby John,** *Ph.D., M.B.A., is Assistant Professor of Marketing at Bentley College, Waltham, Massachusetts. His area of research interest is health care marketing.*

**George Miaoulis,** *Ph.D., M.B.A., is Professor of Marketing at Bentley College, Waltham, Massachusetts. His area of research interest is health care marketing.*

Health care products can be visualized along a continuum extending from more directly (and obviously) oriented health care products to less directly (and not so obviously) oriented health care products (see Figure 1). Thus, health care products include health care services and health care goods (which are more obviously health care oriented products), health-concerned goods/services, and health-related goods/services (which are less obviously health care oriented). (See the Box for some examples of these goods and services.)

Health care services, at the extreme left of our continuum, have benefited significantly from the maturation of the health care marketing literature. We have included these services in our continuum to provide perspective for the reader, as our intention is to focus on the balance of the continuum. For ease of discussion, we will simply refer to the balance of the continuum as "health care products."

## HEALTH BELIEF MODEL

The Health Belief Model is a concept used by preventive health care professionals to predict an individual's propensity to engage in preventive health activity based on the individual's perception of his or her susceptibility (i.e., the threat and severity of potential illness) and the benefits of preventive behavior.[1] The model profiles an individual who will engage in preventive health behavior as one who (1) has minimal levels of relevant health motivation and knowledge, (2) perceives himself or herself as potentially vulnerable to a threatening condition or illness, (3) is convinced of the efficacy of intervention, and (4) sees few difficulties in undertaking the recommended action.

The model suggests that an individual's preventive health behaviors are a function of

- the "benefits-barriers," an analysis of the advantages and disadvantages of the health prevention activity or consumption,
- the perceived threat associated with the condition or illness, and

## FIGURE 1

## THE HEALTH CARE PRODUCTS CONTINUUM

| Health care services | Health care goods | Health-concerned goods/services | Health-related goods/services |

---

**Examples of Goods and Services Along the Health Care Products Continuum**

| *Health care goods* | *Health-concerned goods and services* |
|---|---|
| Analgesics | Healthful/natural foods |
| Vitamins | Bottled water |
| Stomach remedies | Caffeine-free drinks |
| Self-diagnostic tests | Low cholesterol foods |
| Therapeutic skin care | Controlled calorie foods |

| *Health-related goods and services* | *Health care services* |
|---|---|
| Athletic shoes | Health promotion programs |
| Athletic/leisure wear | Quick care centers |
| Self-help books | Physician services |
| Health clubs/spas | Hospital services |
| | Home nursing care |

---

- cues to action, which include mass media and interpersonal communications.

Thus, in terms of predisposition to behavior:

$$(\text{Predisposition to preventive health care behavior}) = f \ (\text{Perceived threats, perceived benefits})$$

In essence, the Health Belief Model asserts that individuals will likely engage in preventive health maintenance behaviors, if the perceived threat of illness and benefits of the behavior are high enough when balanced against the barriers, or costs, of engaging in the preventive behavior. The Health Belief Model also suggests that it is possible to differentiate among individuals based upon their relative propensity to engage in preventive health maintenance behaviors and their perceptions of threats, benefits, and barriers.[1] At one end of the spectrum, there are individuals who do not see any advantage to engaging in preventive health behaviors. For these individuals, the barriers to engaging in preventive health behaviors outweigh the perceived benefits. At the other end of the spectrum, there are individuals who perceive a high level of threat from health conditions or illnesses. These individuals perceive that the benefits of engaging in preventive health behaviors outweigh the barriers.

Thus, the Health Belief Model suggests that one way to segment the market for health care products is based upon the differences among individuals in their perceptions of the benefits and barriers to engaging in preventive health behaviors.[1]

## HEALTH BENEFIT SEGMENTATION

Segmentation analysis is based upon the premise that broad markets that appear to be heterogeneous can actually be divided into smaller homogeneous segments.[2] These smaller segments provide opportunities for developing very specific and efficient marketing strategies designed to elicit particular responses from the target audience.[3]

---

*Segmentation analysis is based upon the premise that broad markets that appear to be heterogeneous can actually be divided into smaller homogeneous segments.*

---

Benefit segmentation[4] is recognized as an important concept used to identify target markets and develop marketing strategies.[2] Benefit segmentation studies can provide critical information for the marketing planning process, including new product and service evaluation; product, service, or program planning; market positioning; and marketing communications development.[2,5,6] Benefit segments remain stable over a long period of time, thereby adding to their usefulness in market strategy planning.[5]

Traditionally, benefit segmentation has been used by packaged goods marketers, but it also has proven to be a useful tool in marketing planning for nonprofit and health care organizations such as hospitals.[7,8] A review of the marketing literature suggests, however, that while researchers have studied various aspects of the issue for the marketing of health-related products and services, no published studies to date directly integrate benefit segmentation analysis and health theory or concepts such as the Health Belief Model.

Marketing researchers have recognized the contributions that benefit segmentation can make in effective health promotion planning[9,10] and have assessed the role of benefits in the Health Belief Model.[11] Consumer psychographic measures relating to health/medical services and attitudinal dimensions have been used to determine homogeneous groupings in a rural setting.[12] Benefit segmentation has been applied to a variety of preventive health issues and has been integrated in a health care education model.[13,14,15] Other segmentation variables used by health care marketing researchers include socioeconomic variables,[16] health role behavior,[17] and physician loyalty.[18] The benefit segmentation approach also has been used to identify segments in the

hospital market[19] and in the ambulatory care pharmacy market.[20] A segmentation approach for the women's health care market based upon demographic, behavioral, family, and personal variables has been proposed.[21]

We draw on an exploratory benefit segmentation study that was performed to determine consumer beliefs, attitudes, and benefits sought from preventive health behaviors. In the study, 175 (87 women and 88 men) in-depth interviews were conducted. This sample reflected a cross section of demographic characteristics, and positive (e.g., exercising) as well as negative (or, at risk) health behaviors (e.g., smoking). The study identified six segments, each seeking different benefits from preventive health behaviors and having different attitudes toward such health behaviors. See Table 1 for a description of the six segments.

The Hypochondriac and the Health Seeker segments are at one extreme. These segments are highly *proactive* in their consumption of health-related products and services, and they are more likely to engage in preventive health behaviors. At the other extreme are the Band-Aider and the Do Not Bug Me benefit segments. These segments are *reactive* to health care needs and likely to seek only therapeutic health care products and services. The Follower and the Self-Sufficient segments are moderately proactive in their predisposition toward preventive health care behavior. Each of the six segments is descriptively profiled in the Appendix.

*Hypochondriacs* actively seek and need recognition. The benefit they seek is assurance that they are really healthy. Hypochondriacs tend to seek excessive medical attention and health-related products and services because they believe that this will ensure good health. They seek attention from health care professionals to satisfy their dependency and recognition needs.

*Health Seekers* strive for a long, healthy life. They believe that preventive health care is the key to achieving this goal. Health Seekers actively engage in positive health behaviors, such as participating in fitness programs, limiting alcohol intake, refraining from smoking, and controlling weight. This group actively seeks health information and participates in preventive medical services, including physical examinations and health screenings. Health Seekers tend to be well-educated professionals.

*Followers* seek the guidance of others who they believe are better informed to advise them about health care issues. They tend to follow the crowd and are not convinced that preventive health behaviors can deliver what is promised. Followers are likely to wait for symptoms to develop before seeking medical attention.

**TABLE 1**

BENEFIT SEGMENTATION ANALYSIS

| Name of segment | Health seekers | Followers | Band-Aiders |
|---|---|---|---|
| Benefits sought | Long life, continued good health. | Want someone else to be concerned about their health, looking for guidance. | Recognition for being hard workers and rarely sick. |
| Category beliefs | Preventive medical services are the key to a longer and healthier life. | Not sure whether preventive services can deliver what they offer, best to follow the crowd. | Preventive care is for other people who get sick a lot. When your time is up, it's up! |
| Health services sought | Very broad range of services; nutritional counseling, exercise programs, hypertension tests, dental, etc. | Generally the annual physical, await symptoms before seeking medical services. | Primary treatment oriented; seek only essential preventive services, e.g., vaccinations |
| Degree of participation | High, very active, continuous. | Sporadic. | Minimal. |
| Occasions of use | Corresponds to particular health needs at various life stages. | Depends on the degree of persuasiveness of the preventive service. | Following work-inhibiting symptoms, accidents, etc. |
| Personality/lifestyle | Rational, open-minded, appreciates "savings" from preventive services. Plan ahead, body conscious. | Other-directed, highly impressionable by "knowledgeable others." | Family-oriented, set in ways; not impressed by wonders of science. |

**TABLE 1**

CONTINUED

| Name of segment | Do Not Bug Me | Hypochondriacs | Self-Sufficient |
|---|---|---|---|
| Benefits sought | Relief from everyday pressures and tensions. Looking for ways to cope with problems. | Tremendous need for recognition, want people to notice them and to assure them that they are okay. | Self-reliance. Home remedies do the job. |
| Category beliefs | Needs to smoke, eat, etc. to deal with tension. It is just too tough to quit. | Do not wait—see the doctor right away. Must get all possible medical attention to make sure everything is okay. | I can take care of myself. Don't trust doctors and hospitals. |
| Health services sought | Annual physical. | Any and all. | Home remedies and over-the-counter drugs. |
| Degree of participation | Seldom. | Excessive. | Nonparticipation in institutional medicine. |
| Occasions of use | To keep employer and/or family off his/her back. | Symptom-of-the-day club members. | Only have remedies. |
| Personality/lifestyle | Easygoing, gregarious on the outside; anxious and very nervous on the inside. | Dependent and lacking self-confidence. Seeks attention from others. | Independent, previous bad experiences with doctors. |

*Self-Sufficients* are independent individuals who tend to rely on home remedies and over-the-counter products to meet their health care needs. Members of this segment are innately distrustful of the traditional health care system. This distrust typically results from negative personal experience with the health care system. Self-Sufficients tend to be older, less educated, and have a lower socioeconomic status than other segments.

*Band-Aiders* seek recognition for their claims of rarely being ill. Seeking and utilizing health care services and products are in direct contrast to the image of robust health they want to project. Band-Aiders believe that pre-

---

Band-Aiders *tend to seek medical attention only after symptoms or accidents occur that inhibit their ability to function normally.*

---

ventive care is for the sickly. This segment tends to seek medical attention only after symptoms or accidents occur that inhibit their ability to work or function normally.

*Do Not Bug Me's* use negative health behaviors such as smoking, drinking, or eating excessively to deal with the stress of everyday life. Typically, the Do Not Bug Me's do not utilize any preventive health care services besides a physical examination to pacify employers or family members. This segment includes a heavy concentration of smokers and obese individuals. These individuals are frequently observed to be easygoing, but are inwardly extremely stressed.

## MARKETING STRATEGY IMPLICATIONS

The benefit segments described in this article provide an opportunity to examine some of the marketing implications for health-related products and services along the health care continuum. This is a useful first step in the evolution of rigorous health benefit segmentation studies for specific health-related products or services (i.e., low cholesterol foods, health clubs, and athletic apparel).

The three fundamental objectives of market segmentation strategies[9] bring the implications of this exploratory study into clear focus:

1. *Identification and comparison of marketing opportunities.* Segmentation enables an organization to examine the needs of each segment against the benefits offered by its own products/services and the benefits of competitive products/services. Segments with low satisfaction levels may represent marketing opportunities.

2. *Finer adjustment of products/services and marketing appeals.* Market segmentation permits the targeting of consumers in homogeneous groups, thus enabling an organization to develop products/services and marketing appeals that meet the specific needs of groups of consumers.

3. *Development of marketing mixes and budgets.* Segmentation allows an organization to develop realistic marketing mixes and budgets based on clear forecasting of the responses of different consumer groups. This permits the allocation of funds to achieve difference goals in different parts of the market.

Table 2 lists the range of health-related products and services, as well as traditional health care services for perspective. A coding scheme of high (H), moderate (M), and low (L) priority identifies the expected response of each of the benefit segments discussed in this article.

The following discussion demonstrates the link between health concepts such as the Health Belief Model and benefit segmentation research in developing effective marketing strategies for health-related products and services. The reader should bear in mind that this discussion presents generic implications of the benefit segmentation analysis for marketing strategy development and that these are examples used for illustrative purposes. Actual behaviors need to be studied for each category of health care product in the preventive health care market to confirm these propositions.

### Vitamins

Hypochondriacs represent a segment with a high potential for vitamins, because by definition they seek any and all medical services believing that maximum medical attention will ensure good health. The consumers in this segment are in a proactive mode, seeking products such as vitamins, self-diagnostic kits, and preventive remedies. This analysis suggests that the vitamin marketer needs to focus promotional efforts on brand preferences rather than product utility for hypochondriacs. Consumers in the Health Follower and Self-Sufficient segments have a significantly lower propensity to use products such as vitamins because by definition these consumers do not believe that preventive health services are needed, or they are self-reliant and await illness before they seek medical attention. The segmentation analysis suggests the vitamin marketer needs to use a different appeal to these segments, stressing product utility. The opportunity may be to show that vitamin usage is not inconsistent with self-reliance and self-help. Consumers in the Health Follower segment may be

## TABLE 2

### MARKETING STRATEGY IMPLICATIONS*

| Product and service categories | Benefit segments | | | | | |
|---|---|---|---|---|---|---|
| | Hypochon-driac | Health Seeker | Health Follower | Self-Sufficient | Band-Aider | Do Not Bug Me |
| Over-the-counter health products | | | | | | |
| Analgesics | H | L | M | M | M | H |
| Vitamins | H | L/H | M | M | L | L |
| Stomach remedies | H | L | M | L | M | H |
| Self-diagnostic tests | H | L | L | M | L | L |
| Therapeutic skin/hair care | M | M | H | H | L | L |
| Health-concerned goods & services | | | | | | |
| Natural | H | H | H | L | L | L |
| Bottled waters | H | H | H | L | L | L |
| Caffeine free | H | H | H | L | L | L |
| Low cholesterol | H | H | H | L | L | L |
| Controlled calorie | H | L | M | M | M | L |
| Health-related goods & services | | | | | | |
| Athletic shoes | L | M/H | H | L | M | L |
| Traditional athletic wear | L | M | L | L | L | M |
| Designer leisure wear | L | L | H | M | M | L |
| Self-help books | H | H | M | M | L | L |
| Health clubs/spas | L | L | H | L | L | L |
| Participatory sports | L | | H | L/H | L | L |
| Spectator sports | L | L | M | M | H | H |
| Traditional health care services | | | | | | |
| Doctors | H | L | H | L | L | L |
| Quick care centers | H | L | M | L | H | H |

*Coding Scheme
  H —High priority segment
  M —Moderate priority segment
  L —Low priority segment

prompted to use vitamins because taking vitamins is a convenient way to engage in preventive health behavior. Consumers in the Do Not Bug Me segment, by definition, are not predisposed to using health care products or services and are not appropriate for health care products such as vitamins. It appears that marketing resources should not be directed to this segment.

### High-performance athletic shoes

This discussion focuses upon the marketing of expensive, high-performance athletic shoes, rather than lower-priced "sneakers" that are often purchased by individuals in the mass market for comfort or status rather than for exercise purposes. The Hypochondriac segment is symptom-oriented, rather than preventive-oriented, and they seek constant reassurance that they are healthy. Exercising with high-performance athletic shoes does not satisfy this need. In contrast, exercise is an important part of the life style of consumers in the Health Seeker segment, and athletic shoes become an extension of themselves and a fulfillment of the health-seeking process. This segment is knowledgeable about athletic shoes and is likely to purchase the right shoes for every sport or fitness activity. The Health Follower segment will follow the Health Seeker segment, because its members want to "look" healthy. The Band-Aider segment is also concerned about projecting a robust image and its members tend to be moderate consumers of high-performance ath-

## FIGURE 2

### *GRAPHIC DISPLAY OF MARKETING STRATEGY IMPLICATIONS

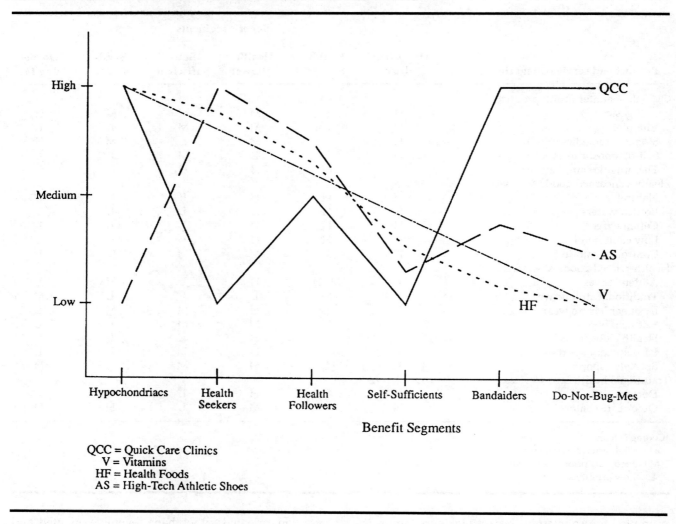

QCC = Quick Care Clinics
V = Vitamins
HF = Health Foods
AS = High-Tech Athletic Shoes

letic shoes. The Self-Sufficient and Do Not Bug Me segments are low priority for the marketer of high-performance athletic shoes, because they are not interested in or do not have time for preventive health behaviors.

### Healthful foods

The segmentation analysis suggests that the Hypochondriac, Health Seeker, and Health Follower segments are most likely to respond to the marketing of healthful foods. Individuals in these segments seek longer, healthier lives, and they are inclined to consume products they perceive as assisting them in achieving this

goal. Health Seekers are the "opinion leaders" for health foods, and they will respond to the message that the consumption of health foods should be part of a preventive health regimen. Health Followers are likely to follow the lead of the Health Seekers. The Self-Sufficient, Band-Aider, and Do Not Bug Me segments are less attractive market development opportunities for health foods. Self-Sufficients may respond to a message that health foods will keep them healthy enough to stay out of the health care system. Band-Aiders and Do Not Bug Me's may respond to health food promotion that stresses convenience and guilt-relief.

## Health clubs

Hypochondriacs have a lower propensity to join a health club because exercise does not provide the constant reassurance they need that they are healthy. Health Seekers tend to have a moderate to low propensity to join a health club because they are independent and do not need the structure of a club to exercise. Health Followers, on the other hand, are the primary target market for a health club for social reasons and because they seek to emulate Health Seekers without having to structure their behaviors independently. Health club marketers often find it difficult to retain Health Followers, however, because they have to be reminded constantly of the benefits of regular attendance. The Self-Sufficient segment is a potential market for health clubs if this service is positioned as a means of self-help so that they do not get caught up in the medical system. The Band-Aider and the Do Not Bug Me segments tend not to be targets for health club services because they are not interested in or do not have the time for preventive health behaviors.

## Strategy implications overview

Figure 2 presents a graphic display of the marketing strategy implications by segment for a selection of health care products. The segments are identified on the horizontal axis and predisposition to use the product on the vertical axis. In general, for products and services with a high predisposition for usage, marketers need to stress benefit differences between brands; for products and services with a low predisposition for usage, marketers need to stress product utility.

• • •

In the last decade, health care marketers have increasingly embraced marketing principles to gain competitive advantages. Marketers of health-related products and services can draw from the vast amount of knowledge regarding consumer health care attitudes and behaviors found in the health education and health promotion literature.

This article represents an exploratory step in integrating marketing and health care theory and practice to demonstrate the potential application for the marketers of health-related products and services. The approach used in the article has demonstrated that more effective marketing strategies can be developed by integrating this health care knowledgebase with the principles of benefit segmentation. The propositions that are presented regarding the appropriateness of the various segments (based on benefits sought) in the preventive health care market need to be confirmed for each health care product. Finally, the ethical issues surrounding the targeting of certain segments (such as hypochondriacs) need to be considered.

## REFERENCES

1. Becker, M.H., and Maiman, L.A., "Sociobehavioral Determinants of Compliance with Health and Medical Care Recommendations." *Medical Care* 13 (January 1975): 10–24.
2. Wind, Y. "Issues and Advances in Segmentation Research." *Journal of Marketing Research* 15 (August 1978): 317–37.
3. Kotler, P. *Marketing Management*. Englewood Cliffs, N.J.: Prentice Hall, 1980.
4. Haley, R.I. "Benefit Segmentation: A Decision-Oriented Research Tool." *Journal of Marketing* 32 (July 1968): 30–35.
5. Calantone, R.J., and Sawyer, A.G. "The Stability of Benefit Segment." *Journal of Marketing Research* 15 (August 1978): 395–404.
6. Young, S., Ott, L., and Feigin, B. "Some Practical Considerations in Market Segmentation." *Journal of Marketing Research* 15 (August 1978): 405–12.
7. Moriarty, M., and Venkatesan, M. "Concept Evaluation and Market Segmentation." *Journal of Marketing* 42 (July 1978): 82–86.
8. Ryans, A.B., and Weinberg, C.B. "Consumer Dynamics in Non-Profit Organizations." *Journal of Consumer Research* 5 (September 1978): 89–95.
9. Mitry, N.W., and Smith, H.L. "Consumer Satisfaction: A Model for Health Services Administrators." *Health Care Management Review* (Summer 1979): 7–13.
10. Zaltman, G., and Vertinsky, I. "Health Service Marketing: A Suggested Model." *Journal of Marketing* 35 (July 1971): 19–27.
11. Oliver, R.L., and Berger, P.K. "A Path Analysis of Preventive Health Care Decision Models." *Journal of Consumer Research* 6 (September 1979): 113–21.
12. Reese, R.M., Stanton, W.W., and Daley, J. "Identifying Market Segments Within a Health Care Delivery System: A Two-Stage Methodology." *Journal of Health Care Marketing* 2 (Summer 1982): 10–23.
13. Bonaguro, J.A., and Miaoulis, G. "Marketing: A Tool for Health Education Planning." *Health Education* (January/February 1983): 6–11.
14. Miaoulis, G. "A Market Segmentation Analysis: Pre-Adolescent Pregnancy Issues." *Journal of Health Care Marketing* 9 (June 1989).
15. Miaoulis, G., and Bonaguro, J. "Marketing Strategies in Health Education." *Journal of Health Care Marketing* 1 (Winter 1980): 35–44.

16. Stratmann, W.C. "A Study of Consumer Attitudes About Health Care: The Delivery of Ambulatory Services." *Medical Care* 7 (July 1975): 537–47.

17. Wortzel, L.H. "The Behavior of the Health Care Consumer: A Selected Review." *Advances in Consumer Research.* Cincinnati, Ohio: Association for Consumer Research, 1975.

18. Berkowitz, E.N., and Flexner, W. "The Market for Health Services: Is There a Non-Traditional Consumer?" *Health Care Management Review* 6, no. 1 (Winter 1981): 25–34.

19. Finn, D.W., and Lamb, C.W., Jr. "Hospital Benefit Segmentation." *Journal of Health Care Marketing* 6 (December 1986): 26–33.

20. Carroll, N.V., and Gagnon, J.P. "Identifying Consumer Segments in Health Services Markets: An Application of Conjoint and Cluster Analyses to the Ambulatory Care Pharmacy Market." *Journal of Health Care Marketing* 3 (Summer 1983): 22–34.

21. Harrell, G.D., and Fors, M.F. "Marketing Ambulatory Care to Women: A Segmentation Approach." *Journal of Health Care Marketing* 5 (Spring 1985): 19–28.

# APPENDIX

## DESCRIPTIVE PROFILES OF BENEFIT SEGMENTS

### Hypochondriacs
*Unhappy Henry*

Henry is a single, 26-year-old sales representative with a major marketing firm. He is a member of the "Symptom of the Month Club," and is unhappy unless he is ill. He seeks attention through his health care behaviors and seizes every opportunity to discuss his current symptoms, see his physician, and try new over-the-counter remedies. Henry travels five days a week on his job, and carries two toiletry cases. One contains his personal toiletries and the other contains his over-the-counter and prescription medications. Henry does not exercise regularly and does not watch his diet. He does not overindulge in alcohol or smoke.

### Followers
*Stressed-Out George*

George is a 45-year-old president of his own company in a major city. He is divorced and has a teenage daughter. George travels two to three days a week, and has a great deal of business and personal stress in his life. He deals with stress by engaging in exercise every day, whether running, playing tennis, or horseback riding. George tends to seek the advice of others regarding health-related issues. He is reluctant to give up his daily self-rewards of ice cream and chocolate cake, but he does try to watch his cholesterol level and does not eat much red meat. His primary concern is to avoid a heart attack, and he is willing to invest a minimum amount of effort to do so.

George owns several pairs of expensive running shoes, but no designer athletic wear. He has an annual physical and takes vitamins every day, but prefers not to take medication when he is ill.

### Band-Aiders
*Macho Brice*

Brice is a 28-year-old construction supervisor. He has a Bachelor's degree in English from a major university and spends much of his spare time reading philosophy; however, he rarely shows this side of his personality to anyone other than his close friends. Brice seeks recognition for being able to work and function despite adversity. He takes over-the-counter remedies when he is sick and continues to work. He cannot understand why other people do not have his stamina (although he is typically recover-

ing from a health problem that did not prevent him from working). Brice drinks coffee all day, and the staples of his diet are cheeseburgers, french fries, and Coke. Although Brice is not overweight, his doctor has warned him that he has an extremely high cholesterol level. Brice is a smoker and has tried unsuccessfully to quit. Brice rarely exercises and owns one pair of Reeboks.

### Health Seekers
*Debra the Health Freak*

Debra is a 37-year-old health care education professor at a midwestern university. She is married with one child. Debra practices what she teaches, and health and fitness are a major part of her life. She believes that positive health behaviors, such as exercise, not smoking, and eating healthy foods are the key to a long and happy life. She is in top physical condition. Her life with her husband revolves around daily running, occasional marathons, and participation in a wide variety of sports activities.

Debra is very concerned about the quality of her running shoes and chooses them carefully. She does not wear designer athletic wear, nor does she take vitamins or over-the-counter drugs. When Debra does get sick, she continues running until she gets better or until the illness is so disabling that she cannot run.

### Self-Sufficients
*Independent Stella*

Stella is a 65-year-old widow of first-generation Greek ethnic background. She retired with a pension after 25 years as an assembly line worker, and now works part-time. Her life experiences have made her distrustful of the medical community, which she perceives as an overpaid bureaucracy. She believes that Medicare, Blue Cross, and other health insurance companies do not give people all the benefits to which they are entitled. Stella avoids traditional medical care and physicians as much as possible and relies instead on home remedies.

### Do Not Bug Me's
*Career Mom Claire*

Claire is a 35-year-old vice president with a Fortune 500 company. She is married and the mother of a one-year-old. Claire struggles every day to balance the pressures of her career and her family life. She eats too much, smokes too much, and does not have time to exercise.

When Claire is challenged about her eating and smoking, she responds with "Don't bug me, I have all I can do to cope with my job and my family." Claire is very concerned about her appearance, however, and she buys only the best apparel for herself and her family. She owns designer athletic clothing, but only wears it when travelling or relaxing. Claire is knowledgeable about and conscious of healthy foods, but because of the demands on her time, her family consumes mostly prepared meals and foods.

# Index

# About the Editor

Montague Brown is a consultant and Director of Strategic Management Services, Inc., a management consulting firm in Washington, D.C. Brown is Of Counsel with the law firm of Calligaro and Mutryn and is also Editor of *Health Care Management Review.*

Dr. Brown's practice focuses on strategic issues and policies including integration of delivery systems, managed care, strategic alliances, delivery networks, and joint ventures.

Dr. Brown holds an AB and an MBA from the University of Chicago, a Doctor of Public Health and a Juris Doctor from the University of North Carolina. He has held research and teaching positions at the University of Chicago, Northwestern University, Duke University, and the University of Kansas.